Advance Praise for

Functional Maternity

"Functional Maternity beautifully explains the many physiological changes that occur during pregnancy and the vital role of nutrition and lifestyle in supporting the body's ability to adapt to them. This is an excellent read for prenatal practitioners or anyone seeking a higher-level understanding of functional medicine as it relates to maternity care."

—Lily Nichols, RDN, CDE, author of *Real Food for Pregnancy* and *Real Food for Gestational Diabetes*

"The potential of functional medicine to inform maternity care shines through in this text. Written in a clear, informative style, it provides a valuable guide for healthcare practitioners and those interested in optimizing their nutritional health during pregnancy and beyond. As an acupuncturist involved in integrative maternity care, the collaboration between health practitioners is a foundation of practice. Dietary self-care is also regarded as an essential foundation for health within Chinese medicine. This text with its evidenced-based approach takes this concept further, providing an important bridge into the realities and possibilities of what functional medicine has to offer as part of maternity acupuncture and obstetrical care."

—Debra Betts PhD, LAc, TCM Practitioner, Adjunct research fellow (NICM) University Western Sydney, author of *Essential Guide to Acupuncture in Pregnancy & Childbirth*

"'Using Functional Medicine and Nutrition to Improve Pregnancy and Childbirth Outcomes,' is a massive subject to research and undertake. This is what Sarah Thompson has done. This author has challenged conventional medicine to open their obstetrical training to consider the nutritional care of their patients. This entire book is a challenge to physicians to do more than just instruct their patients to watch their weight gain and prescribe a prenatal vitamin. As chronic disease rises in our population, there is little doubt that our dietary patterns are flawed. The research and content of this book enhance your knowledge on how nutrition, specific vitamins, and minerals facilitate the enzymatic pathways for a healthy mother's body to function."

—Raymond W. Deiter, DO, FACOOG

"This book is a collection of heart-warming stories linked with biochemistry and the added personal touch that makes the information palatable and memorable. The goal of helping other women in their journey through motherhood was not lost even when handling dense topics like metabolic pathways. I look forward to referencing this book when looking for nutritional treatments for maternal health issues. All mothers may benefit from practitioners reading this book."

—Dr. Jo Nell Shaw DC, ND, CACCP

"Sarah Thompson, L.Ac, is that rare acupuncturist who also has a passion for western research. With infectious enthusiasm, she has thrown herself into really understanding optimal nutrition for moms-to-be during preconception and pregnancy. This book is perfect for any health practitioner who wishes to deeply understand functional nutrition for mother and baby. Sarah bridges the gap in current nutritional thought by increasing the reader's knowledge of nutrition and health. She understands that true health for mom and baby is more than just calories and macronutrients. Sprinkled with fun anecdotes explaining Sarah's path to this field, this book will answer questions you didn't know you had but will be glad you got answered."

—Rachel Blunk, LAc, FABORM, Acupuncturist, and Author of *Waiting on Pins and Needles*

"As a midwife working with homebirth and birth center clients, I have never encountered a better resource than Sarah. She is well versed in what she does, and her incredible knowledge not only helps our clients but also helps further my own and my staff's knowledge beyond what any of our medical training did. I am beyond grateful for Sarah and her exceptional mind! You will often hear me say, 'I want to be Sarah when I grow up!' This is how much we love her! I highly recommend her book and services to any woman at any stage in their life."

—Althea Hrdlichka CPM, LM, RM, Founder of Tender Gifts Midwifery & Birth Center & Mother's Life Tea LLC

"Working in an underserved community, it's a must that we find ways to improve maternal outcomes; *Functional Maternity* highlights, educates, and fascinates us in helping women succeed in their overall well-being and the journey we call motherhood."

—Amber Rivers MSN, WHNP-BC

"*Functional Maternity* is a groundbreaking book that has the potential to improve pregnancy and birth outcomes. This evidence-based information is perfect for practitioners to best meet this special population's changing needs from preconception to labor and delivery. It is also written in such a way that the layperson can digest the complex topics."

—Kelsey Sweet, DC

"This is the book I didn't even know I'd been waiting for my entire life! If only I'd had access to it during my own pregnancies. It has already become an indispensable resource in my doula business and is something I'll be recommending all my clients read."

—Kate Finley, Birth and Postpartum Doula

Functional *Maternity*

Using
Functional Medicine and
Nutrition to Improve Pregnancy
and Childbirth Outcomes

SARAH THOMPSON
LAc, CFMP, DOULA

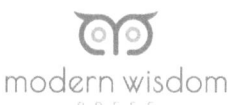

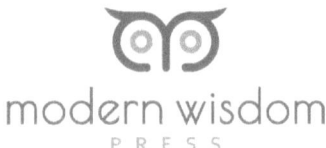

Modern Wisdom Press
Boulder, Colorado, USA
www.modernwisdompress.com

Copyright © Sarah Thompson, 2021
Visit the author's website at www.functionalmaternity.com

All rights reserved. No part of this publication may be reproduced or transmitted in any form or by any means, mechanical or electronic, including photocopying or recording, or by any information storage and retrieval system, or transmitted by email, without permission in writing from the author, except as provided by United States of America copyright law. Reviewers may quote brief passages in reviews.

Published 2021
Cover Design: Melinda Martin
Author's photo courtesy of Shawna Cruz Photography

DISCLAIMER
Neither the author nor the publisher assumes any responsibility for errors, omissions, or contrary interpretations of the subject matter within.

MEDICAL DISCLAIMER
The purpose of this book is to provide educational and information resources; it is in no way a substitute for medical care. The content is not intended to be a substitute for professional medical advice, diagnosis, or treatment. Always seek the advice of your physician or other qualified health provider with any questions you may have regarding a medical condition.

Functional Medicine is a physiological, systems-based approach to medicine. The focus of diagnosis and treatment is on finding root, underlying causes and connections between biological systems, not symptom management. Professionals who are certified in functional medicine do so as a certification off their medical licenses. Medical licenses or healthcare professions that are approved for functional medicine certification include certified nutrition specialists, dentists, optometrists, podiatrists, mental health professionals, occupational therapists, pharmacists, physical therapists, physician assistants, registered dietitians, registered nurses, nurse practitioners, midwives, chiropractors, acupuncturists, MDs, and DOs. Functional Medicine is not a licensed profession.

This book is dedicated to:
My daughters.
My motivation to try. May their future be brighter.

My grandmother.
She inspires me, even though she is gone.

Contents

Introduction 1

Part One	THE CHALLENGE 7
Chapter 1	A Society Of Lost Women 9
	Women Are Looking for Answers 10
	Practitioners Are Looking for Answers 11
	There Are Answers 12
	Why No One Is Listening 14
	Collaboration 17
Chapter 2	Why Me? 21
	The Imposter in the Room 21
	The A-ha Moment 24
	What I Learned from My Traditional Chinese Medicine Training 26
	Bridging Two Worlds 28
Chapter 3	Why Maternity Functional Medicine 31
	What Is Functional Medicine 31
	You Can't Reverse Physical Damage 33
	Standard American Nutrition Versus Functional Nutrition 34
	Respecting Dietary Culture 36
	It Starts in Childhood 38
	Insufficiency Versus Deficiency 42
	The Nutrition Connection 43
	Nutrition in Disease 45
	Why Specializing Matters 47

Part Two	Functional Maternity: A Different Approach 51
Chapter 4	Preconception Nutrition for Baby And Mom......................53
	Fetal Programming..53
	DNA Methylation 55
	A Word on Unmetabolized Folic Acid......................................60
	Folate or Choline in Methylation...63
	Histone Modification..64
	Placental Development 66
	You Are Your Mother and Your Grandmother 68
	Nutrition and Physical Degeneration 69
	A Cultural Approach to Phytates...72
Chapter 5	Metabolic Changes Throughout Pregnancy..............................75
	The Krebs Cycle 76
	Oxidative Stress...79
	Understanding Carbohydrates...83
	Glucose Metabolism Changes Throughout Pregnancy..............85
	Lipid Metabolism and Ketogenesis..86
	Importance of Cholesterol...87
	Oxidative Stress, Coenzyme Q10, and Fat Protection 89
	Protein Metabolism..91
	Anabolism, Catabolism, and Metabolic Regulation 94
Chapter 6	The Story of Hormones...95
	Steroidogenesis..96
	Adrenal Hormone Synthesis 99
	Vitamin K and Steroid Synthesis Regulation 103
	Vitamin D and Steroid Synthesis Regulation.........................104
	Vitamin D Metabolism in Pregnancy 106
	Progesterone..107
	Estrogen..110
	Testosterone 115
	DHEA-S..115
	Cortisol...117
	Hormonal Interactions that Sustain Pregnancy......................120

Chapter 7	Thyroid Physiology 121	
	How the Thyroid Works 124	
	Thyroid Hormone Activation 128	
	The Iodine Debate...129	
	Environmental Halogens and Thyroid Hormones 133	
	Thyroid Antibodies – Autoimmune Disease in Pregnancy 134	
	Thyroid Hormones in Pregnancy..137	
PART THREE	APPLYING NUTRITION AND FUNCTIONAL MEDICINE TO MATERNITY HEALTHCARE 137	
Chapter 8	Nausea In Pregnancy..141	
	Metabolic Factors...143	
	Hormonal Factors..145	
	Bacterial Dysbiosis – The Case of H. Pylori..............................149	
	Nutritional Factors..151	
	Genetics...154	
	Ginger Versus Peppermint: Which Is Best for Nausea Symptoms? 156	
Chapter 9	Anemia In Pregnancy...157	
	Birth of a Red Blood Cell...161	
	In Pregnancy We Double 163	
	Shifts in Iron Metabolism 164	
	Inflammation and Iron Deficiency 167	
	A Cultural Approach to Oxalates..168	
	Anemia Is More than Just an Iron Deficiency 169	
	Anemia in the Vegan Diet 172	
	Lost Mothers..174	
	A Case of Anemia..175	
Chapter 10	Depression and Anxiety 177	
	Getting to Know the Nervous System 180	
	Can Cholesterol Be Too Low? 183	
	Nutrition in the Tryptophan Pathway 184	
	Nutrition in the Tyrosine Pathway 187	

	Nutrient Power	189
	Depression as a Sign of Inflammation	190
	Anxiety Is the Physical Manifestation of Stress	192
	Pregnancy Depression & Anxiety and DHEA	193
	Assessing Depression and Anxiety in Pregnancy	194
Chapter 11	Gestational Hypertension	193
	Diet and Hypertension	198
	Anemia and Hypertension	200
	Electrolyte Balance and Dehydration	201
	Nutritional Associations to Preeclampsia	204
	Epigenetics, Placental Development, and Preeclampsia Risk	206
	Maternal Vascular Changes in Preeclampsia	207
	Oxidative Stress in Hypertension and Preeclampsia	208
	Mitochondria, CoQ10, and Preeclampsia	212
	Know Your Scope	213
Chapter 12	Functional Childbirth	211
	Old Discoveries, New Applications	216
	A Quick Look at Labor Physiology	217
	The Wonderful, Amazing Cervix	220
	Collagen Remodeling	222
	Nutritional Deficiencies and Cervix Remodeling	224
	Prostaglandins and Cervical Ripening	226
	The Other Prostaglandins	227
	Dietary Fats and Prostaglandin Formation and Function	228
	Hyaluronic Acid – The Forgotten Component of Cervical Ripening	231
	Oxytocin and Protein	229
	Oxytocin Physiology in Labor	236
	Oxytocin and the War on Prenatal Vitamin A	238
	Are You the Key Master?	242
	What About Baby?	243
	An Illusion of Control	244

Chapter 13	Why the Method Of Birth Matters	241
	The Catecholamine Surge	241
	Possible Impact of Scheduled Birth on Baby's Brain	242
	The Microbiome	243
	Mom's Diet and Microbiome Health	245
	Group B Strep and Antibiotics in Labor	247
	Birth Method and the Microbiome	249
	Health Risks in Cesarean-delivered Babies	250
	Cesarean Risks for Mom	251
Conclusion	Take the Next Steps	253
	Using this Information in the Clinic	253
	The Death of Philosophical Debate in Medicine	256
	Don't Stop Here	258
Appendix A	Prenatal Dietary Reference Intakes	260
Appendix B	Glossary of Terms	288
Notes		291
Index		329
Resources For Continuing Your Journey		355
Acknowledgments		361
About the Author		362

Introduction

If you have navigated the maternity world as a pregnant mother or even as a birth professional or practitioner, you will know very quickly that little emphasis is given to the mother's nutritional health.

Questions at prenatal appointments are not driven toward prevention or nutrition but are used to determine the health of the baby and assess for possible complications that could lead to the need of medical interventions, such as medications, induction, or surgical delivery of a baby safely.

The little attention given to maternity or even prenatal nutrition is often simplified to, "Are you taking a prenatal vitamin?" As you will see in this book, there is no prenatal vitamin that gives the necessary nutrients needed for a mother to function throughout each trimester. So many changes occur, maternally, that a single prenatal vitamin is more likely to leave the mother insufficient in different nutrients at various stages of gestation and possibly with more different nutrients at other times. This is because a prenatal vitamin is designed to grow a baby, not support a mother functionally.

Often, the discussion on nutrition during pregnancy ends there.

Maternity nutrition is much more complex than a standard set of nutrients that can be put into a pill with one purpose: to grow a baby. Maternal demands through gestation vary so greatly from person to person and from trimester to trimester that it would require someone specifically trained in this specialty to deliver the information required to facilitate a functional pregnancy.

OB/GYNs and midwives are strategically placed to be able to offer a glimpse of this biochemical uniqueness yet are often poorly trained in nutritional approaches and are unable to support their patients in this way.

They need help.

Over the years, I've worked with physicians, nurses, midwives, doulas, and women all over the world who are searching for answers to their nutrition and pregnancy questions. Functional medicine has given me the skills I need to truly help these women thrive.

Nearly every patient who has come to see me in late gestation or postpartum has said, "I wish I had found you sooner. No one had discussed with me how important nutrition was." If we were discussing how important nutrition was to these ladies, we might just have seen our negative maternal health statistics come down.

This is where we, as practitioners and women, have a unique opportunity to change maternity statistics. By understanding the unique needs and demands the mother's body undergoes in pregnancy, we can help facilitate the natural processes that build upon each other throughout pregnancy to end in a functional labor. If we are to change the current state of health in America, we need to start at the beginning. Birth is the beginning, for both the mother and the future mother-to-be. To be able to provide the best care in these phases of life, specialized focus in continuing education is a must, just like any other medical specialty.

When I first started writing this book, I had several people ask why I titled it *Functional Maternity*. Why not Functional *Pregnancy* or Functional *Prenatal Nutrition*? The reason they were asking was that they really didn't know what I meant by maternity. You see, the care of women has been lost in our care of pregnancies.

I recently sat down with some family friends, a group of successful businessmen. I was surprised by their curiosity about my book. They were all first-generation Americans with a strong cultural influence. Even as men, they were receptive and strongly believed in the natural methods of birth and the importance of diet in childhood for overall health. After our conversation, they all congratulated me on being the one to present this information and how important they thought it was. I did not expect that from a group of older male businessmen. They were ready to order a copy for their daughters and granddaughters.

What it showed me is that everyone is concerned, everyone knows that nutrition is important, but not many people are talking about it. I do not pretend to have all the answers, but I do believe that nutrition is a crucial part of healthcare that has been neglected.

If you Google "maternity nutrition", you'll find hundreds of articles that talk about pregnancy nutrition, but all of them are geared toward the growth of the baby, not the function of the mother.

Prenatal is defined as "care of pregnancy." Prenatal nutrition is focused on the growing baby and nutrients needed to pass the placenta to help a fetus become a healthy baby, not the functional health of the mother.

Maternity is defined as "care of the mother." Maternity functional medicine takes nutrition a step further by looking at the intricacies of maternity physiology and how the body compensates for the fetal demands. Changes that require a different set of nutritional needs than that of the growing baby. Nutritional demands that, if not met, could change pregnancy and labor outcomes for the mother.

This is an area of nutrition that has failed mothers. Our focus, medically and nutritionally, has been on the growth and delivery of a healthy baby and not on the health and function of the mother.

In this book, I'm going to show you the utterly amazing world of functional medicine, and how this deep knowledge of nutrition and system interconnection has the power to change the course of maternity healthcare. To not only help women during their current pregnancies but just maybe save future women from the increasing risk of maternity complications by creating healthier pregnancies and healthier daughters.

To help you better understand this all-encompassing approach to supporting maternity, I'm presenting the information in three parts.

In Part One, I will outline the shortcomings of the standard approach to maternity and why functional medicine is needed. I highlight the burning questions you have and help introduce you to the answer. You will get a deep look into the connections between nutrition and birth statistics and begin the process of using nutrition to improve pregnancy health. This will set the stage on which the rest of the book's topics play out by explaining the faults of the current system and the need for collaborative work between conventional and adjunct professionals.

In Part Two, we'll talk more specifically about how to apply functional medicine in support of mothers and babies. I'll take you on a journey into a more complex understanding of how hormones and systems work to support the pregnant mother and her growing child. This information is crucial in accurate differentiation and treatment of the conditions we will discuss in Part Three. I'll illustrate the complex topics of metabolism, steroid hormone formation and function, as well as thyroid function and other aspects of physiology that can affect pregnancy health and function.

In Part Three, we'll dive more deeply into applying nutrition and functional medicine to all phases of maternity. I'll build upon the information I presented in Part Two by applying this information to specific and common conditions that affect pregnancy health and childbirth outcomes, such as nausea in pregnancy, hypertension, and the functional processes of childbirth.

Finally, I will guide you through the intake process and give you the tools necessary to begin assessing, diagnosing, and treating these complaints in your clinic.

Whether you are a seasoned practitioner, birth worker, or expectant mother, this book will become an essential resource over time that will help you learn to do the following:

Introduction

- Recognize unique patterns of maternal health and the effects nutrition has on the increased risk of pregnancy-related complications.

- Create dietary protocols for gestational hypertension, pregnancy nausea, and many other common conditions in pregnancy.

- Use nutrition and diet to increase natural birth success.

- Be confident in guiding others through their pregnancy journey with research-backed nutrition advice.

- Practice on the cutting edge of advanced specialized functional medicine.

- And so much more.

My hope is that *anyone* who works with pregnant women or is preparing for pregnancy can use this book as a maternity and prenatal nutrition resource for improved pregnancy health success.

Welcome to the journey.

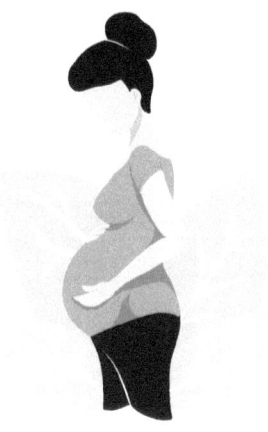

Part One
The Challenge

"Childbirth should be a natural event that occasionally needs medical help, not a medical event that sometimes happens naturally."

- KEMI JOHN

A society of lost women • Why me? •
Why maternity functional medicine

Chapter 1

A Society Of Lost Women

Maternity healthcare in America has become heavily medicalized over the last few centuries as I'm sure you've seen through your own experiences in the birthing world. I am not saying that conventional medicine isn't amazing. Without the vast discoveries and medical advances, we as humans would not have the life expectancies that we enjoy in modern times. There are many birthing women who do, in fact, need these interventions.

As we have advanced, our medical sciences with new techniques and procedures, we have lost our connection to the natural biology and preventative nutrition that cultures before us knew. An overuse of these lifesaving techniques also comes with risks and possible complications and should be reserved for only true emergency scenarios.

For the last several decades medical researchers, professors, physicians, midwives, doulas, mothers, and women like you have begun to sound the alarm and raise questions as to whether our medicalized approach to pregnancy and childbirth is to the benefit of women. They are beginning to question why we are seeming to need more intervention in birth.

The changing environment of natural medicine and the increasing interest in alternatives to the conventional model of care abounds in all aspects of health—none more than in maternity support and care. Women are beginning to question the care they are receiving through these standard practices and are seeking more natural ways to experience birth.

The natural birth world is exploding with those seeking ways to encourage natural and functional experiences that leave women empowered. The increasing demand for midwives, doulas, and other pregnancy support personnel is testament to the desire of women to seek support and knowledge in their pregnancy and to the desire of practitioners to seek ways to provide additional support for these women.

I have not found a medical modality that has all the answers. There is not one view of maternity healthcare that is better than the other, we need each depending on the situation presented. Chiropractors offer structural support to keep the mother's body aligned. Acupuncturists offer a traditional Chinese medicine (TCM) approach to biochemical changes and can help modify dysfunctional patterns. Mental health specialists can help with the psychological changes that occur from the transition into motherhood. Doulas offer emotional and physical support and guidance through labor and encourage a mother in her journey. Midwives offer low-risk moms a less aggressive approach to prenatal care. And conventional western physicians need to be available if true emergencies arise.

The different views on maternity care have remained mostly separate and at odds. Conventional medicine argues that natural therapies give false hope to birth outcomes while the natural modalities condemn the interventions of conventional medicine, stating that all women have the capacity to birth naturally. Because of this division in care, women and practitioners alike are wrought with questions.

Maternity functional medicine offers a link between the conventional western medicine ideas and the alternative and support practitioners, answering many of the questions consistently raised by mothers and practitioners.

Women Are Looking for Answers

A physician I know once told me that patients come to him because they want "something." It doesn't have to be the 100 percent cure, but they want to know that they are doing everything they can and that you have an answer for them. The worst thing you can tell a pregnant mother is, "There is nothing we can do." The reality is, there is always something that he can do. If not he and his services, he can refer to someone else who might offer some support or answers.

Pregnant women have questions—lots of questions. As the rates of pregnancy complications continue to rise, mothers are becoming afraid of childbirth and are losing trust in the medical system. They do not want to be a statistic if they can help it. They are looking for answers to help them support themselves physically and psychologically. I remember, over a decade ago, being a pregnant woman asking the questions. It is a hard place to be because deep down you know there is more that can be done, and there is more than what you are being told.

Many women are looking to nutrition and nutritional support to help them achieve their ideal pregnancy. Nutrition is confusing, and as women become more aware that nutrition is a foundational key to proper health, the more confused they seem to be. They have more questions about prenatal nutrition than ever before. These women are asking the questions but not receiving answers. Physicians are not equipped with the training or skills to be able to answer these nutrition questions. So, these women are turning to social media for advice from their friends, followers, and want-to-be nutritional professionals, setting themselves up for less helpful nutrition advice from multilevel marketing schemes and people with anecdotal information that may be more dangerous than helpful.

Humans are a combination of physical and psychological components, with interconnected systems that are dependent on proper nutritional intake. We must be able to support them in all aspects of health, and if we are not capable of providing this sort of support, then we need to refer to the specialists who can.

Practitioners Are Looking for Answers

Whether you are a conventional medicine provider, an alternative medicine provider, or a birth support professional, we have all sought out our professions because we wanted to have the best tools in our toolbox to treat and prevent disease and support pregnant women. Each professional has chosen the path that called to them in their desire to help birthing women.

I've never met medical or birth professionals that took this path because they wanted to abuse pregnant women. They each believe they have the answers and genuinely want their clients and patients to achieve birth success. It's just that their idea of birth success is different.

I am trained as a birth doula. My acupuncture and functional medicine practice has been, primarily, a fertility and pregnancy-based practice. It seemed like a great addition to follow my patients from fertility struggles to childbirth success and beyond by being present at their birth and guiding them through their transition into motherhood. It also helped me open doors to connections with a variety of birth professionals. Through the years, I've been blessed to have OB/GYNs, certified nurse-midwives (CNMs), and homebirth midwives as colleagues, references, and partners in patient care. Many of these professionals are going on to do their own functional medicine training, many in my mentorship and coaching programs.

Specialized education in functional medicine is on the rise. Those of us in this field have seen the beauty and benefits of functional medicine. We were looking for answers for our patients and have sought out the knowledge to help them and ourselves. Physicians and alternative medicine practitioners alike have been drawn to the science behind the medicine because it helps answer our questions and our deeper questions into function and nutritional connections. Functional medicine not only answers the questions we have but also gives us the skills to be able to help answer the questions our patients have.

There Are Answers

You are here because you have questions and are looking for answers. Whether you are a mother or a practitioner, I have been you.

When I first started my acupuncture practice in 2005, I worked for an interventional pain management specialist. It wasn't until I became pregnant with my own child that I started to think about women's health and pregnancy. I started researching pregnancy and childbirth. I had always been aligned with more natural techniques and as I became more educated on the current state of pregnancy statistics, I, like many mothers, did not want to fall into these statistical groups. It was scary. Natural birth, not so much. Vaginally birthing a child scared me less than the idea of inductions, epidurals, and cesareans.

It was then that I came across the book *Nourishing Traditions* by Sally Fallon.[1] Now, I had studied nutrition in undergraduate and graduate school, and what she was presenting was completely different than what I had been taught. I was intrigued.

Everything she wrote about in her book was a modern interpretation of a much older book, *Nutrition and Physical Degeneration,* by Dr. Weston A. Price. Every great functional medicine practitioner will agree that this one book, lost in time, has set the foundation of how they approach their practices and nutritional advice.

I give credit to this book and its timing in my life for igniting my obsession with prenatal and maternity nutrition and the effects dietary habits have on childbirth outcomes and future generations.

Dr. Weston Price was a dentist who practiced in the early 1900s. Today he is known as the "Isaac Newton of Nutrition" for his advancement in nutritional studies. Dr. Price made several connections in practice between the "civilized" diet of the times and the increase in dental cavities and overall poor health of those populations. He had to know *why*? He traveled the world studying different traditional cultures. These cultures, with their ancestral diets, had little to no cavities, beautifully straight teeth, and as Dr. Price notes, were less likely to have complications in birthing.

The early 1900s was a dangerous time to have a baby if you lived in "civilized society." During that time, the maternal mortality rate was 1 in 100 (wow!). From the time of Dr. Price, medical discoveries, improved nutrition, and other advancements decreased the mortality rate, and it decreased until the 1990s when it began to slowly rise again. In 2000, we saw a dramatic shift—in the wrong direction. While the rates in the rest of the developed world decreased substantially, the U.S. maternal death rate and the rate of preventable complications went up.[2] As of 2017, the maternal death rate in the U.S. did drop slightly but has remained stable with no change. According to some studies, 50 percent of the maternal deaths in America are preventable because they are highly associated with chronic preventable diseases associated with poor nutrition.[3]

Women and birth professionals alike are looking for answers as to why these statistics have risen sharply and continue to rise. As the data connecting nutrition to these complications continues to pile up, the professionals we consider the most trusted in our healthcare may not be the best resources for nutritional advice.

Why No One Is Listening

Nearly every woman that comes into my office leaves saying, "I feel like you actually listened to what I had to say." Every woman who leaves the office of any type of medical professional should feel this way. Even if the practitioner doesn't have all the answers, every mother deserves to be heard, understood, supported, and educated.

The focus of prenatal care has been put on the health of the baby, not the health of the mother. In this, we have neglected women emotionally and physically. Pregnant women have become lost in the system of baby care.

The worst thing you can say to a mother who is experiencing a horrible pregnancy or has had a traumatic birth is, "At least you have a healthy baby." This is not support; it is ignoring the physical and emotional pain this mother has gone through. We have invalidated her questions, concerns, beliefs, and her journey to motherhood.

The reality is that most practitioners say this not because they are heartless or cold but because they truly do not have the training to provide the necessary support to these women. Physicians were not given the nutrition education that would give them the skills to support these women through pregnancy by addressing their symptoms, nor are they therapists trained in emotional trauma. They carry the burden of primary care, with the general public feeling they should be able to provide the answers. That is a lot of pressure.

My father is a physician, and I grew up in a medical household. Many of my close friends are medical professionals, and none of them knows a lick about nutrition. Yet surveys show that most Americans believe their physician is a trusted source for nutrition information.[4]

Prior to the 1950s, nutrition was considered a medical discipline, and as the science of cellular medicine and technology grew, the focus on nutrition declined. Dr. Weston Price and Dr. Francis Pottenger were the beginning and end of an era in nutrition research and exploration into disease. Between the 1950s and 1980s, medical schools lowered their curriculum on nutrition, with some schools completely doing away with courses altogether. In the 1980s, a new spark into nutrition began as we saw an increase in diet-related diseases. A comprehensive report prepared by the National Academy of Science-National Research Council in 1985, *Nutrition Education in U.S. Medical Schools*, recommended that medical schools incorporate separate courses in nutrition of at least 25 hours and reinforce this in the clinical experience.

Since then, little has changed. Twenty-five hours of coursework is nowhere near enough training in nutrition therapy, and with the advances in nutrition research we've seen in the past decades, it is inadequate at best.

In 1981, 26 percent of medical schools offered a separate nutrition course. Currently, 71 percent of medical schools fail to provide the minimum recommendations for nutrition education, 36 percent provide fewer than half the recommended number of hours.[5] The majority of coursework available to physicians is preclinical (meaning all textbook, no practical application) and averages 14.3 hours total. Of those schools that do provide clinical experience in nutrition, this clinical practice accounts for, on average, 4.7 hours total! Meaning, primary care physicians most likely have fewer than five hours of clinical experience in nutrition before graduation.

A physician and I had a conversation once about his nutrition training in medical school. He was lucky enough to have attended one of the few medical schools that offered the clinical nutrition curriculum. His coursework had focused on IV nutrition therapy for patients on life support and those unable to feed themselves. He joked that it wasn't very practical to his family practice clinic. Funny/not funny as these are the trusted sources of information for many Americans. These are the people we are supposed to go to for medical help and support, and they are missing a large part of how the body functions and they know it.

More than 50 percent of graduating medical students rate their nutrition knowledge as inadequate, and physicians report that they have not received adequate training to give them the ability to counsel their patients on nutrition.

A 2008 survey of resident physicians found that, although 77 percent agreed that nutrition assessment should be included in routine primary care visits and 94 percent agreed it was their obligation to discuss nutrition with patients, only 14 percent felt physicians were adequately trained to provide nutrition counseling.[6]

Multiple surveys of residents, fellows, and practicing physicians assessing specific nutrition knowledge found mean correct responses ranging from roughly 50–66 percent. Meaning, in all the surveys, the physicians scored an average of 58 percent. Wow! People, that's an "F". So, the professionals we've been told to trust the most with our health are scoring an F on nutritional surveys.

This may not get better either. Time is not limitless, and medical school is composed of a specific amount of time. The advances in medical technology and science are growing by the day, and these subjects outweigh nutrition in medical curriculum. For schools that do want to improve their nutrition programs, they are unable to find suitable professors. Physician nutrition specialists are far and few between and bringing in non-physician faculty is difficult.

The truth is that many physicians may never be that source. For them to obtain the knowledge they need, they will need to pursue continuing education and certification in programs, such as the Institute for Functional Medicine (IFM), or clinical nutrition.

Again, this takes time, and the average physician is overworked, with little time to devote to extensive new studies. According to a 2018 survey produced by The Physicians Foundation, 80 percent of physicians across all specialties reported being at full capacity or overextended, and 40 percent of physicians reported feelings of burnout. This survey is done every other year and the newest—the 2020 survey—isn't any better, with an increase to 58 percent of physicians experiencing burnout.

Our physicians can't do it all, and we cannot expect them to. Collaborative practitioners such as midwives, nutritionists, and functional medicine providers can come together to support physicians and, in turn, help mothers become healthier.

Together, we can improve our stark maternity statistics.

Collaboration

Megan and John were like many couples today, who not only wanted a healthy baby but also had desires for their birth experience. Their first child was born via cesarean due to a failed induction after Megan's blood pressure rose sharply at the end of her pregnancy. Their physician had told them it was a good thing they were under medical supervision because this could have taken her or her baby's life.

Megan believed her physician but was not convinced that her symptoms could not have been caught early or treated differently—maybe even prevented. She also had guilt that maybe she had done something to cause the issues in her pregnancy. She had shown signs of preeclampsia earlier in her third trimester, such as pitting edema and headaches. But because her blood pressure had not risen and she was not losing protein in her urine or gaining excess weight, her physicians did not see a problem—yet. She asked questions regarding what she could be doing to feel better or prevent the possible complications. She was told there was nothing she could be doing, that these were just "a part of pregnancy" and may or may not lead to something bigger. They would watch her symptoms, and if they became concerning, they would induce.

After her traumatic delivery, in her mind, she wondered what she could have done differently.

With her second child, they decided to go a different route. They chose a midwife in the hospital system experienced with vaginal birth after cesarean (VBAC) deliveries. She hired a well-known local doula when she read studies showing that women with doula support had better birth outcomes with decreased rates of cesarean delivery. She hoped that these changes might give her a different way to prevent the same outcome but with the medical support available if she did need intervention.

Even with midwifery care, she started to experience similar symptoms to what she had with her first pregnancy, pitting edema and headaches. Her midwife started watching her urine for protein and taking her blood pressure. At 33 weeks, she had a small spike in blood pressure. Their midwife told them that if her blood pressure continued to rise, they would need to transfer care to an obstetrician (OB), and that there was a chance they would need to deliver via cesarean again if symptoms continued to rise.

Megan and John were referred to me by their doula. They came to see me at 34 weeks. When I first saw Megan, she was exhibiting pitting edema, mild headaches, and her blood pressure in-office was 134/82. No laboratory tests (labs) other than a basic complete blood count (CBC) that showed borderline anemia at 30 weeks had been done. I decided to run a few more, starting with a comprehensive metabolic panel (CMP), magnesium, and vitamin D (calciferol).

Her CMP showed extremely low levels of potassium as well as an increase in her liver enzymes. Her magnesium was low, and her vitamin D was low—all nutritional and chemical prerequisites to preeclampsia.

I connected with their midwife, and we discussed what I thought might be going on and consulted on a protocol and plan to treat the presenting deficiencies in hopes of correcting them before symptoms became worse.

We looked at her supplement regimen. She was taking a prescription prenatal that she had received from her midwife with only five ingredients: 400 IU of vitamin D, 1.7 mg riboflavin, 2 mg pyridoxine hydrochloride (pyridoxine HCl), 1.4 mg of folic acid, 8 mcg methylcobalamin. This was the approved prescription prenatal for their multi-practitioner practice that was recommended to every patient.

Megan's midwife was intrigued about what I was able to see in her lab work and was even more interested to see how the changes I made would affect what she thought was an inevitable outcome.

Megan's diet was good but not great. She ate a standard American diet and followed many of the national nutrition guidelines. She ate low-fat dairy, avoided high-fat foods, ate grains at most meals, snacked on fruits, ate her vegetables (but typically only at dinner and as garnishes at lunch). She avoided excess refined sugars, baked goods, and sodas. She felt like she was doing a good job.

We changed up her diet, adding in more dietary fats, had her eat whole eggs every day, increased her vegetable intake, added in nuts and seeds, increased electrolyte-rich foods like coconut water, cucumbers, and watermelon, cut down on her refined grains, and gave her some better supplements. Within a week of starting the dietary "tricks," her edema had improved.

We retested her metabolic panel at 36 weeks and saw improvements in her electrolyte values and a slight decrease in her liver enzymes. We decided to test them again the following week. Again, we saw improvements. Megan's blood pressure improved as well and came down to normal levels.

Megan was able to have a beautiful, natural hospital VBAC birth with her midwife and doula, all because we looked at her symptoms from a functional view that could be changed, not an inevitable condition that would be controlled with medical intervention.

Medical intervention is the norm, not because conventional medicine is not good at catching and treating medical conditions as they arise, but because we have failed to train our primary professionals in nutritional importance and fail to work collaboratively in patient care.

We have a defensive position against the other side, and this approach is becoming detrimental to the health of the women we serve. Functional medicine could be the tie that binds us as a collaborative system that works together in patient care—giving our physicians the support they need, mothers the care they deserve, and together improving our national birth statistics.

Chapter 2

Why Me?

I had coffee with a colleague several months ago to connect after COVID-19 shutdowns and touch base on where we both were in business. He is a psychotherapist who specializes in wilderness therapy, which, if you are not familiar with, you should explore—it's fascinating. I was about midway through writing this book at the time and he asked how it was going. I was honest, as I usually am (probably to a fault).

I told him the information part was easy. I could talk about how amazing functional medicine is, how it can be applied to maternity care, and why it is important all day long. What I couldn't seem to do was talk about myself. Everyone was telling me I needed to sell myself as the expert in my book, but I just didn't know how.

He said, "You're an imposter."

Excuse me?

"You don't belong."

He was right.

The Imposter in the Room

What he had meant in this conversation was not that I didn't belong, but that I personally believed I didn't belong.

Apparently, this is common. So common that psychotherapists have a term for it: "imposter syndrome." People who have become good at their trade but still feel they are not ready to be "the expert."

One of the great things I took from my medical education was, so I had always thought, that I am just the facilitator of the medicine and it is the medicine itself that heals. When I graduated from traditional Chinese medicine, they told us, "We've given you enough to get started, but you are not a master; go out and learn more." So, my entire career, I've felt that I'm still learning and not yet a master.

I'm nothing special; in the scheme of things, I'm a nobody. I'm not a famous doctor with a fancy medical degree and titles from Yale or Stanford who worked for the Centers for Disease Control and Prevention (CDC) or some other prominent medical group. I'm not a biochemistry PhD who studied nutrients in applied science. I am none of these, so why do I think I can sit at the same table as some of these great minds? Basically, what is my experience to give me the confidence to be the one to write this book?

I've struggled with this for years, literally years, as I've thought about writing this book! *Why me?*

All I've done is find other people's studies, compile and connect them, and share this knowledge with patients and colleagues. Anyone could do this. I kept wondering when some great mind out there would write a book on all the cool things I had found. It wasn't until patients, birth professionals, midwives, and physicians themselves started telling me I should write a book that it actually hit me that maybe I'm the person to do it.

When I was a kid, I was obsessed with dogs. Trust me, there is a point.

I was that kid who read every book I could find on the different dog breeds. I wanted to know everything I could about the evolution of dogs, how humans were able to engineer different breeds for different jobs, and the breeds' genetic predispositions to diseases. You name it, I probably knew it. I also took pride in being able to identify different breeds of dogs out in public or on TV and in movies. I found books on extinct breeds of dogs and studied their ancient history. Literally, if there was a book on it, I bought it, read it, highlighted it, and wrote notes in it, and I engulfed myself in the knowledge of dogs. I still have them; it's embarrassing.

Yeah, I was the awkward kid—still am. You know those "me at a party" memes? I start talking about pregnancy, nutrition, or, to this day, dogs, and I've lost everyone.

All right, Sarah, what does any of this have to do with maternity?

My point here is that I am, by nature, a "how and why" person as are most of those scientists who are exploring hypotheses and physicians who continue their education in specialized fields and those professionals seeking out functional medicine. We are full of questions and yearn for answers. We just chose different paths and professions to do so.

Even as a kid I had to know everything I could about what I was passionate about. I asked questions and searched for answers and seemed to gravitate to the road less traveled. If I couldn't find the answer, I dug deeper. Just as I do now. I oddly enjoy studying.

After years of tolling and some great colleagues who help me work through my own fears and insecurities, I've discovered something important about myself. I am not the imposter in the room. I have every right to sit at the table and be the voice to share this knowledge. Not because I discovered it but because I brought the voices of thousands of scientists around the world together in a collective that can now have a voice.

Instead of asking, "Why me?" I should be asking, "Why not me? If not me, who?"

I am still not a master. "People who think they know everything know nothing." I am still studying and exploring. I am continuously looking for the next article or study because we do not know everything about the body, and scientists are discovering new things daily. We are just fledglings in the understanding of the body. This is just another step in increasing the reach of the studies that connect nutrition with disease and nutrition as the real savior of future women.

The A-ha Moment

Anyone who has known me long enough will know that when I was younger, I had zero interest in kids, pregnancy, or the whole family thing. I had goals, career goals. And was going to be happy as a dog mom. I wanted to do sports medicine and pain management and kick ass. I started off learning everything I could about what I was newly passionate about. I took additional courses in orthopedics and trained with one of the most world-renowned orthopedic acupuncturists in the world. I even got a job working with a pain management physician in my hometown to increase my experience and knowledge in chronic pain treatment.

Nothing about pregnancy and women's health was on my radar.

I had always studied and respected the role nutrition played in health, and with my pain patients, we discussed how diet could help them recover, heal, or decrease their pain.

When I first started my journey into maternity care, I was pregnant with my first baby. (Surprise!) It was fascinating; Why had no one told me how amazing women's health and reproduction was? Ha! I was enthralled with pregnancy and this tiny human I was creating. How could I make her (we didn't know she was "her" at the time) the healthiest person I could? How could I make myself the healthiest mother I could be? A-ha! I needed to know more.

Enter a new obsession.

I chose to work with hospital-based midwives, and I began asking them questions. Lots of questions. Even with my midwives, what I was eating never came up. With my base in traditional medicine, nutrition, and my newfound love for Dr. Price, I was concerned about the lack of acknowledgment of nutrition in my care. I had no idea it was this way. How could no one be addressing what I was or was not eating throughout my pregnancy, and how could they expect me to navigate this on my own?

I transferred primary care three times during my first pregnancy because I found their attention lacking. I landed on a wonderful midwife who gave me resources and guided me more through my pregnancy than those before but not through everything.

I found and read every book I could find on prenatal nutrition, just like the dog thing, but nothing and no one seemed to be able to answer my questions. They just told me, "Don't eat oysters," and "Drink low-fat milk." I was baffled by the lack of science-based information on prenatal nutrition. Even with my background, I was confused; I could only imagine how a mother without any nutritional training must feel.

I started subscribing to medical journals; they are not cheap. The answers to the questions I was asking were there, in articles, journals, and books, but nowhere had the information been consolidated. It was scattered, spaced, and required composition to pull together. I had binders of notes and diagrams that I had put together connecting the dots of different articles. So many brilliant minds in the past have quotes about asking the right questions, and they are right. Many of the answers I was searching for required me to ask or, in this case, search for the right questions and keywords.

Then I had a double a-ha moment. Why was no one talking about this?

My obsession didn't end with the birth of my first child. If anything, it only intensified. The more women I met and talked to, the more I felt women needed support and help. This was my purpose, this was my path, and *this* is what I was supposed to do. I was supposed to help women achieve not only better births but also better pregnancies and, thus, postpartum health through nutrition.

What I Learned from My Traditional Chinese Medicine Training

People always ask me how and why I got into traditional Chinese medicine (TCM) as a career path when I'm, obviously, obsessed with the western physiology side of health. It does seem like an odd path, and it wasn't something that was even on my radar until I was in college.

My original path was veterinary school. Remember the dog thing? Seemed like a logical decision. I worked in vet clinics from the time I was 14 years old through my graduate degree. It was through this love of animals that I found acupuncture.

During my undergraduate degree, I worked in two different veterinary facilities that provided acupuncture for animals. The first was an equine vet in my home state of Oklahoma. He worked primarily with racehorses, and acupuncture was a technique that he used frequently for muscle injuries. It was intriguing but didn't quite spur my interest at that point. I really didn't see the beauty in acupuncture until I transferred to Colorado State University (CSU). There, I worked at the CSU Veterinary Teaching Hospital and was able to observe acupuncture treatments done on a variety of conditions. It was here that I finally saw how amazing acupuncture could be.

Animals don't understand placebo; they either get better or they don't. You can't tell a dog, "Today I'm going to needle your hip and it's going to relieve the pain of your dysplasia," and the dog says, "Thanks, doc, I feel great." The dog either gets up and walks or it stays in the same condition it was before the treatment. I watched animal after animal have these amazing changes in their health and demeanor. I had to know more. I had to know *how* this medicine worked. So, to the dismay of my parents, I left the idea of veterinary school and pursued a degree in TCM.

Most people consider the acupuncture degree to be a subpar medical degree. Heck, until recently, we didn't even have the option of a doctorate. Just so you know, we study anatomy and physiology, pharmacology, biochemistry, and pathology, just like any other medical profession. We also study the TCM view of the body, which is vastly different. Different doesn't mean wrong.

You must understand that many of the physiological discoveries made throughout the centuries through TCM were made in a time where they didn't use modern science to describe and justify their findings. Over the course of centuries, ancient TCM physicians discovered organs and their functions, well before European medicine. These TCM physicians just described them in a way that makes no sense in our modern medical terminology. They used the things they saw around them to describe what they saw in the body. Epilepsy, for example, is a wind condition, as it shakes the human body as the wind shakes a tree. Progesterone is the hormone of the luteal phase, and progesterone is considered a yang hormone. Yang in TCM represents heat in the body. When progesterone is high, like in the luteal phase or pregnancy, the body temperature is higher, and thus, there is more yang.

One of my favorite things about living in this time in history is the physiological discoveries being made on a regular basis that make me say, "Hey, that's the exact theory as the TCM theory on disease progression, just in modern terms and with research backing." For someone like me, reading these journals and finding these connections is thrilling.

But that's not the only thing I learned from my TCM training. The most important thing I took from my medical school was the idea of differentiation and that within a disease are multiple patterns. Identifying the correct pattern is essential to correct treatment.

This is, basically, the same idea as functional medicine: the idea that there is a deeper, more root cause of a condition and not just a single superficial symptom. In TCM, all the organs are connected and work together, each a cog in the system. If a cog breaks or gets rusty, the whole system begins to breakdown, just like in functional medicine. Functional medicine, to me, is the scientific verification of TCM theory.

Within each disease, there are different patterns of symptoms. Consequently, you'll see lists of symptoms associated with medical conditions, but a patient will only have a few of them, and the next patient will have a different set. These represent the different patterns in disease progression.

Bridging Two Worlds

How did a conventional medicine-raised Oklahoma girl like me fall into alternative Asian medicine?

My mother was born in Seoul, Korea, and my grandmother was culturally Korean. So, even though I am a corn-fed Okie, I grew up in a multicultural home. My grandmother is a huge part of who I am. Her Korean traditions were a big influence on my childhood and upbringing. As a young child I even spoke a little Korean, but those days are long gone. I loved hearing her stories from Korea—some beautiful and some sad. These stories were my history, my ancestry, and my culture even though I was American. Her house was always filled with amazing Korean dishes, and she fed us a lot! Seriously, Korean grandmothers don't like skinny grandchildren.

Maybe it was my maternal heritage and connection to my ancestry that gave me my interest and desire to learn more about traditional cultures and ancient medicines. Either way, I've always felt drawn to the ancestral cultures of other countries, tribes, and peoples before the influence of western society. So much innate knowledge, lost.

When I was pregnant with my first child, my grandmother was full of cultural advice on pregnancy, birth, and postpartum care. To me, it was beautiful. If we had lived in another time, she could have been my midwife, doula, and childbirth support. She knew it and lived it. She told me specific foods to eat: not just ingredients but how to prepare them, what temperature I should eat them at, and special meals that throughout cultural history were endemic to childbirth.

Traditional cultures have long understood the nutritional value of certain foods during pregnancy and infancy in the health of both mother and baby, and not that long ago so did western medicine. Although I had studied nutrition in college, the knowledge my grandmother gave me was more informative than anything I read in my studies.

When I first discovered Dr. Weston Price and his book, I ate it up (pun intended). It bridged my cultural heritage with my scientific mind. It seemed to be the missing link between the two schools of thought on nutrition in my life.

I have always felt I was a bridge between two cultures for many reasons, but one big one has always been diet and the culture around food and nutrition. Much of what Dr. Price presented reminded me of the foods and traditions that my grandmother had brought with her and instilled in us. Beliefs with no scientific backing that had been passed down from mother to daughter for generation upon generation. Much of this food culture was counter to what the standard American nutrition guidelines told us, and it never made sense to me.

I've always been drawn to understanding the science of western-based nutrition. I am very analytical in nature and do not do well with abstract theory, so I went to traditional Chinese medicine school, which is all theory. Makes sense, I know. I lean on studies that help to give a deep picture of how the body functions at the foundation of health. That desire to know is strong, but I also feel connected to my heritage as do many people I've met on my journey.

Functional medicine helps connect the cultural food knowledge with scientific nutrition studies. It is the perfect link for the two worlds when used correctly and may be the resource we need to bring back traditional pregnancy rituals with scientific backing.

Chapter 3
Why Maternity Functional Medicine

Maternity is, arguably, the most important specialty in any profession. As professionals who specialize in maternity care, we are in a position of responsibility. What we do doesn't just affect the women in our office, but the next generation.

Pregnancy and childbirth are crucial transitional times for women. Women become mothers and they change physically, emotionally, and spiritually. They do not remain the same person they were before; in a way, they are reborn. The actions and methods of this transition are crucial to the health of this new woman from then on. If her transition is functional, she is poised for health success; if it is dysfunctional, she will need support and recovery to maintain all aspects of health.

How a mother eats and drinks, as well as her lifestyle choices, not only affect her health but also the health of her unborn child and future generations through genetics. We are not only supporting women but paving the way to reduce preventable disease at the source: fetal development.

All women should be given the opportunity to benefit from functional medicine during preconception, pregnancy, and beyond.

What Is Functional Medicine

I have gravitated toward functional medicine because it connects what we know culturally and traditionally with medical science. We are lucky to live in a time we can begin to connect the two.

Skeptics out there have argued that the definition of functional medicine as "root cause medicine" eludes the question of "What is functional medicine?"

I kind of agree with them. If we want to defend our medicine, we need to do a better job of explaining what we do.

Here goes.

Functional medicine takes western medicine and combines it with clinical nutrition. It also considers how the different systems of the body work together to create overall body function.

We are a big engine with lots of moving parts, not independent but interconnected. If you remove a cog, the engine does not function the way it is designed. Each cog moves another cog, that cog moves another, and so on. Functional medicine looks at how these cogs are connected and what grease is needed to lube the connections. When a cog is broken, we use science-backed techniques to repair the damage so that the system works correctly. We don't just put gum on it and say done.

Science has shown us that there are connections between the gut and the brain. The microbiome of the gut—the bacteria we have or don't have—has a profound effect on the production and function of neurotransmitters. Depression can be caused by gut dysbiosis, manic behavior by the *Clostridium* family and its toxic byproducts.

Oxidative stress is a causative factor in numerous medical complications including some found in pregnancy. These are examples of what functional medicine addresses. By looking at these biochemical connections, we can correct the problem and restore system function, not just treat the presenting symptoms.

Functional medicine does not neglect that medications have their place in care. For many, they are lifesaving necessities. Some may not be able to remove their medications, but we can support them more effectively and prevent the common side effects associated with many medications by understanding how they affect the cogs in the system.

You Can't Reverse Physical Damage

There is no magic pill. Functional medicine is the next step in patient care, but it cannot treat everything.

I am an asthmatic. I wasn't diagnosed until my mid-twenties. I had a bad upper respiratory infection that became bronchitis and required a trip to the hospital. Factor in a group B strep lung infection from infancy (another story for another chapter), and I damaged my lungs enough to create chronic asthma.

When I was first diagnosed, I was put on three different medications and was told this was my new life: "There is nothing more we can do." I didn't really like that much as I had just finished my degree and was all about alternative medicine. I thought I could cure the world. I was determined to get myself off *all* my medications. I was going to be an example. I did exercises to improve my lung strength, acupuncture, chiropractic, etc., and was able to remove *one* medication. That wasn't enough. I saw a natural medicine physician who had me do food allergy testing. This didn't make any sense to me at the time because I knew what had caused my asthma and it wasn't food. She really didn't explain to me why it was important, but I was desperate and wanted more relief (daily meds are not my thing). I got the results back and was surprised to see pears as my biggest allergen.

Now, what made pears interesting was that, at the time, I was renting a house on a pear orchard. I ate pears and breathed in pear pollen daily; my whole world was pears. The combination of living in an allergen-saturated environment with the addition of a cold virus and some childhood history was the perfect storm to cause my lungs to trigger severe inflammation and permanent physical damage. When my lease was up, I moved and my exasperated asthma symptoms got better. By identifying triggers that increased immune responses and avoiding them—sorry, cats—I have been able to decrease the inflammation in my lungs.

In time, I got off my daily medications, but you cannot reverse damage. My lungs are still weak, and I will always have weaker lungs from the experiences I have had. I must carry an emergency inhaler and that is okay; I've made amazing progress that I was told I would never achieve.

This is what functional medicine does. It is not a cure; it is a way of helping your body be the best it can be with the genetics, experiences, and damage that has occurred. Prevention is always easier than treatment, so the sooner we can start working with people on their diet and lifestyles, the more likely they are to be able to decrease their risk of disease and complications.

The next question then becomes: What form of nutrition are we using in functional medicine?

Standard American Nutrition Versus Functional Nutrition

The politically correct nutrition platform is what you see in hospitals, schools, nursing homes, and in the government's USDA recommendations to Americans regarding food intake. These guidelines are rooted in poorly done, corrupt research studies that aided the food industry agenda, not actual nutrition science. The guidelines focus heavily on carbohydrates (all whole grain sources are created equal), reducing fat intake (specifically saturated fats), limiting cholesterol-rich foods, adding more polyunsaturated fats, avoiding red meat, and limiting salt.

These guidelines were put in place with the great intention of helping Americans navigate nutrition easily. Sadly, Americans are more confused about nutrition than ever. These outdated guidelines are still being pushed to Americans while the research contradicts what we have been told for generations.

The western nutrition approach was based on nutritional studies that had accrued between the 1950s and '80s. These studies were very analytical and scientific with not much focus given to overall composition. Also, they were often biased and funded by corporations looking to promote their agenda.

It was during this time that the nutrition guidelines that we use in America were formulated.

If you want to know the politics behind this, read *Food Politics* by Marion Nestle. Talk about eye-opening. Moving on.

Traditional and ancient cultures didn't have modern science to validate their diet or explain the effects these foods had on the body. They used what they knew to describe what they saw, and what they knew was nature. Every traditional and ancient culture described health, medicine, and food based on the things they saw around them: wind, water, earth, fire, metal, bitter, hot, sour, sweet, etc. Such is the way diseases and pathology are described in TCM. It doesn't make it not accurate; it just makes it different.

Dr. Price would have conversations with medicine men from different cultures and discuss disease in terms of presentation. One of my favorite stories in his book is the retelling of his experience in Canada where many people had scurvy. It was being treated unsuccessfully by the local western physicians, who at the time did not know that vitamin C deficiency was the cause. He spoke with a traditional medicine man, and after describing the symptoms the medicine man told him to eat a specific organ meat from a specific animal to treat the presenting symptoms. This traditional medicine man did not know what vitamin C was, but he knew that if you ate this organ (high in vitamin C, by the way), it would cure the symptoms associated with a specific pattern described in terms they knew based on the world around them.

Dr. Price was bringing light to the knowledge that traditional cultures had known for millennia into terms that could be rationalized by the new scientific mind.

Relying on science doesn't mean we negate past experiences and history. It is a way of validating what we have known throughout generations. Food preparation techniques that have long stood the test of time are now being shown to increase nutrient density. These traditional cultures did not know why they were doing it other than it did not make them sick when they did.

Much of the functional medicine community has latched onto the paleo diet, autoimmune paleo diet, or some other ancestral-titled diet. I think these diets offer people a quick way to feel better but don't really consider true cultural and traditional diets as we know them. It is easier to tell people to avoid a food group than to teach them how to use it properly. It is well-established that many healthy and traditional cultures have used grains, legumes, nuts, seeds, and other food types removed in these extreme diet programs.

I believe all whole food types have a place in the diet except for special conditions. It is teaching people to use them properly that is difficult. America is a culture of no culture. We are a group of descendants of cultures from all over the world. Those who are more recent transplants still maintain much of their heritage and food culture, but as time goes on, it is lost, leaving us with lost traditions that had helped us navigate the foods around us and gave us the ability to use them in ways that decreased antinutrients and increased nutrient density.

I feel blessed to have had a strong base in Korean food culture growing up. I grew up in a region not known for its overall health or dietary habits. My saving grace was that my family often ate traditional Korean meals with vegetables and whole food ingredients being ever-present. Don't get me wrong; we also ate our fair share of spaghetti and fried chicken too, but my mother and grandmother always had kimchi and seaweed snacks for us and made it a point to have a variety of vegetables. You know that scene from the movie *My Big Fat Greek Wedding* when the main character is reminiscing about her childhood, and she is sitting in the cafeteria by herself with her traditional Greek moussaka for lunch and the other kids make fun of her? Yeah, that was me with kimchi and seaweed.

Respecting Dietary Culture

Confusion about nutrition seems to be, in part, associated with our loss of food culture. Around the world, cultures have unique and regional cuisines that incorporate whole and natural food sources. These food customs are passed down through generations and are based on experiences and ancient analysis of these foods and how they affected health. America is lacking in food culture. Our blending of cultures and our history of development have led to a culture that is highly dependent on processed, easy, and bland foods, in general.

I had a patient who came to see me after seeing another functional medicine practitioner in my community. He had a big practice with multiple functional nutrition coaches and pushed programs. She was of Indian descent. She and her family primarily ate Indian cuisine.

After consulting, he gave her his recommendation and game plan and hooked her up with one of his coaches. The program did not consider her cultural heritage. The meals and foods they had planned for her were highly smoothie-based and she didn't own a blender, and they were all American-based meals. Nothing about it was something she could do because it would have required her to throw out her pantry, culture, and food heritage and relearn a completely new American-style cuisine.

When she came to me, her first question was if I was going to make her drink smoothies and stop eating her cultural foods. No. Part of what functional medicine should do is acknowledge what traditional cultures have developed over millennia. These other practitioners and coaches should have been able to take what this woman was already doing and make it better.

When I work with my patients, I never give out generic meal plans because they don't work. What I do is a technique I call "red-lining." I have them keep a one-week food journal so I can see what they are eating on a regular basis. I assess the cultural cuisines they may be consuming, meals they gravitate toward, and I take what they are doing and make it better by modifying and adding to what they have given me. I add in nutrient-dense recipes related to what they presented and give them ideas for substitutions.

Because of this technique I can work with anyone around the world, which I do, considering their local and cultural foods, and still have the same results, without making them drink smoothies twice a day. My respect for their food culture is important and stems from my own family heritage.

Therefore, when I look at nutrition and the diets of those I treat, I am not looking at different diet programs like paleo. These diet programs are not universal and often disregard cultural and traditional food preparation and dietary habits. They also do not consider the personal uniqueness of the patient. It is another generic program, and, I would argue, an extreme diet that limits many nutrient-dense whole foods.

Much of food culture around the world is designed around the health of pregnant mothers and the growth of children. Much care and focus have been given to these special times in life. Many societies reserve special foods for these groups, knowing that the nutritional intake of a mother impacts the health of her offspring.

It Starts in Childhood

Remember when I said that by specializing in maternity, we affect more than the woman in the office? We have generations of women whose mothers and grandmothers have been neglected nutritionally, whose childhoods, where diet affects adult health predispositions and genetic expression, were bathed in modernized kids' meals containing chicken nuggets and hot dogs, devoid of nutrient density.

We have failed women before they even knew they were women.

Back to the 1930s, Dr. Weston Price spoke highly of his colleague Dr. Kathleen Vaughan and her book *Safe Childbirth*. Dr. Kathleen made great connections between the prenatal diet, prepuberty life, diet of female children, and how these nutrition and lifestyle patterns affected the development of their pelvic shape and ability to birth. Of Dr. Vaughan's findings, Dr. Weston Price said,

> *"Dr. Vaughan presents such an array of facts and data that the book must impress every reader. It is of vital importance that her conclusions be considered, for in my opinion our methods of bringing up our girls and the habits of our women with many of the customs of 'civilized' life must be radically readjusted."*

Sitting in a school lunchroom with a group of parents, teachers, and my kids' elementary school principal, I learned a valuable lesson about the state of the school nutrition programs.

At the time, my kids were attending an expeditionary charter school. I probably set myself up for failure here, but I envisioned this school, with its mission and educational style, to somehow be better than the local school district in many regards to their school health and nutrition programs and philosophies. Yes, they were part of the district school lunch programs, but they had a school vegetable garden. We packed our own lunches, so I wasn't too concerned at first. I assumed that the parents and staff were probably of the same mindset as me.

Like most school classrooms, celebrations for holidays and special events that include food and drinks were common. Most of the teachers sent great lists of items to bring, keeping the fun items and healthy items in balance. I was at this PTO meeting for the first time because I had a concern. One of the teachers had been rewarding the students with Coca-Cola, including mine, and I was not okay with this. We are not soda drinkers by the standard soda description. A sparkling water or quality root beer from time to time, sure, but my kids had never had real soda, especially Coca-Cola.

As I voiced my concern, I was met with a startling comment by the principal: "I got into education to teach kids skills, not nutrition." He ended it by saying it wasn't his job to police the teachers in their food rewards. He wasn't wrong, but he wasn't right.

How do most of us get our nutrition knowledge? It sure isn't from our physicians, we've established that. Do you remember how you learned about nutrition when you were growing up? I sure don't.

I remember my physician father following diets he thought were the best for us as a family. I still remember him saying things like, "It's pure protein," when talking about healthy foods and encouraging us to eat them.

According to the CDC, the education system plays an important role in helping students establish healthy dietary habits.[7] In fact, it is the primary source of nutrition education for Americans and should be part of the comprehensive health education curriculum in each school.

Yet students in America receive fewer than eight hours of nutrition education each school year, well below the 40–50 hours required to change behavior.[8] In addition, the number of schools providing the required hours of nutrition education dropped from 84.6 percent to 74.1 percent from 2000 to 2014. Why all schools are not mandated to teach nutrition is beyond me.

In 1947, Congress passed the National School Lunch Act to provide all children, whose families could not afford it, a school lunch. Today, nearly 100,000 schools across the country provide lunches for children, feeding 29.6 million students per day. Furthermore, 21.8 million of these students qualify for the free or reduced lunch prices, meaning their families' income falls at or below 130 percent of the poverty level and up to 185 percent above the poverty level. And 12.54 million students are using the free or reduced-price breakfasts as well.[9]

The following guidelines are listed on the CDC website from the 2015–2020 Dietary Guidelines for Americans recommendations for children ages 2 years and older:

- Eat a variety of fruits and vegetables.
- Eat fat-free and low-fat dairy products.
- Eat a variety of protein foods.
- Eat oils.
- Eat whole grains.

Those are your highlighted nutritional guidelines for children. Thank you, government.

The USDA is responsible for the execution of these guidelines in the school lunch programs, and they are falling short. Data from the National Health and Nutrition Examination Survey (NHANES) showed that, on average, all school children fell short of the Dietary Guidelines for Americans. On a scale of 1–100, the average Health Eating Index for 2005 (HEI-2005) score was 58.

The guidelines do state that a vegetable must be offered at each lunch, but the definition of what constitutes a vegetable is vague and includes french fries, relish, pizza sauce, and ketchup.

Research from the University of Michigan identified school lunches as a direct link to the increasing childhood obesity rates. According to the research, those who regularly had school lunches were 29 percent more likely to be obese than those who brought lunch from home.[10]

Childhood chronic diseases are on the rise, and just like their adult family members, most of these conditions are preventable with proper nutrition. One in five children over the age of six is obese, and the rate of type 2 diabetes diagnosis in children aged 10–15 rose five percent between 2002 and 2012.[11] It is no wonder why when you look at a standard breakfast and lunch menu provided by a government-funded school in America.

Most foods served in school cafeterias are highly processed, and school districts are forced to party with big food industry leaders, such as Tyson and Pepsi, due to low food budgets. If you have kids and you've ever visited their school cafeteria, you have seen this firsthand. PB&J sandwiches may be listed on the school lunch menu, but what they really are is prepackaged Smuckers Uncrustables. For breakfast, you may see "assorted muffins" on the menu, but what they really are is Otis Spunkmeyer Double Chocolate Muffins with 35 grams of sugar per muffin.

For many kids, their education system is the only place they can receive nutrition education, and for many American children, the school nutrition program is their primary source of calories for their entire day. Children do not learn by what they are told, they learn by their experiences. When their nutritional experiences tell them that these are acceptable choices, this is what they learn. In the communities with the least nutrition education and the most dependence on the school nutrition system we see the most childhood health problems and, in adulthood, higher rates of maternity complications and death.

Insufficiency Versus Deficiency

We have been told for generations that, due to efforts to fortify grains and nutrition education programs, nutritional deficiencies in the United States are rare, and that those Otis Spunkmeyer muffins are fine because they have added vitamins and minerals and are made with whole grains. Well, I hate to be the bearer of bad news, but this is a myth. In all actuality, nutritional deficiencies and insufficiencies are significantly more common than you think.

Insufficiencies in nutrients have long been left out of the nutritional deficiency picture, often left untreated until severe deficiency symptoms are present. To explain this, I am going to use vitamin D.

The term "insufficient" means a mild decrease, and "deficiency" means greater decrease. When we look at serum levels of vitamin D, we see that the normal reference range for this value is large, 30–100 nanograms (ng)/mL. Vitamin D insufficiency, by western standards, is defined as blood values below 30 ng/mL; deficiency is defined as 20 ng/mL or lower. This definition is calculated by analyzing bone growth and formation. With serum levels below 20 ng/mL, we see signs of bone malformation. Those with values above 20 ng/mL seem to be fine.

Vitamin D does so much more than help move calcium into bones. We need large amounts of vitamin D for pancreatic function, ovarian and reproduction function, the immune system, and so much more. Science is slowly catching up to the idea that many of our serum nutritional values, like vitamin D, are off.

A 2011 report published by the Endocrinology Society recommended that the deficiency value be raised to 20–30 ng/mL, and insufficiency value be raised to between 30–40 ng/mL, making the functional range of serum vitamin D 40–60 ng/mL.[12][13] This change was spurred by an analysis of studies showing that even those with serum vitamin D levels between 30–40 ng/mL still had markers for bone loss and other vitamin D-associated functional insufficiencies such as depression.

In addition, the current recommended daily intake for vitamin D in pregnancy is 600 International Units (IU), yet studies show that a mother needs to consume 4,000 IU, the upper limit of dietary intake, to meet the demands of pregnancy.[14] Fewer than this and she could fall into the insufficiency and deficiency ranges that are associated with a list of pregnancy complications.

The Nutrition Connection

Since the 1960s, the CDC has conducted a series of surveys to assess different health topics among the American public. In 1999, these surveys became focused, primarily, on nutrition and health across the United States. This survey system is called the NHANES. Data are released every two years.

A very telling portion of these surveys is the "What We Eat in America" components. It is conducted jointly between the USDA and the Department of Health and Human Services (HHS), the overseeing body of the CDC, to analyze actual dietary intakes. This information is then compared to the Dietary Guidelines for Americans, which are already flawed and found to be lacking. What we see from these studies is the following:

- 80 percent of Americans are not consuming the *minimum* recommended servings of vegetables per day.
- 75 percent of Americans are not consuming the *minimum* recommended servings of fruits per day.
- >40 percent of Americans are not consuming the *minimum* recommended servings of whole grains per day.

- \>40 percent of Americans are not consuming the *minimum* recommended servings of protein per day.
- 75 percent of Americans are not consuming the *minimum* recommended servings of healthy fats per day.
- \>65 percent of Americans are consuming *more* than the recommended limit of servings of added sugar per day.
- 70 percent of Americans are consuming *more* than the recommended limit of servings of saturated fats per day.
- 90 percent of Americans are consuming *more* than the recommended limit of servings for added sodium.

Percentage of dietary intake below the recommended daily intake level		
Nutrient	Girls Age 14–18	Adults Age >19
Vitamin D	98 %	95%
Vitamin E	99%	94%
Magnesium	90%	61%
Vitamin A	57%	51%
Calcium	81%	49%
Vitamin C	45%	43%
Vitamin B6	18%	15%
Folate	19%	13%
Zinc	24%	12%
Iron	12%	9%
Thiamine	10%	7%
Copper	16%	5%
Cobalamin	7%	4%
Riboflavin	5%	2%
Niacin	4%	2%
Selenium	2%	1%

Table 1: Based on the data collected by the CDC 2016 HNANES

The data also show that when we apply this to age and sex, children and young adults are consuming less nutrient-dense foods than any other group, with consumption of vegetables being worse in boys ages 9–13 and young women ages 14–18. The data point to adolescent girls as having the highest rates of nutritional insufficiencies and deficiencies at the ages in which their maturing bodies need adequate nutrition intake for future reproductive function.

Data on outright nutritional deficiencies are limited, mostly because many nutrients are not accurately measured in blood work and finding ways to assess nutrient function is limited and evolving. Considering the data that show Americans are not consuming even close to the minimum nutritional requirements set forth by the Dietary Guidelines for Americans, which is already subpar, we can assume that many are low in nutrients that can affect overall body function—especially in pregnancy where the nutrient requirements increase and change with physiological changes.

Nutrition in Disease

The connection between nutrition and disease is not new—not by a long shot. Throughout all known human history, great emphasis has been given to nutrition across the world.

Plato, the great fifth-century B.C. Greek philosopher, was a known proponent of moderation, frequently saying that excess food intake led to disease and ailments. Many of the dietary philosophies he propounded closely follow the now known Mediterranean Diet that is associated with the best all-around health benefits. That seems fair since Greece is a Mediterranean country. Other cultures, too, took nutrition seriously. In Chinese culture, entire schools of medicine were devoted to understanding the complex relationship food had on the body and disease, with the earliest writings coming from 200 B.C.

The history of modern nutrition science is a bit younger, with the first vitamin being isolated in 1926. The discovery and connection of vitamins to serious diseases of the time were undeniable and ushered in a period of great nutrition excitement. This was the era of Dr. Price and his colleagues, who studied and compared nutrition in both industrialized and traditional societies. Their advances in nutrition research led to food fortification programs that decreased severe nutrition malnutrition and associated disease. This excitement waned with advances in medical technology and the development of medications and vaccines.

The 1970s saw a great shift in nutrition research and theory as rates of cardiovascular disease and diabetes began to increase. Research linking both high fats and high sugars to cardiovascular disease battled one another for legitimacy. In the end, the fat researchers won, thanks to politics and money. Thus, the standard American dietary guidelines promoting low-fat, high-carb diets were born. In 1980, the U.S. National Academy of Sciences Food and Nutrition Boards reviewed the studies and concluded that evidence against fat was insufficient.

Jump ahead to the 2000s and these dietary guidelines have only slightly changed, still touting low fat and high carb diets with fortified foods. Finally, research has started to grab onto this idea that these dietary patterns are fueling the growing rates of chronic disease.

Chronic disease is on the rise, with nearly half of all Americans having at least one preventable chronic disease.[15] The connection between these chronic diseases pre-pregnancy and the development of them in pregnancy are highly connected to dietary and lifestyle choices.

Yet, when you do a search in PubMed for "Nutrition in Pregnancy Disease," the studies you find are focused on the nutritional deficiencies, dietary patterns, and their effects on the growing baby yet not on the health of the mother. Yes, making sure babies are healthy is a priority, and protecting these innocent lives from future health problems as a complication from this maternal disease is prudent. But shouldn't we also work on addressing the mother's health and reducing the effects of the disease by focusing on her nutrition when nutrition is a primary driver of the disease?

Some of the most disturbing increases seen, statistically, in maternal health are the rise in chronic pregnancy-associated diseases, such as gestational diabetes and hypertension. Studies are beginning to link these diseases with nutrient intake and dietary patterns as well as lifestyle and childhood health.

In 2003, the *Journal of Nutrition* published an article stating current concepts in the pathogenesis of preeclampsia included endothelial dysfunction, inflammatory activity, oxidative stress, and predisposed maternal factors, providing targets for nutritional investigation.[16]

A 2019 study published by the *British Journal of Obstetrics and Gynecology* found that the standard western diet increases the risk of developing gestational hypertension, while a diet higher in seafood and vegetables reduced the risk.[17]

In addition, when we look at these data, there is a strong correlation between maternity complications and racial groups, specifically non-Hispanic Blacks. The reason the rates among non-Hispanic Black Americans are so high is under serious debate. Many theorize that it is because medical care in areas with denser minority populations is poor. Some theorize that there is racial neglect by medical staff. While these may be just and accurate causes of the increased rate of maternal death among minorities, I pose a different theory.

Nutrition.

Why Specializing Matters

You cannot know everything about everything.

Functional medicine has been wonderful for so many people. The medical understanding of how the body is connected and the role nutrition plays at a biochemical level to create function is the basis of all functional medicine. I love functional medicine, and it is the key to helping so many prevent and overcome chronic diseases. Functional medicine certification gives you the base, but courses and studies that focus primarily on maternity give you mastery.

Everything in the body is connected, but there is uniqueness in maternity, as there are in other times in our life, that requires more specialized focus and education. This specializing in no way takes away from the beauty of whole-body functional medicine but considers the flow of the different stages of life.

Different phases of life offer different metabolic and system function differences. Pediatrics, maternity, menopause, geriatrics—at all these times in our lives the body is not the same, and it does not function the same. Just like everyone is biologically different with individual needs, so are they at different phases of life.

Nutrition needs change throughout our lives. With specialized medicine, we can focus on these individual times in the journey of life with better focused healthcare. There is nothing wrong with—and I believe we benefit from—having specialized medicine, with the understanding that the whole body is connected.

We have seen functional medicine break off into specialties such as neurology, psychiatry, fertility, and oncology. I would argue that maternity is the most important specialty for not only the individual patient but also humanity.

The nutritional health of the mother, the genetic expression and epigenetic possibilities that can occur when a mother is not nutritionally sound along with the method of birth all play into the foundation of health for the infant and its health into childhood and adulthood. Maternity and birth are the absolute foundation for the future health and prevention of chronic disease. If we really want to reverse the increasing rates of preventable disease in our society, we must start at the beginning with birth.

I had another functional medicine practitioner reach out to me with a question about a patient he had who was pregnant. He had run a functional lab panel on her, most of it unnecessary (one of my big hang-ups with many functional medicine practitioners, but that's a whole other topic). He was calling because her copper levels were elevated, and he was concerned about copper toxicity and how he could chelate and help her detox during pregnancy. Woah, time out! He, obviously, had no training in maternity care and really had no business working with this woman. Copper levels naturally elevate in pregnancy. Her levels were within normal ranges for her gestation, and he was about to put her through the ringer for a misdiagnosis based on non-pregnancy lab values.

Pregnancy is a unique time in human physiology. The body undergoes some amazing changes that outside of pregnancy could elicit disease and damage. I have not seen a single class or functional medicine program discuss these changes. By not doing so, we have given functional medicine practitioners zero skills in working with pregnant mothers, a demographic that arguably needs functional medicine the most.

Specializing in maternity care gives you bigger, more advanced tools in your toolbox. Understanding how bloodwork values change in pregnancy provides a key component to proper use of functional medicine in pregnancy. Many values that would be considered abnormal prior to pregnancy are completely normal during pregnancy.

This is only one example of how maternity care differs and how having advanced training in the care of pregnant women is crucial for proper treatment.

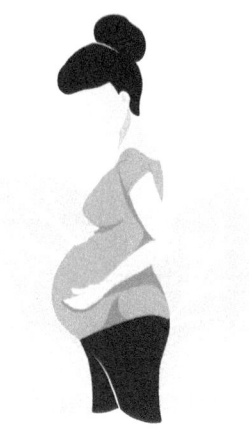

Part Two

Functional Maternity: A Different Approach

"When we learn how to work together versus against each other, things might start getting better."

- Alex Elle

Preconception nutrition for baby and mom •
Metabolic changes through pregnancy • Steroidogenesis •
Thyroid Physiology

CHAPTER 4

Preconception Nutrition for Baby And Mom

Whether we are discussing prenatal nutrition or maternity nutrition, we are always aiming for a healthy baby; we just want a healthy mom as well.

A healthy pregnancy begins before conception ever happens. I have a saying in the clinic: "We are preparing for preparing." Each phase of pregnancy is influenced by the trimester before. The nutritional focus we are putting on each phase is to support the changes required in the current trimester to ensure that the next phase is functional. The preconception phase of pregnancy is, in the scheme of things, the most important phase, as it sets the stage for the health of both the mother and the baby during pregnancy and beyond.

Fetal Programming

During the initial weeks of pregnancy, as the embryo becomes a fetus, deoxyribonucleic acid (DNA) is sequenced and patterned, creating the characteristics of the new baby. The preconception health of mom and dad will affect the success of the first weeks of pregnancy and the fetal programming that dictates the genetic expression of the new baby.

I have a fantastic handout I give to my preconception couples that explains, in-depth of course, ovarian and testicular function, health, and the role of nutrition. This handout is downloadable from my website (www.functionalmaternity.com.) Back to fetal programming.

In 1990, British epidemiologist David Barker hypothesized that poor nutritional habits during pregnancy influenced genetic expression and was directly related to the origins of cardiovascular disease, diabetes, and an increased risk of chronic disease later in life. This "Barker's Hypothesis" was the beginning of the understanding of epigenetics. These changes in genetic and metabolic programming occurred at certain points in fetal development.

Studies have since connected maternal and fetal nutrition with what we now call genetic programming, or epigenetics. So far, research has been able to highlight specific genetic changes, through fetal programming, that increase the risk of maternal, fetal, and placental health issues.[18]

Some of the interesting connections that have been found include studies that link maternal malnutrition with an increased presentation of obesity in children. Meaning if a mother was malnourished and her baby was born underweight, this baby was *more* likely to become obese later in life. This phenomenon was first seen in Holland after the 1940s famine.[19] Mothers during this time were consistently malnourished and the children born during this time were more likely to become obese in adulthood. Interestingly, we also see that the children born to mothers who are obese are also more likely to become obese in adulthood.[20]

The idea that overnutrition and undernutrition can change fetal genetics to express a higher risk for excess weight gain has been replicated in animal studies as well. These changes have been associated with the expression of genes associated with abnormal metabolism, mitochondrial dysfunction, and an increased response to stress.[21] [22]

It is well-established that babies born to women with gestational diabetes have hyperinsulinemia, which are excessively high levels of insulin, during gestation and often in the hours after birth. Newer research is linking this condition to more permanent changes in the child's glucose metabolism, making it more likely for them to have insulin resistance and metabolic syndrome in adulthood. We also see that this can occur in women with controlled gestational diabetes as well.[23]

If we continue down our current path, with rates of gestational diabetes increasing yearly and knowing that maternal gestational diabetes genetically programs babies to be more insulin-resistant and increases their risk of gestational diabetes, we will continue to see these statistics rise. If we can prevent gestational diabetes in women by addressing the functional physiology of pathology, we may be able to reduce the cases of gestational diabetes in future generations.

So far, the recognized key mechanisms involved in epigenetics are DNA methylation and histone modification. These processes regulate gene expression in the initial stages of cellular growth, at conception, and are heavily influenced by maternal nutritional intake.

DNA Methylation

Methylation is a hot new term in the health world. Most of you have heard of methylation at this point, and most of you are already familiar with methylenetetrahydrofolate reductase (MTHFR) and its role in folate methylation. For some of you, this is a new concept.

Methylation really means the addition of a methyl group somewhere in physiology. When we are talking about DNA methylation and fetal programming, we are talking about the need for methyl groups to regulate DNA expression in fetal development.

Methyl groups inhibit the expression of genetic mutations, basically keeping the DNA in sequence and protecting its coding. In 2012, this epigenetic process was identified as a key factor in fetal programming.[24]

Methyl groups are found, primarily, in the foods we consume: one-carbon nutrients, a.k.a. our B vitamins and choline. For dietary B vitamins to be used in cells, there are several complicated processes that need to occur, requiring a functional mother and adequate nutrition.

Deep breath.

Dietary folate and choline are the two main methyl donors used in the body to create the primary DNA methyl donor, the compound s-adenosylmethionine, but you know it best as SAMe (also known as AdoMet in Europe).

Making SAMe is quite the process.

It starts with the dietary consumption of folate and choline, as well as other nutrients such as riboflavin-B2 and magnesium, which are also important for the steps in these cycles to work flawlessly.

Folate is naturally present in many food sources and is essential for the nucleic acid synthesis and other vital biological processes in the body. Dietary folate is metabolized into tetrahydrofolate (THF) in the liver. The first step in making folate usable in the methylation cycle is to transfer carbon from the amino acid serine to THF. This reaction is catalyzed by the enzyme serine hydroxymethyltransferase (SHMT), a vitamin B6-containing enzyme. (See Figure 1.)

The outcome of this reaction is 5,10 methylenetetrahydrofolate, which is, in turn, transformed into 5-methyltetrahydrofolate (5-MTHF) via the enzyme methylenetetrahydrofolate reductase (MTHFR), a vitamin B2-containing enzyme. This step and the required riboflavin are now becoming an area of focus in methylation management. 5-MTHF is the primary methyl donor for the reaction in the methionine cycle that produces SAMe.

MTHFR has taken the spotlight in genetic variant identification and treatment. An estimated 30 percent of all people carry at least one variant in the gene that expresses this enzyme.

Recent observations obtained from women undergoing in vitro fertilization (IVF) who carried the C677T MTHFR SNP showed that these women generated preimplantation embryos with high rates of genetic variants and decreased embryo viability.[25] This single-nucleotide polymorphism (SNP) and, to a lesser extent, the A1298C MTHFR SNP are known to affect the amount of folate that enters the methionine cycle. Ten percent of people are homozygous for these variants. This is a serious genetic mutation that affects fertility and pregnancy outcomes. Research seems to point to a more prominent effect on folate methylation in those who are homozygous carriers and to a lesser extent in those with a single variant. This is an important consideration when addressing recurrent miscarriages and many pregnancy complications.

Folate, Folic Acid & Choline

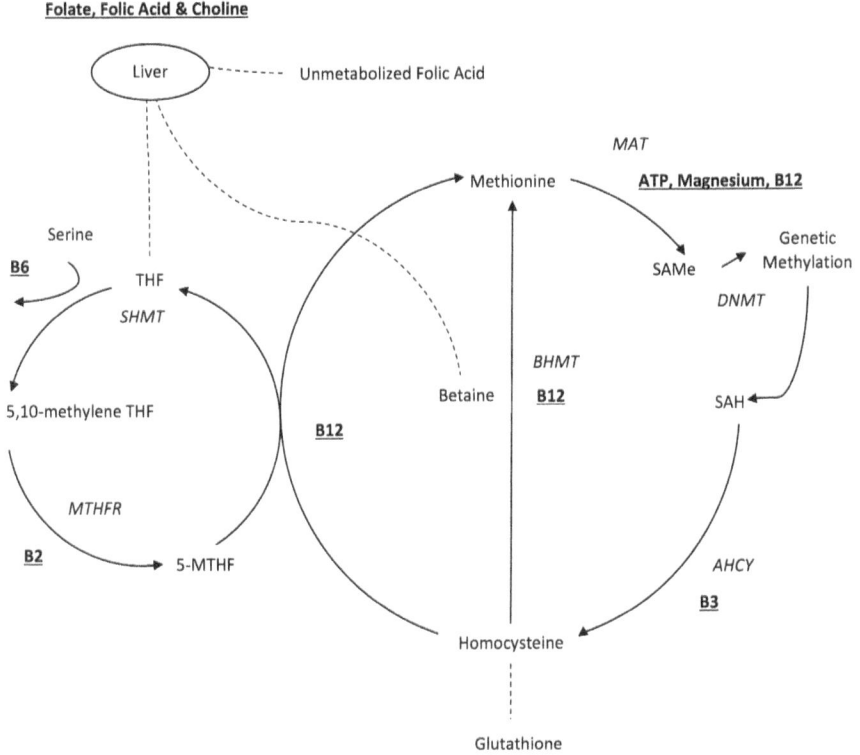

Figure 1: The folate and choline cycles that create SAMe for genetic methylation. 1) Dietary folate is metabolized into THF in the liver, 2) *THF + Serine + SHMT + B6 = is 5,10 methylenetetrahydrofolate, 3) 5,10 methylenetetrahydrofolate + MTHFR = 5-MTHF, 4) Methionine synthase + 5-MTHF + Zinc + B12 + Homocysteine = Methionine, 5) MAT + ATP + Magnesium + B12 = SAMe, 6) DNMT transports SAMe to cells, removes a methyl group, and leaves behind SAH, 7) SAH + Adenosylhomocysteinase + B3 = Homocysteine – Choline is oxidized in the liver to make TMG, which can also be used. TMG + BHMT + Homocysteine + B12 = Methionine.*

Once folate has been converted to methylfolate it functions in the methionine cycle. To enter the methionine cycle, it needs zinc and vitamin B12 (cobalamin). Several genes code for an enzyme called methionine synthase that requires B12 to function correctly.

Methionine synthase + methylfolate + zinc + B12 + homocysteine = methionine.

Did you see that? I just snuck that little homocysteine in there.

Homocysteine is a byproduct of DNA methylation. Yep, we are making a repetitive cycle here. Homocysteine is not a good chemical on its own. It is associated with several diseases, including gestational hypertension.

Once methionine is produced it is then bound to adenosine triphosphate (ATP), energy produced in glucose and fat metabolism (more in Chapter 5) to create SAMe. The enzyme s-adenosylmethionine synthetase (SAMe synthetase) fuels this reaction. This enzyme requires magnesium and cobalt—not something you ever think about in nutrition—for function and is activated by potassium. So, electrolyte balance is especially important to the formation of SAMe.

Now that we have SAMe, how does it get used in DNA methylation?

DNA is made up of a combination of nucleotides. These are the building blocks of DNA. Each nucleotide consists of an amino acid base bound to a sugar (deoxyribose in DNA) and a phosphate group. (See Figure 2.)

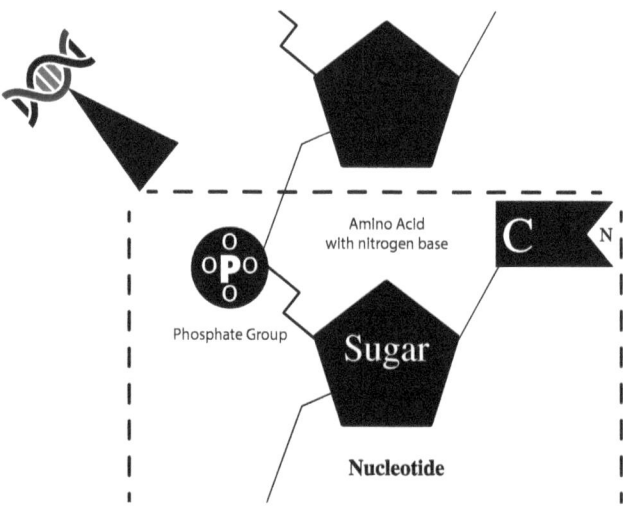

Figure 2: Nucleotide structure. SAMe deposits a methyl group into the nitrogen base.

A bunch of nucleotides strung together make the strands of DNA. The DNA sequences in the newly formed embryo are a combination of nucleotides from both mom and dad. These newly formed strands need to be activated—or not activated—for genetic expression, cellular development, and basic life expression of our new baby.

The addition of a methyl group to the nitrogen ends of the amino acids in the nucleotides is catalyzed by DNA methyltransferase (DNMT). DNMT is stimulated by cortisol, which rises at different phases in gestation to stimulate important functions in fetal growth.

Certain environmental chemicals, such as bisphenol A (BPA), can inhibit DNMT function. BPA is a chemical found in the production of plastics and resin in industrial manufacturing. These plastics are everywhere in our lives—water bottles, baby bottles, sippy cups, plastic storage containers, canned food, etc.—and they wreak havoc on our bodies in many ways, one of which is the genetic expression of embryos.[26]

After DNMT transports SAMe to deposit its methyl group, adenosylhomocysteine (AdoHcy or SAH) is left behind. The enzyme adenosylhomocysteinase converts SAH into homocysteine and adenosine. This reaction requires vitamin B3 (niacin).

Unmetabolized homocysteine is toxic. The body is pretty cool and has multiple pathways of recycling homocysteine into usable compounds, such as the antioxidant glutathione and methionine. Recycling it back into methionine is crucial for overall health.

There is a secondary pathway of breaking down homocysteine to methionine and thus the formation of the SAMe required for fetal genetic methylation: betaine-homocysteine methyltransferase (BHMT), a zinc-containing enzyme.

Betaine is a methyl donor that is consumed in the diet and produced in the liver through the breakdown of choline, which also comes from the diet. Choline is oxidized in the liver to make the betaine needed for homocysteine metabolism. Betaine is also known as trimethylglycine (TMG). It enters the BHMT pathway where a methyl group is removed and connected to homocysteine to create methionine, which is ultimately converted to SAMe and SAMe to homocysteine, and the cycle continues. (See Figure 1)

For fetal programming to occur the way it is supposed to, mothers and fathers need to consume adequate amounts of these nutrients prior to conception. The nutrients are stored in the egg and sperm and upon conception begin to transcribe the fetal genetic code. Most miscarriages are due to faults in the genetic coding and can occur before a mother even knows she is pregnant. I could probably write a whole other book, or at least a few good chapters, on the importance of male preconception health as well because it is just as important as that of the mother. Please check out my eBook download *Functional Fertility - Improving the Health of Your Eggs & Sperm for Better Conception Success* on my website.

This is an amazing and exciting time in science as more and more research is being published about epigenetic expression and other influences on genetic expression in fetal development through adulthood.

A Word on Unmetabolized Folic Acid

Folic acid and folate are different forms of vitamin B9. The name folate comes from the Latin word "folium," which means leaf. Interestingly, it is found in high amounts in green leafy vegetables.

Folic acid is the form found in most supplements, especially the prescription prenatal vitamins often given in doctors' offices and in fortified foods. It has been recommended as the best source of vitamin B9 for generations.

Food-sourced folate is naturally bound to proteins. Before it can be absorbed these proteins need to be removed. These proteins are called glutamate residues, and dietary folate can have up to seven of these stowaways that need to be reduced to one before it can be absorbed.

This breakdown is quite the process. At best, only about 50 percent of dietary folate is absorbed.[27] In addition, natural folate is heat-sensitive and can be destroyed in cooking.

Folic acid is synthetically reduced to be a single glutamate-containing compound, has a better absorption rate, at about 85 percent, and can tolerate high heat. When you compare it to the absorption rate of natural folate and natural folate's sensitivity to heat, it would seem to be the better option.

Interestingly, studies show that natural folate, not folic acid, is more functional in the body. But studies comparing dietary folate and folic acid are, well, interesting.

There is no doubt that folic acid is more stable and better absorbed than naturally occurring folates, raising blood levels of the unmetabolized folates quicker. It's once these two compounds enter the body that we see some stark changes in how they function. The liver is the primary organ of folate metabolism and partial storage. Once absorbed, folates are transported to the liver to be methylated into 5-methyltetrahydrofolate (5-MTHF), the form required for DNA methylation to occur. Natural folate does this well, which is why you see serum folate levels rise and decrease quickly after consumption. Synthetic folic acid on the other hand, not so much.

Concern is starting to be raised about the negative effects of high-dose folic acid, simply because it does not metabolize well (methylate) in the liver, and thus we see high serum levels of folic acid, but it is unmetabolized. No one is arguing that these unmetabolized folates exist or that folic acid saturation is needed to have a functional effect on the body, which leads to excessively high levels of unmetabolized folic acid. The argument now is what does this mean? And does it cause damage? Because these unmetabolized folic acid compounds are considered "inactive", many believe they are benign. Others are beginning to paint a slightly different picture.

NUTRIENT HIGHLIGHT: CHOLINE

Choline is a dietary nutrient similar in structure to B vitamins. Your body can produce a small amount of choline on its own, but not enough to fulfill all of your daily needs, especially in pregnancy. Dietary intake is also required.

Choline plays a role in various body functions, including cell membrane structure, genetic methylation, metabolism, and mental health.

There are two different forms of choline found in the diet: a water-soluble form and a fat-soluble form.

Water-soluble choline is absorbed through the small intestines and transported to the liver for storage. There it is phosphorylated into a fat-soluble form (phosphatidylcholine) as needed to make up cell membranes, phosphatidylcholine.

The active fat-soluble choline forms are more prominent in the diet. These dietary nutrients are absorbed directly into the bloodstream and go to work throughout the body without needing to be processed in the liver.

Several factors determine choline need and the risk of deficiency. During pregnancy, there is an increased demand for choline, with most of it going to the developing baby.

A study from 2017 suggested that only 8.5 percent of pregnant women were meeting the choline demand in pregnancy, or over 90 percent of women were deficient. As of this year, few prenatal vitamins contain choline.[28] There is also concern that the current recommended levels for choline in pregnancy are too low and that, due to the increased demand in the third trimester, this should be changed.

The current adequate intake (AI) values for choline in pregnancy is 450 mg/day. In 2017, the American Medical Association announced their support of increasing prenatal supplements to contain the 450 mg/day of choline. Sadly, most prenatal supplements, including the top-selling brands, do not contain any choline.

A 2015 article published in the *Journal of Clinical Nutrition* may have found an interesting connection that affects DNA methylation. The study fed folic acid-saturated diets to mice. One group was homozygous for the MTHFR mutation, and the other group was heterozygous (or not functionally variant). What they found was interesting. The high-dose synthetic folic acid supplementation induced a pseudo-MTHFR homozygous presentation by reducing the activity of the MTHFR enzyme. These mice also developed enlarged livers associated with non-alcoholic fatty liver disease.[29]

A 2012 study published in the *Journal of Pediatric Biochemistry* reported that folic acid supplementation during pregnancy was associated with an increased risk of autism in the developing baby.[30]

A 2017 review found enough evidence between unmetabolized folic acid and autism to elicit a warning on its use.[31]

Folate deficiency is highly associated with neural tube defects (NTDs). NTDs occur when the neural tube (the precursor to the central nervous system (CNS) that includes the spinal cord) doesn't close properly in early development. Supplementing with both folate and folic acid has been shown to reduce the risk of NTDs. The concern now is that the synthetic folic acid, due to its poor metabolism, may be causing other problems in the CNS during this crucial developmental phase.

These new discoveries make us rethink the folic acid supplements and fortification that is hugely popular in the United States and now around the world.

Folate or Choline in Methylation

So, which methyl donor vitamin is better: folate or choline?

Well, we need both. Different cells prefer different methyl donors. We also see that in those who are homozygous for the 677CT MTHFR mutation, there is an increased sensitivity to betaine in all cells. So, the old treatment plan of just giving high-dose methylfolate for these women may not be the optimal treatment approach.

This is an individual question and something that, as trained maternity functional medicine practitioners, we should be able to help a mother determine and assess through proper testing and presentation.

This process is the foundation of a baby's genetics, and methylation is essential in expressing the genetic predispositions this new person will carry into adulthood. Without proper methylation to silence damaged DNA and stabilize the genomic code, we see the expression of certain negative genetics in future adulthood, such as cancer and genes associated with chronic disease. But it's not the only process that affects genetic expression.

Histone Modification

Histones are basic proteins that help to package and condense DNA into a complex called chromatin. The proteins look like a cylinder with multiple tails extending to enwrap the DNA strands, holding them secure and tight. The way in which these tails function is influenced by methylation, acetylation, phosphorylation, adenylation, and ubiquitination.[32] The structure of the chromatin is heavily influenced by these factors, which change the way the DNA is expressed.

A little walk back in time to organic chemistry, that is, *if* you took organic chemistry. If not, no worries, I'll help you catch up.

DNA is negatively charged, due to its large amount of phosphorus. Histones should be positively charged to allow for a tightly coiled DNA strand. Methylation increases this tightness, stabilizing the DNA strand and preventing genetic expression. Acetylation, on the other hand, opens the genetic code by creating a repelling negative charge.

We've already discussed, probably a bit too much, the methylation process. We see SAMe methylation occurring on the tails of the histones as well, increasing and stabilizing their structure to protect DNA.

Acetylation provides the opposite. Histone acetyltransferases (HATs) are enzymes that acetylate histone tails, or deposit acetyl groups to the protein ends. These enzymes contain a compound called acetyl coenzyme A (acetyl-CoA), which contains vitamin B5 (pantothenic acid).

Acetylation is not all bad and is important for the genetic expression that must occur for the new baby to develop properly. Too much, though, and without balance and we see the genetic expression of damaged or negative genes. Other enzymes called histone deacetylases (HDACs) remove the acetyl group. When functioning normally, histones are acetylated to increase expression and then deacetylated to stabilize the DNA strands again. There are 18 known HDAC enzymes that use either zinc or vitamin B3 (niacin) to function[33], making zinc and B3 essential for stabilizing DNA after transcription.

Just like everything in the body, balance is key. The body needs both inflammation and anti-inflammation properties, the same way it needs the balance of methylation and acetylation to open and close the ability of DNA to transcribe genes. Although it is a bit more complicated than just methylation and acetylation, these two actions are the primary drivers of histone modification.

Histone modification is dependent on several different nutrients, including vitamins B3, B5, B6, B9, B12, zinc, magnesium, manganese, calcium, and coenzyme Q10 (CoQ10). The histone modification process is highly influenced by maternal dietary patterns, not just nutrient intake.

Animal studies have shown that maternal diets that are high in saturated fats and fructose—so, the standard American diet—are associated with marked fetal liver dysregulation.[34] These dietary influences on histone modification have become a base for the fetal origins of adult disease.[35]

Studies have also shown that preconception maternal diet is essential for the correct genetic expression in the early stages of conception. Malnutrition, especially in the nutrients required for proper methylation, and deacetylation can lead to increased histone acetylation that opens the genetic code, allowing the expression of negative genes associated with fetal and adult diseases, such as increased appetite and metabolic dysfunction.[36] [37]

Similarly, changes in histone modification were seen in mice who were overfed. Overnutrition, or an excess intake of calories at a single meal, was associated with increased fetal insulin resistance.[38]

These processes don't just affect the development of the embryo but also the genetic expression and formation of the placenta.

Placental Development

The placenta is the organ that sustains most of pregnancy after about the tenth week of gestation, providing oxygen, nutrients, and hormonal signals. In those first few months, the growth and genetic expression of the genes in these cells will set the stage for the predisposition of disease as well as the health of the baby and the mother throughout the remainder of pregnancy.

Histone modification and DNA methylation become especially important when we are looking into the proper development of the placenta. The healthy development of the placenta is essential for both maternal and prenatal health. Several gestational diseases have been connected to dysfunctions within the placenta, including preeclampsia and maternal depression. Establishing a healthy placenta begins before conception, with the proper nutrients being stored within the sperm and eggs.

The trophoblast cells make up the outer lining of the newly formed embryo, and as the embryo embeds into the endometrial lining, these cells begin to change to form the placenta. A specialized trophoblast cell, called a cytotrophoblast, changes the structure of the maternal uterine blood vessels, making them larger.

We see in studies that these trophoblast cells contain receptors for vitamin D, and these cells both produce active vitamin D and respond to vitamin D levels.[39] Vitamin D is a fat-soluble vitamin that takes time to increase in the blood.

Supplementation therapies often take months to correct deficiency, hence the importance of correct vitamin D intake in the preconception diet. If the placental trophoblast cells are unable to function correctly, the placenta may develop poorly and increase the risk of fetal and maternal complications.

The growth of the placenta does not stop at 12 weeks but continues to grow throughout gestation. Like the growth and development of the baby itself, the placenta accelerates its growth at specific times in gestation. To stimulate this growth, the cytotrophoblast cells produce placental insulin growth factor (PIGF). PIGF stimulates the growth of both the baby and the placenta throughout pregnancy. Receptors for PIGF are found on the placenta and these receptors respond to both insulin and PIGF. PIGF specifically stimulates anabolic processes in the mother to increase nutrients needed for fetal growth. During mid- to late-gestation, the maternal serum levels of PIGF rise to facilitate the final growth spurt of the baby and placenta.

Interestingly, from working with patients all over the world, I have found that standard blood work panels in other countries run PIGFs. Lower levels of PIGF are indicative of a poorly functioning placenta and are associated with an increased risk of cardiovascular conditions such as hypertension and preeclampsia. Many countries use this to predict the possibility of developing these conditions to treat the conditions early. Studies also show that is a promising tool at predicting preeclampsia risk.[40]

Another key nutrient in the correct development of the placenta is zinc. Mouse studies have shown that zinc-deficient diets lead to smaller and weaker placentas and babies.[41] When analyzed, they found changes to the placental morphology. The placental morphology was also associated with changes in vascular function, increasing the risk of hypertension, preeclampsia, and other dysfunctional patterns associated with a decrease in placental blood flow.

The health of the placenta has been indicated as a primary driver of maternal disease, and if we are to help our mothers, we need to start by helping the initial growth phase with proper preconception nutrition. The effect maternal diet has on the health of the placenta doesn't stop in the first trimester. The continued dietary choices can create both positive and negative changes to the placenta's ability to grow and function. By focusing on nutrients that help the placenta function properly, such as magnesium, vitamin D, zinc, vitamin E (tocopherol), and vitamin C, we can help prevent the diseases associated with poor placental function.

You Are Your Mother and Your Grandmother

The diet of the mother and the father before conception is essential to a successful pregnancy. But sometimes we are our genetics, and dietary patterns cannot influence ancestral history. Newer research is pointing toward a connection between maternal stress responses and epigenetic changes in fetal development that can last generations.[42]

Stress is another factor that influences epigenetics. Crazy, right? The emotional and physical stress a woman experiences in her pregnancy creates a genetic ripple effect through the generational line, subsequently affecting her children and grandchildren.

Post-traumatic stress disorder (PTSD) is often associated with wartime survivors and soldiers, but we also see PTSD in traumatic birth experiences. We also see that many of the preventable diseases we are discussing increase stress responses in the body and can also affect genetics in the same way.

Research has just begun to elucidate the connections between trauma survivors and the genetic stress in their future children. Timing must be right for this to occur. A woman must be in the early stages of pregnancy when the trauma occurs to have an influence on the genetic expression of stress response in future generations.

These changes transfer through generations, especially among female children. You need to imagine that a pregnant woman, if she is carrying a daughter, is also carrying her granddaughter in the egg that is developing inside the female fetus. All the eggs this child will ever have will develop while she is in utero. The dietary habits, stress responses, and environment of the mother not only influences her pregnancy and her child, but also her grandchild.

Most of the research and the things I discuss in this book culminated into a pattern of familial dysfunction due to several different factors. Stress is a component of the whole picture that must be addressed as much as the nutritional components.

Nutrition and Physical Degeneration

In Dr. Price's book, he looked closely at the physical changes that occurred in families and birth order. He made connections between traditional societies, diet, and how this impacted not only the birth outcomes but also the health of the children born.

He found that birth order made a difference in the physical profile of children. When he examined people of native tribes, he found that children born while the mother was living a traditional life and consuming traditional foods were more robust and had fewer health problems. Children born once the mother was moved to government rations were weaker with more dental and physical changes.

In his book, he often quotes another researcher at the time, Dr. Kathleen Vaughan, and her book, *Safe Childbirth*. Dr. Price wrote,

> "The difficulty encountered at childbirth in our modern civilization has been emphasized by Dr. Kathleen Vaughan of London. In her book, 'Safe Childbirth,' she states that faults of development more than race modify pelvic shape. In the Foreword to her book, Dr. Howard A. Kelly, Professor Emeritus of Gynaecological Surgery, Johns Hopkins University, says: "Dr. Vaughan presents such an array of facts and data that the book must impress every reader. It is of vital importance that her conclusions be considered, for in my opinion our methods of bringing up our girls and the habits of our women with many of the customs of 'civilized' life must be radically readjusted."

Later, he also wrote,

> "Dr. Vaughan's work places emphasis on the necessity that the human body be properly built, especially that of the mother-to-be. She shows clearly that the shape of the pelvis is determined by the method of life and the nutrition. In all primitive tribes living an outdoor life childbirth is easy and labor is of short duration. She shows that this is associated with a round pelvis and that the distortion of the pelvis to a flattened or kidney shape, even to a small degree, greatly reduces the capacity and therefore the ease with which the infant head may pass through the birth canal."

What Dr. Vaughan discovered in her work with traditional cultures was that the nutrition of the mother and the nutrition and life of the child as it grew was more indicative of narrowing pelvic formation than race. This accounts for the changes Dr. Price noted as well.

> "One of the outstanding changes which I have found takes place in the primitive races at their point of contact with our modern civilization is a decrease in the ease and efficiency of the birth process. When I visited the Six Nation Reservation at Brantford, Ontario, I was told by the physician in charge that a change of this kind had occurred during the period of his administration, which had covered twenty-eight years and that the hospital was now used largely to care for young Indian women during abnormal childbirth.

> "A similar impressive comment was made to me by Dr. Romig, the superintendent of the government hospital for Eskimos and Indians at Anchorage, Alaska. He stated that in his thirty-six years among the Eskimos, he had never been able to arrive in time to see a normal birth by a primitive Eskimo woman. But conditions have changed materially with the new generation of Eskimo girls, born after their parents began to use foods of modern civilization. Many of them are carried to his hospital after they had been in labor for several days."[43]

NUTRIENT HIGHLIGHT: ZINC

Zinc is the second most abundant mineral in the body, next to iron. Zinc is an elemental mineral that makes up the structure of over 100 known enzymes and is a cofactor for over 300 other enzymes. It is required for the function of the immune system, protein metabolism, healing, DNA synthesis, and cellular division. The body does not have the ability to store zinc, so it needs to be consumed in the diet daily.

Zinc is possibly the most important nutrient for conception and pregnancy. It is essential for the enzyme-catalyzed reactions that ignite embryonic development.

During conception, when the sperm enters the egg, there is a literal spark that occurs, like a firework. Studies in IVF have found that when the sperm and egg meet, there is a firework reaction that occurs. By analyzing these zinc-catalyzed sparks, physicians can determine which embryos are the strongest and most likely to survive transfer.[44]

Like most minerals, zinc is poorly absorbed and the form in which it is consumed makes a difference in how the body processes it. We see in studies that zinc absorption is better when it comes from foods high in protein and from animal sources.[45] In fact, the amount of protein in the food source and meal directly dictates the amount of zinc absorbed.

As foods are digested together, complex proteins are broken down into amino acids that bind to minerals like zinc. These chelated forms enhance the absorption.

Phytates in foods are the biggest inhibitors of zinc and other minerals' absorption.

Maternity functional medicine is not going to change structure, at least not for the mothers we are currently working with. But it could help save the lives of future mothers, by giving them the genetic nutrition and support they need in utero and in the early stages of life to help their bodies function properly.

So, both prenatal nutrition and maternal nutrition are crucial. If we want to make changes that begin to decrease the current statistics that are rising each year, we need to start treating each mother nutritionally not only for her current health and well-being but also with the knowledge of prevention. If we can change the genetic expression and the birth method of new daughters, then we can begin to change their pregnancy and birth fate and that of their children, and so on.

A Cultural Approach to Phytates

Phytate is the storage form of phosphorus. Foods that are high in phosphates are primarily the reproductive portions of plants, a.k.a. seeds. This includes grains, seeds, nuts, and legumes. Each of these is in hibernation form waiting for the right environment to release the germ inside. To protect the nutrients needed to germinate, these seeds contain phytates that inhibit proper digestion of the seed and keep the nutrients safe for when it is ready to grow. Removing phytates increases absorption.

Legumes and grains have been staples of the human diet for tens of thousands of years. They are a natural part of a healthy diet. Hunter-gatherers collected the seeds of many plants, stored them, and used them. Traditional cultures, just like the ones Dr. Price wrote about and analyzed for their health, consumed many of these seed foods. I always tell patients that many of the extreme healthy diet fads limit these foods because it is easier to tell you to avoid them than to teach you how to use them.

There are accounts of the Aztec tribes using and soaking their legumes before boiling. Many people I've met from around the world have a cultural tradition of soaking legumes before they are cooked. Soaking starts the germination process, not enough to see a sprout, but enough to break down the phytate into phosphorus and release the stored minerals.

Other traditional techniques used to prepare legumes include the fermentation seen in Asian cultures, such as in the making miso, tempeh, natto, and doenjang.

Grains are another seed food that we have forgotten how to use. Some will say that the older, more traditional methods of harvesting and storing grains would have allowed for the sprouting process to begin. Maybe? Sprouting in storage could have happened, but the goal was to store grains in a cold, dry spot so that they would last—not sprout—and grow. It was more the method of preparation that made a difference. Traditional breads came from soured dough, and whole grains were soaked, just like legumes, before cooking.

There is modern research that supports this idea. Several studies show that zinc absorption from whole wheat flour is low, but when the same flour is soured the zinc absorption increases substantially.[46] Souring dough and letting grains ferment is an ancient and traditional practice around the world. Our ancestors knew from trial and error how to use their seed food sources to maximize health.

I have fond memories of my grandmother washing rice. Washing rice was one of the first jobs I was given at her house as a kid. It was tedious, and I would frustratingly ask when she was going to cook it because, well, I was hungry. She would tell me that washing the rice made it good for the stomach. In her words and her time, she didn't know why, she just had been told—like her mother before her—that you wash the rice. I still do this, and when I'm lazy and I try not to, I can hear her voice in my head, "Aigo, why you no wash rice?" and I buck up and wash the rice.

Chapter 5

Metabolic Changes Throughout Pregnancy

Pregnancy is amazing, and the changes that a mother's body goes through to facilitate the growth of life is a miracle of nature. Metabolic changes, from anabolic to catabolic and back again, occur at varying stages of gestation. To understand these changes and how they affect the pregnant mother, you must first understand the basics of cellular metabolism.

Cellular metabolism is the process by which the body turns dietary fuel into energy.

This is one of my favorite topics to discuss with all my patients no matter what condition they are coming in for. This is the metabolic cycle that gives us life, and if my nine-year-old can learn it so can my patients. When my oldest daughter was in third grade, she had to do a project for her class. They called it an expedition. She could pick any topic, research it, make a poster of the information she gathered, and do a presentation in front of her class. The day she got the assignment, she came home and told me she wanted to know how food gave her energy. Proud mom moment!

I, of course, totally geeked out. I set her up in my office in front of a whiteboard and went to town. I was about halfway through my lecture when I saw her eyes glazing over. Hmmm, she wasn't quite ready for full-out biochemistry at nine. Fair enough.

I started over and started smaller. I drew pictures and used a car analogy: The fuel was the calories, the sparks that ignited the calories were enzymes, and the byproducts were energy and pollutants. In the end, not only did my daughter learn all about mitochondria and the citric acid cycle, but I learned a few valuable lessons about how to talk to my patients.

You see, most people do not have a degree that required them to take biology or biochemistry. Shocking, right? Most people see nutrition and health as children do, with confusion and in basic terms. So, as any patient of mine, or anyone who has done one of my courses will know, I love analogies and I love drawing things out. I use not-so-scientific terms to describe overly complicated concepts to pretty much everyone.

By the way, she rocked her presentation.

The Krebs Cycle

Our body is made up of billions of cells. The cell is the smallest unit of life. Cells, in the human body, are not all the same and each is designed for specific tissues and specific functions. What they all have in common is that they contain little organelles called mitochondria. These are the engines of the cells, and this is where cellular metabolism occurs.

Mitochondria also contain their own DNA, which is passed from mother to child through the egg cells. Remember all that methylation and acetylation stuff and how it can program metabolism in future generations?

This cellular metabolic cycle goes by several names: cellular respiration, the Krebs cycle, the citric acid cycle, and the tricarboxylic cycle. It is a series of complex enzymatic reactions that produce energy in the cells. This energy is called adenosine triphosphate (ATP). Calories from carbohydrates and fats serve as the primary fuel sources for these reactions. Proteins are only used as energy in emergency situations because they require extra steps in the liver before they can be added to the cycle.

To be used in cellular metabolism, carbohydrates are broken down into their base molecule: glucose. This glucose is then transported to the individual cells by insulin. Insulin binds to specific receptors on the cells that allow insulin and glucose to enter. Glucose is then broken down into pyruvate before entering the mitochondria and the Krebs cycle. Each molecule of glucose gives us two pyruvate molecules, meaning two spins on the Krebs cycle wheel.

In the mitochondria, the pyruvate molecule is further broken down into acetyl-coenzyme A, the same acetyl-coenzyme A that is an acetyl group donor for histone acetylation. Acetyl-coenzyme A is the first molecule to enter the actual Krebs cycle.

Once acetyl-CoA enters the system there are eight steps in the cycle of energy production, each requiring a different enzyme and each enzyme requiring a different array of nutritional requirements. (See Figure 3.)

When I first learned this cycle in school, an important part was never taught: the understanding of how individual nutrients influence the formation and function of these enzymes. This is a crucial part of functional medicine training and something many of you are seeking. Seems key to understanding metabolism, doesn't it?

Of all the dietary nutrients, the biggest influencers of the Krebs cycle are the B vitamins. B vitamins are water-soluble vitamins—perfect for a system that requires water to function. Any deficiency in these vital mitochondrial nutrients can compromise the entire system:

- Any enzyme that has the term "decarboxylation" (which means it causes a release of carbon dioxide) in its name requires vitamin B1 (thiamine).

- Many of the enzymes in the Krebs cycle are flavoenzymes, meaning they have vitamin B2 (riboflavin) in their structure.

- Nicotinamide adenine dinucleotide plus hydrogen (NADH) is synthesized from niacin-vitamin B3-containing NAD and is the cofactor for several enzymes in the cycle.

- Vitamin B5 (pantothenic acid) is required for coenzyme A formation and fatty acid oxidation.

- Vitamin B7 (biotin) is the cofactor for enzymes required for fatty acid metabolism into acetyl-CoA.

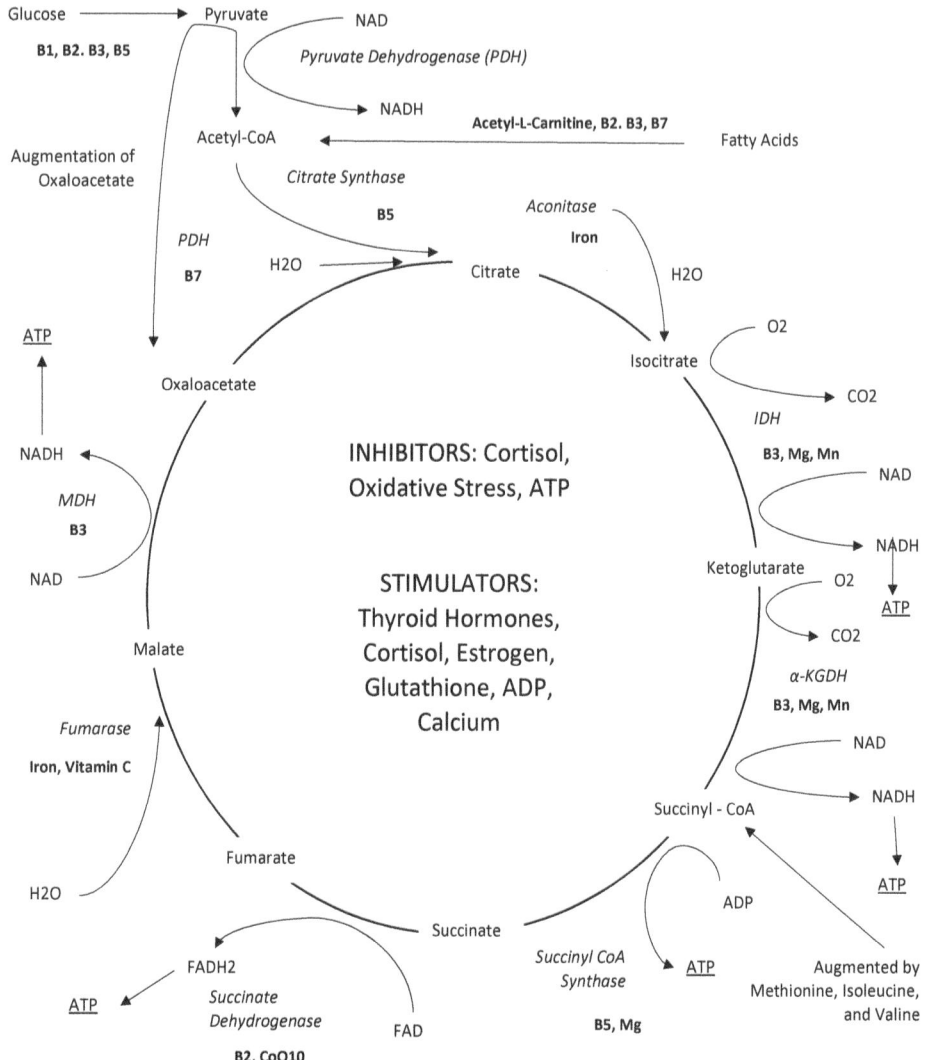

Figure 3: Krebs cycle with nutrient cofactors. 1) acetyl-coenzyme A + oxaloacetate + citrate synthase + ATP + magnesium = citric acid, 2) citric acid + (iron and sulfur containing) aconitase + water = isocitrate, 3) isocitrate + oxygen + isocitrate dehydrogenase + B3 + Mg + Mn = α-ketoglutarate, 4) α-ketoglutarate + oxygen + ketoglutarate dehydrogenase + B3 + B1 + lipoic acid + (B5-containing) coenzyme A = succinyl-coenzyme A, 5) succinyl-coenzyme A + succinyl-coenzyme A synthetase - phosphate = succinate + AT, 6) succinate + oxygen + (CoQ10-containing) succinate-coenzyme Q10 + B2 = fumarate, 7) fumarate + water + fumarase = malate, 8) malate + oxygen + malate dehydrogenase + B3 = oxaloacetate.

This system is also extremely sensitive to environmental toxins, chemicals, and natural pollutants. Aluminum, for example, has been shown to disrupt this cycle by decreasing the activity and expression of key enzymes needed for the cycle to function.[47]

Oxidative Stress

As I've already stated, the Krebs cycle is like an engine. The fuel is dietary carbohydrates and fats, and these are moved through a system that ignites and changes this fuel to produce heat and energy to give life to the machine—us. Like any other engine, this machine also produces pollution.

Several of the steps in this cycle produce the byproduct carbon dioxide. Many of the reactions are oxidizing reactions that also produce other byproducts called reactive oxygen species (ROS).

The body has created a wonderful system of balances to keep these pollutants in check. Antioxidants neutralize oxidative particles in cells to prevent them from causing damage in the body. The antioxidants your body makes through biological processes and the antioxidants you eat in your diet help to reduce oxidative stress.

Over 125 clinical diseases have been linked to oxidative stress, such as cardiovascular disease, cancer, and, in pregnancy, miscarriage, preterm labor, intrauterine growth restriction (IUGR), and preeclampsia.

The mitochondria also house some DNA, which has been known to mutate under oxidation. When the mitochondria replicate, these mutations also replicate. So, when the damage occurs in one mitochondrion, it is passed down to future mitochondria and you get generations of organelles that carry diseased DNA.

Another thing we see is that when a cell cannot convert calories into energy the cell goes into a process called apoptosis (cell death), a natural way of clearing out dysfunctional cells. When the body is riddled with oxidation, we see lots of apoptosis.

NUTRIENT HIGHLIGHT: VITAMIN B5 (PANTOTHENIC ACID)

Vitamin B5 (pantothenic acid) is the precursor to acetyl-CoA. Like all B vitamins, B5 is water-soluble and must be consumed in the diet daily. Unlike many vitamins, there is no upper limit for vitamin B5 supplementation or intake as there have been no known toxic side effects found.

Acetyl-CoA is required for every metabolic process in the body, with its primary role being an acetyl-group donor in acetylation reactions, like those in genetic expression.

B5 has also been shown to play an important role in the production and regulation of adrenal hormones. Primarily due to acetyl-CoA and its ability to increase sensitivity to adrenocorticotropic hormone (ACTH) by the adrenal cells.

The bioavailability of vitamin B5 is estimated to be 50 percent of dietary intake.

Some level of oxidative stress is a normal part of aging. As we get older, our innate production of antioxidant enzymes goes down and the mitochondria become weaker. This is a natural progression that occurs with age and one of the key factors to why we see an increase in oxidative stress-associated maternal disease in older mothers.

When we see oxidative stress and aging cells before their time, this is disease.

So, what would cause an imbalance in the ratio of oxidative compounds and antioxidants? Well, a couple of things:

- **Environmental Toxins** - I put this first because it is quite common to see a buildup of other ROS from environmental pollution, pesticide use, heavy metal exposure, viruses, bacterial infections, etc. This puts additional stress on the cells. The natural production of antioxidants is unable to keep up with the growing amount of toxicity and the ratio becomes imbalanced and disease occurs. This can also include smoking—one of the reasons that smokers tend to age quicker—and the long-term use of certain medications.

- **Nutritional Insufficiencies and Deficiencies** - This is my second because it is more common than you think. Each step in the Krebs cycle requires vitamins and minerals to function. In addition, the formation of endogenous antioxidants often requires multiple vitamins and minerals to be formed and to function. A deficiency in any individual or group of nutrients could cause a dysfunction in the system and increase oxidative stress.

- **Genetics** - Certain genetic mutations are known to increase the risk of oxidative stress, and oxidative stress is more likely to cause an expression of negative genetics. It's a vicious cycle.

- **Poor Diet** - You would think this would fall into the category of nutritional deficiencies, but there are other dietary aspects that can increase oxidative stress. Consuming refined and processed sugars, refined and processed trans-fats, processed foods full of chemicals, and overall junk food can increase oxidative stress by adding in chemicals and compounds that increase oxidation. Pair that with nutritional deficiencies and diets low in antioxidants and you have a recipe for cellular oxidation, a.k.a. the standard American diet.

Long-term oxidative stress increases cellular inflammation, weakens metabolism, damages DNA, and causes apoptosis. Certain organ systems are more likely to be affected by oxidative stress:

- **Cardiovascular** - The heart and blood vessels are sensitive to damage, and changes in how the system functions can be life-threatening. High blood pressure, atherosclerosis, migraines, and stroke have been linked to oxidative stress.

- **Neurological** - The brain is overly sensitive to oxidative stress. Neurons are the biggest user of glucose, and their mitochondria are working overtime to provide enough energy for these cells to create rapid fast signaling. Dementia, Alzheimer's disease, Parkinson's disease, depression, anxiety, chronic fatigue, essential tremors, autism, and attention deficit disorders have all been linked to oxidative stress.

- **Immunology** - The link between the immune system and oxidative stress has been well-established through the diagnosis and treatment of cancer. It can also be seen in the progression of autoimmune disease.

- **Metabolic** - It would seem to be a no-brainer that oxidative stress affects the mitochondria, where metabolism occurs, and would have an impact on metabolism. Oxidation of cells can cause excess hunger with low energy and weight gain. It can also be a cause of type 2 diabetes, insulin resistance, and other conditions associated with poor metabolism.

- **Hormones** - The organs that produce hormones (ovaries, testes, and adrenal glands) are also highly affected by oxidative stress. Oxidative stress raises cortisol and has the same reactions in the body as elevated cortisol due to perceived stress. The ovaries and testes produce the hormones necessary for reproduction, and oxidative stress is highly associated with infertility in both men and women.

- **Pregnancy** - Many of the growing complications in pregnancy have a link to oxidative stress. The placenta is very vulnerable to oxidation. When the placenta shows signs of oxidation, it cannot function properly. Preeclampsia, gestational diabetes, IUGR, childbirth complications, and postpartum depression have all been linked to oxidative stress.

Understanding Carbohydrates

Sugar is now the villain of the dietary world. We are a society of extremes and when a study links a macronutrient to a health factor, we quickly create a war against it and eliminate it altogether. Remember the whole no-fat craze? But we need glucose to function. Carbohydrates are not the enemy, and there are many extreme diet programs that remove all carbohydrates.

Carbohydrates are broken down into simple sugars through the digestive processes. These simple sugars are glucose, fructose, and galactose (from dairy). The war on carbohydrates currently lumps them all into a group of "avoid." Not all carbohydrates are created equal; there are good and there are bad. I believe all foods have their place in the diet and that extreme diets cause nutritional deficiencies. There are complex and simple carbohydrates, and they are a bit different.

Simple carbohydrates are the individual sugars. Digestively, these sugars do not need to be broken down and are absorbed instantly. Metabolically, they provide an instant energy source that is often described as a sprinter: super fast, super intense, and with a quick drop followed by fatigue.

Complex carbohydrates are, in scientific terms, polysaccharides, meaning they are several different sugars bound together, typically, three or more. Digestively, these carbohydrates take longer to break down. Metabolically, they provide a steadier stream of glucose energy because the bound sugars take time to break down, at least, generally. There are some "complex carbohydrates" that work more like simple carbohydrates because the protein, fiber, fats, and other components have been stripped from the source and the starch can be instantly broken down. They are often paired with more simple carbohydrates: white bread, cakes, pastries, etc.

Finding the middle ground is important. There are always exceptions to the rules. Naturally occurring sugars, both simple and complex, have their place. Choosing quality over quantity and making sure that they are paired correctly with other macronutrients is important.

Simple carbohydrates, like those found in fruits and raw, unfiltered honey, are paired, naturally, with other compounds that slow the metabolism of these sugars. They are also found, generally, in smaller and more controllable quantities. These are the types of sugars and sources our body needs.

Refined sugar has been stripped of the compounds that would naturally be found with them such as fiber, proteins, vitamins, minerals, and other phytonutrients. Anytime you isolate a compound, it has the potential for excess because there is no balance.

Complex carbohydrates, like those found in whole grains and starchy vegetables, can also be either good or bad, based on the quality. Choose whole grains and whole vegetables and avoid processed complex carbohydrates like cereal and white flour that has been stripped of important components.

Glucose Metabolism Changes Throughout Pregnancy

No matter the source, glucose is the building block of all other sugars; fructose is even converted to glucose in the liver. Glucose is the sugar that raises blood sugar, and it is the sugar form that is used in the cells for energy conversion.

During the first trimester, cells are quickly dividing to create the fetus and placenta. This requires quick, instant, fast energy: glucose. To compensate for this rise in demand for glucose, the mother's body increases her production of insulin. This increase in insulin helps transport glucose to the quickly growing tissue to provide energy to help the cells proliferate and differentiate. This is a big change in the mother, with some women increasing their insulin production up to 15-fold what it was prior to conception.[48]

For some, the rise in insulin lasts well into the second trimester, not coming down to preconception levels until 16–18 weeks. After this rise, there is a period of stabilization, with the maternal blood sugar levels being slightly higher than preconception. Once the placenta and maternal blood vessels have bound together, the bloodstream becomes the primary source of nutrients for the growing baby, and glucose is still a big part of growth and development.

As the placenta grows larger, it begins producing higher and higher amounts of lactogen, an insulin-blocking chemical, so that by the third trimester, most of the glucose in a mother's bloodstream is being diverted to her baby for rapid growth before delivery.

Lactogen binds to the insulin receptors on the mother's cells and prevents insulin from bringing glucose into her cells for energy so that the glucose can be taken to the fetus. Lactogen function is heavily influenced by the presence of zinc.[49] This is a crucial metabolic shift that must occur to ensure that the baby grows enough weight for birth and life outside of the womb.

During this time, the mother's cells rely heavily on fatty acids for her own cellular energy.

Lipid Metabolism and Ketogenesis

There are two metabolic phases of lipid breakdown in pregnancy: the anabolic phase of the first two trimesters and the catabolic phase of the third trimester.

During the anabolic phase, there is an increased conversion of glucose to triglycerides for storage in the body fat. The enzyme lipoprotein lipase (LPL) increases to help build adipose tissue. This is done to give the mother reserves that she will need to use in the third trimester when lactogen increases and postpartum for breastfeeding (preparing for preparing). It is a normal part of pregnancy physiology for a mother to gain body fat in the first trimester. Excess weight gain, though, is associated with later complications. It is all about quality over quantity and staying in the bell curve of functional normal.

The transfer to the catabolic phase happens in the third trimester. As the placenta produces lactogen, the need to break down stored body fat as energy triggers the catabolic switch. There is a decrease in the LPL enzyme. Triglycerides that were stored in the first trimester are hydrolyzed into acetyl-CoA to be used in the Krebs cycle for energy production. To break these fatty acids down, an ample amount of B vitamins and acetyl-L-carnitine are required.

Maternal ketogenesis ramps up in the third trimester and the placenta readily accepts these ketones with no barrier. They have a purpose and help with fetal brain development, but too much and there can be issues. If a mother is malnourished or undereating, ketogenesis is accelerated more to provide a substrate for fetal brain development in the later stages of gestation.

The unrestricted and rapid transfer of ketones across the placenta can pose a significant risk. Extended periods of maternal ketosis are highly associated with an increased risk of neurological changes and stillbirth.

The keto diet is one of the most popular diets today. Women are using this extreme diet for weight loss and to help them conceive. I will be honest, I'm not a fan and wouldn't recommend it unless you have specific medical conditions that can benefit from this high-fat and low-carb diet. Some studies show that ketogenic diets in pregnancy are associated with developmental issues in babies.[50]

Importance of Cholesterol

The synthesis of cholesterol happens in the liver and requires acetyl-CoA—yep, that guy again. In our society, we have a war on cholesterol, just as we have a war on pretty much everything we don't understand.

Every cell in the body requires cholesterol and understanding the functions of cholesterol can help you truly identify underlying conditions associated with rises in serum lipid values.

Cholesterol in the serum is generated from the diet, bile reabsorption, and production by the liver. Cholesterol in the diet inhibits liver production of cholesterol. Synthesis can also be influenced by insulin, thyroid hormones, adrenal hormones, reproductive hormone deficiencies, epinephrine, pituitary gland, and carbohydrates in the diet.

There are two main types of cholesterol we measure.

- **Low density lipoproteins (LDL)** - the functional cholesterol that is being transported from the liver to the periphery to do a job.
- **High density lipoproteins (HDL)** - the used cholesterol that is being transported back to the liver for processing into bile for excretion.

Without adequate cholesterol, a mother's body cannot make steroid hormones, including vitamin D, or heal damage, and the growing baby cannot develop properly.

Estrogen rises throughout pregnancy, slowly climbing until the onset of labor. Cholesterol is the foundation of all the steroid hormones, and, as estrogen rises, it signals the production of cholesterol, specifically LDL, and inhibits the clearance of triglycerides—all things needed to sustain the increasing levels of steroid hormones that outside of pregnancy would be a signal of severe disease.

Babies need significant amounts of cholesterol for cells to proliferate and differentiate during development. It has been estimated that there must be a net accumulation of 1.5–2.0 grams of cholesterol for each kilogram of tissue added to the growing fetus.

The fetus and placenta are responsible for the production of steroid hormones dehydroepiandrosterone (DHEA) and estrogens. As the fetus and placenta grow, this demand increases. This increase is essential for the cascade of reactions that needs to occur to trigger the processes of a functional childbirth.

Triglycerides are a storage form of calories, specifically, sugars and unused fats. Generally, elevations in triglycerides are found in those who overconsume dietary sugars and fats or binge eat. In pregnancy, this rise in triglycerides is triggered by rising hormones and helps the mother store body fat for the third trimester and breastfeeding and aids in the growth of the baby.

During pregnancy, we see a rise in serum cholesterol and triglyceride values. This is normal and necessary for the actions listed above. This rise happens in the first trimester and these values stay elevated throughout pregnancy.[51]

In fact, by the end of pregnancy, cholesterol levels are up 50 percent and triglycerides have doubled.

Low cholesterol in pregnancy can have negative implications on pregnancy outcomes. Mothers whose cholesterol is not adequate for the demands of pregnancy are more likely to deliver preterm and have infants with poor weight gain.[52]

High levels can also cause issues and are linked to an increased risk of gestational diabetes and preeclampsia. Elevated cholesterol and triglycerides in early pregnancy have been associated with an increased risk for spontaneous preterm delivery. This is more associated with preconception maternal health and elevated cholesterol and triglyceride levels prior to conception and less associated with elevations that occur during gestation.[53] Studies have also shown that excessively high serum trigliyceride values in the third trimester are more indicative of larger babies than the standard glucose screenings.

Understanding how lipid panels change in pregnancy is important for diagnosing abnormal presentations. Yet rarely are lipid panels used in maternal diagnostics. This is mostly due to inconsistencies in what is and isn't normal in pregnancy lab values and a poor understanding of cholesterol in and out of pregnancy.

Oxidative Stress, Coenzyme Q10, and Fat Protection

Coenzyme Q10 (CoQ10) is not just a cofactor of Step 6 in the Krebs cycle; it is also a potent fat-soluble antioxidant that can reduce oxidative stress. Lipid peroxidation is a complex series of reactions that degrades fats, basically making them go bad. Rancid fats, whether caused by oxidative stress or poor-quality fats in the diet, cause disease. CoQ10 has been shown to protect the fats in the body, like the phospholipids that make up cell membranes, the membranes of the mitochondria, and LDL cholesterol.

During pregnancy, serum levels of CoQ10 rise in conjunction with rises in cholesterol levels. Studies have theorized that this rise in maternal CoQ10 is protective against oxidative stress and helps to balance the inflammatory effects of late gestation metabolic changes and hormones.[54]

NUTRIENT HIGHLIGHT: COENZYME Q10

Coenzyme Q10 (CoQ10) is a fat-soluble antioxidant that is synthesized in the body and found in the diet. Structurally, it is akin to vitamin K. CoQ10 comes in two primary forms: ubiquinone and ubiquinol.

Ubiquinone is a fully oxidized form while ubiquinol is a reduced form. Both forms are found in the diet, but ubiquinone is the most abundant. In the body, dietary ubiquinone from meat (specifically organ meat), fish, eggs, nuts, seeds, and a few vegetables, is reduced to ubiquinol, which is the functional form. Synthesis of CoQ10 is a three-step process that requires acetyl-CoA. Certain microbiome yeasts, specifically the saccharomyces species, also synthesize CoQ10 in the gut. The importance of this in human physiology has not yet been elucidated.[55]

The concentration of CoQ10 is highest in organs with high rates of metabolism, such as the heart, kidney, liver, spleen, pancreas, adrenals, testes, ovaries, and placenta.[56]

Because the body can create CoQ10, it is not considered an essential dietary nutrient. However, as we age, our bodies produce less, and a decrease in CoQ10 production is associated with several age-related conditions. Women who have reached a certain age and become pregnant are termed geriatric pregnancies (how rude) or advanced maternal age (AMA) pregnancies. Studies do show that women who conceive after a certain age are more likely to have complications in pregnancy and childbirth. Knowing that CoQ10 decreases with age, we can use this to evaluate maternal health and prevent complications with proper diet and supplementation when necessary.

Studies have already shown that CoQ10 supplementation helps protect the mitochondria of eggs during IVF therapies in women of advanced maternal age.[57] Few studies, however, have been done on the direct effects of age-related decreases in CoQ10 and other maternal complications seen in older mothers.

Although studies on CoQ10 in the protection of eggs and sperm in fertility have made headlines, the studies connecting CoQ10 to pregnancy complications have not. There have been some interesting studies linking dietary intake of CoQ10 to oxidative stress-associated diseases, such as preeclampsia[58], cholestasis[59], and gestational diabetes.[60]

Protein Metabolism

Proteins are responsible for nearly every function in the body. Collagen, keratin, and elastin are structural proteins that give strength and stability to our cartilage and bones. Actin and myosin are contracting proteins that allow our muscles to contract and relax. Transport proteins move minerals, hormones, and other components around in our bloodstream. Globulins make up hemoglobin in red blood cells. Insulin and thyroid hormones contain proteins in their structure. Neurotransmitters are synthesized from proteins. Antibodies and cell receptors require proteins. Lastly, amino acids are the base for the enzymes we will discuss a lot in this book.

Proteins are complexes of several amino acids, and it is the individual amino acids that we are discussing. The structure of proteins is not a long chain of linked amino acids but a tight ball, as the amino acids pull into each other.

Although there are hundreds of amino acids found in nature and biology, only 21 are required for human life. Twenty-one? Those of you who know a little about nutrition are saying, "Wait, Sarah, there are only 20 amino acids, right?" Until recently, you would have been correct, but the body is still full of mystery. Selenocysteine is considered the twenty-first amino acid.

Selenocysteine is part of a few rare proteins used in the translation of messenger RNA (mRNA). As the name would suggest, selenocysteine contains selenium, making it unique.

Of these 21 amino acids, nine are essential, meaning they need to be consumed in the diet because the body does not have a way of synthesizing them.[61] There is also a group of amino acids called conditional amino acids, meaning the body can make these, but they also need to be supplemented by dietary intake.

The remaining amino acids are synthesized in the body solely.

Essential Amino Acids	Conditional Amino Acids
Histidine	Arginine
Isoleucine	Cysteine
Leucine	Glutamine
Lysine	Glycine
Methionine	Ornithine
Phenylalanine	Proline
Threonine	Serine
Tryptophan	Tyrosine
Valine	

Table 2: List of essential and conditional amino acids.

Breaking down proteins begins with stomach acids and digestive enzymes. This starts by denaturing protein, breaking them down into the individual amino acids. Once absorbed into the bloodstream, they are transported to the liver to be synthesized into new protein complexes and distributed to the tissues for use.

The synthesis of amino acids into usable protein complexes, such as enzymes, requires a healthy and stabilized genetic code. Genetic mutations in the code can cause hiccups in the production of these complex proteins, such as in the case of MTHFR mutations.

Zinc is essential for several actions of protein synthesis, protein complex structure, and protein function. I always love the connection between zinc and protein; zinc requires protein for absorption and proteins need zinc for synthesis and function. Knowing this, we can use protein metabolism values and certain enzymes to assess zinc levels and function.

Proteins can be used in cellular metabolism, but all amino acids contain nitrogen that must be removed by several lengthy and energy-consuming processes in the liver. Thus, this is only really seen in emergency metabolic situations or when dietary consumption is greater than the demands of the body. Amino acids cannot be stored and are either recycled into new amino acids or broken down into ketones, pyruvate, acetyl-CoA, or one of the intermediate chemicals in the Krebs cycle. This process produces ammonia, which the liver neutralizes by converting it to urea (urine).

The demand for proteins during pregnancy increases, peaking in the first and third trimesters when fetal growth and maternal hormone production is highest. Changes in hormone production stimulate changes in protein synthesis. These hormones speed up protein synthesis, recycling, and, in the third trimester, ketogenic metabolic changes. Serum protein levels dip in the third trimester as these demands increase, but too low and this is a sign of malnutrition in pregnancy and can be a cause of complications.

Albumin is a type of transport protein that is measured in metabolic panels. This type of protein is a carrier of vitamins and minerals, hormones, and enzymes, and helps to keep fluids in the bloodstream and out of the tissues (think edema). Remember that cool relationship between zinc and protein? Well, you can see it in albumin as well. Zinc deficiency contributes to low albumin levels and low albumin levels lead to zinc deficiency. Low albumin is a risk factor for several maternal complications including edema, hypertension, and preeclampsia.[62]

Monitoring protein intake and protein metabolism blood values can help to assess how the mother's body is functioning. By understanding the components that go into the regulation of proteins, we can use these values to assess maternal function, change dietary habits, and, in turn, prevent complications associated with poor protein intake and metabolism.

Anabolism, Catabolism, and Metabolic Regulation

All the metabolic changes that happen in pregnancy are tightly controlled by the different steroid hormones. These hormones are produced by the mother, placenta, and the fetus, and, in turn, are influenced by more nutritional factors.

Steroid hormones, thyroid hormones, enzymes, and other factors change throughout pregnancy to create anabolic and catabolic states. These changes in metabolism are crucial parts of the pregnancy process for the mother as well as the baby. Anabolic metabolism is the construction of larger molecules from smaller components. This is a time of increased appetite for substrates, storage of fat, and increased energy output, as well as an increase in all the other functions that go into facilitating these needs. Catabolic metabolism is the breakdown of larger molecules into smaller components.

Anabolism is the use of smaller glucose, fatty acid, and amino acids to make larger compounds such as phospholipids and enzymes. Catabolic is the breakdown of larger proteins and stored fat into smaller amino acids and fatty acids for energy.[63]

Pregnancy is divided into three phases of metabolic change:

1. First and second trimester – Anabolic Phase 1
2. Third trimester – Catabolic Phase 1
3. Fourth trimester/postpartum – Catabolic Phase 2 into Anabolic Phase 2

The placenta is the primary driver of these metabolic changes throughout pregnancy. Among the hormones produced by the placenta, the growth factors, steroid hormones, and neuropeptides fuel these changes in maternal metabolism.[64]

Chapter 6

The Story of Hormones

Many of you are practitioners, birth workers, and well-educated women who may already have a good base in the different hormones associated with pregnancy and labor. I want to take that base and expand your knowledge just a bit. I remember, in my obstetrical acupuncture training, learning about the different hormones—what they did and why they were important. But I'm a "why" person and slightly obsessed with understanding how nutrition affects biochemistry, so I needed to know how and what nutrients were required for these actions and functions.

These were things that I had never been taught, and no physician or midwife I knew had either. I thought at first that maybe there weren't any real connections. Then, as I dug deeper, I found studies that linked nutrients to hormone biochemistry. I mapped the pathways, the enzymes, and their cofactors. I found articles and books discussing nutrient interactions with hormones, with increased and decreased function. I was onto something. Honestly, others were onto it first, but I had not found a concise resource of this information. There were no books or even chapters in books that covered the information I was looking at.

The story of hormone production and function throughout pregnancy and postpartum is a complicated one. One hormone triggers the production of another, which, in turn, regulates the synthesis and secretion of yet another, while on top of all that there are cellular and structural changes occurring throughout the mother's and baby's bodies. It is like watching a multi-season drama on Netflix, but it is important to understand these detailed interactions if we are going to help mothers achieve their natural birth goals.

So, here goes.

Steroidogenesis

Steroidogenesis is the synthesis of cholesterol into steroid hormones: progesterone, cortisol, DHEA, estrogen, testosterone, and, arguably, vitamin D. This occurs in several different organs and tissues, but the most prominent ones are the adrenal glands and reproductive organs.

Cholesterol, if you remember from Chapter 4, is the foundation of all steroid hormones, including vitamin D. The conversion of cholesterol into hormones requires a plethora of oxidizing enzymes, mainly the cytochrome P450 (CYP) enzyme system and hydroxysteroid dehydrogenases (HSDs). Throughout pregnancy, these enzymes increase from two-fold to 13-fold.

Like all enzymes, the ones used in steroidogenesis are activated and influenced by nutrient cofactors. So, as the production of these enzymes increases, so do the requirements for their nutrient cofactors.

All CYP enzymes have iron in their chemical makeup. Iron deficiency can be associated with a decrease in the formation of these enzymes and, in turn, a reduction in the production of steroid hormones. These enzymes' catalyzed actions are considered monooxygenase reactions that depend on an electron transfer from nicotinamide adenine dinucleotide phosphate hydrogen (NADPH), which is a vitamin B3-containing enzyme) via flavin adenine dinucleotide (FAD) adrenodoxin reductase (riboflavin compound) and adrenodoxin (iron- and sulfur-containing), leaving behind reactive oxygen species.

Antioxidants, such as beta-carotene CoQ10, vitamin E, vitamin C, superoxide dismutase (SOD), catalase, and glutathione peroxidase parallel steroidogenesis and protect the cells from the oxidative stress damage of the CYP enzymes.[65]

The transfer of cholesterol into the mitochondria of a cell is the first step in steroidogenesis, requiring steroidogenic acute regulatory (StAR) protein. Yep, this too happens in the mitochondria of the cells, which is another reason why maintaining adequate and healthy cellular energy production and reducing oxidative stress is so important. In the inner membrane of the mitochondrion, cholesterol is converted into pregnenolone, the mother of all other steroid hormones, by the CYP11A1 (side chain cleavage) enzyme, which I prefer because it tells you what it does and helps you understand the chemistry behind it. It's just longer to spell out, and I like the consistency of the CYP genetic identification.

Like all members of the cytochrome P450 enzyme family, CYP11A1 produces free radicals that increase oxidative stress if not neutralized and metabolized correctly.

Cytochrome P450 Enzymes		
Genetic Name	**Common Name and Alternative Names**	**Nutrition Regulation**
CYP11A1	side chain cleavage enzymes 20,22-desmolase 20,22 lyase	Upregulated with MK-4 Upregulated with vitamin D3
CYP17A1	17,20-desmolase 17,20 lyase 17α-hydroxylase 17α-monooxygenase	Upregulated with vitamin D3
CYP21A2	21-hydroxylase 21-monooxygenase 21α-hydroxylase 21β-hydroxylase	Downregulated with vitamin D3
CYP11B1	11β-hydroxylase 11β-monooxygenase	No Known Affect
CYP11B2	aldosterone synthase 18-hydroxylase 18-monooxygenase	No Known Affect
CYP19A1	Aromatase estrogen synthase	No Known Affect

Table 3: The cytochrome P450 enzymes in steroidogenesis go by many names.

Did you know that the corpus luteum means "yellow body" in Latin? Do you know why? It is because it is so rich in red/yellow-colored antioxidant carotenoids.

Studies show that a deficiency of beta-carotene in the corpus luteum inactivates CYP11A1, damaging the first step in steroidogenesis. Supplementing with beta-carotene reactivated the enzyme.[66] Being the very first step in the entire process of making steroid hormones, it is exceedingly important to make sure that the first step is a functional step by working with the nutrients required for this reaction to occur.

Pregnenolone itself is not a true functional hormone, according to science (but there is debate), and its primary role is to be the precursor for the synthesis of all the other steroid hormones. The production of pregnenolone is highly dependent on the availability of LDL cholesterol, stress, and the age and health of the cell. (Remember that whole age-related oxidative stress thing?) (See Figure 4.)

This enzyme is not only important to remember solely for its role in the initial step in steroidogenesis but also because it is important for the formation of vitamin D metabolites in the adrenal glands, skin, and placenta. In the placenta, the CYP11A1 enzyme helps to synthesize the vitamin D metabolites required for fetal and placental function and growth as well as the other steroid hormones that are required throughout gestation.

Each cell in the body expresses all or some of the enzymes required for steroidogenesis. There are multiple reactions that can occur, depending on the cells, to get to the desired hormone end production. There is no one way to make a steroid hormone, but they all start with pregnenolone.

The Story of Hormones

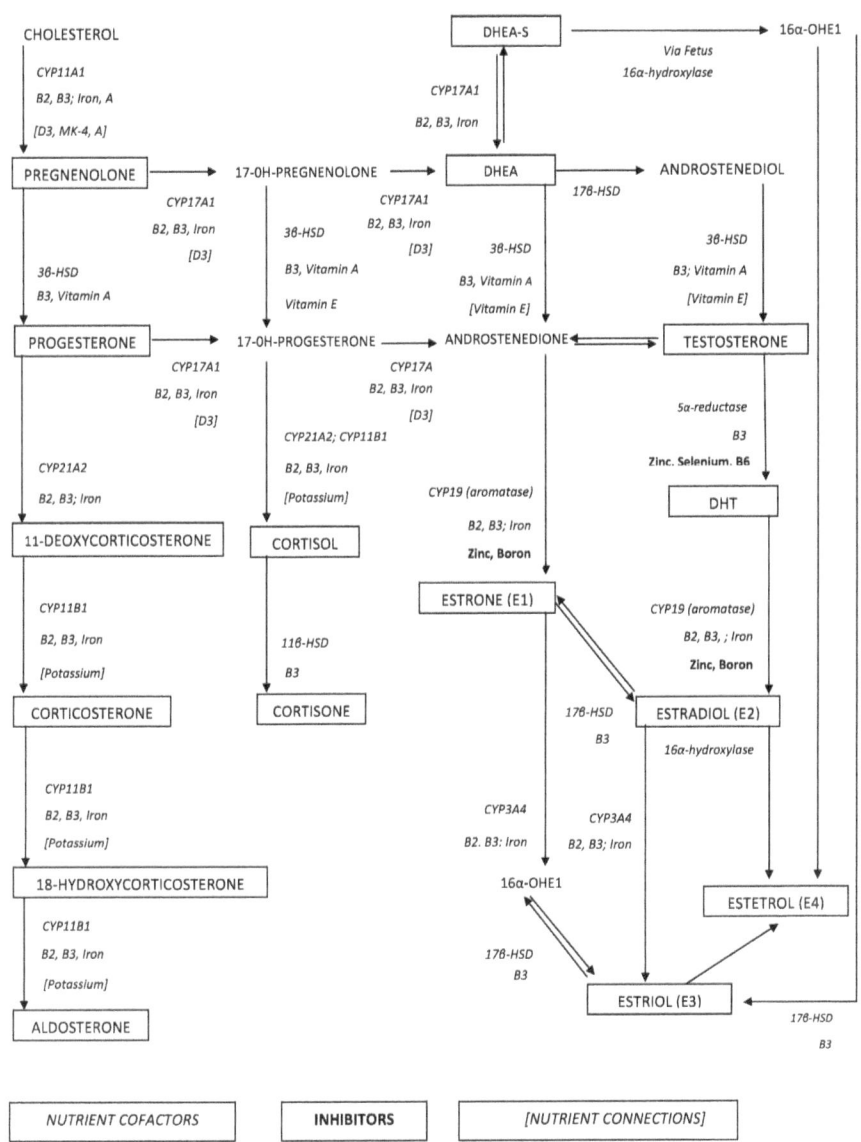

Figure 4: Each enzyme in the steroidogenesis process requires nutritional cofactors and is influenced by nutritional components.

Adrenal Hormone Synthesis

3-beta-hydroxysteroid dehydrogenase (3β-HSD) is the only non-cytochrome P450 enzyme in the corticosteroid pathway and the enzyme that converts pregnenolone to progesterone. This enzyme is highly stimulated by thyroid hormone and adrenocorticotropic hormone (ACTH) from the pituitary gland. ACTH is one of the primary triggers in the production of cortisol from the adrenals, and elevations in thyroid hormone, such as in cases of hyperthyroid disease, can increase stimulation of this enzyme. (Remember this thyroid connection for later.)

The adrenal gland itself is cool, consisting of multiple layers. It is really two glands in one, each section having derived from different embryological tissues in fetal growth. The two functional portions of the adrenal gland are the outer cortex and inner medulla. Each of these portions of the gland produces different hormones and function slightly differently, all based on the genetic expression of specific enzymes in each section.

The cortex produces corticosteroids and androgens and is divided into three regions:

1. Zona glomerulosa
2. Zona fasciculata
3. Zona reticularis

The outermost region of the adrenal cortex, the zona glomerulosa, synthesizes aldosterone but no cortisol or androgens because its genetics do not express the CYP17A1 enzyme that is required to synthesize 17OH-pregnenolone and 17OH-progesterone. The CYP11B1 enzyme that regulates aldosterone production is tightly regulated by ACTH and potassium levels. Aldosterone regulates fluid and electrolyte balance.

The zona fasciculata is the primary source of cortisol. As I mentioned before, there is an expression of the CYP17A1 enzyme required to convert pregnenolone and progesterone to 17OH-pregnenolone and 17OH-progesterone in this region of the adrenal. Part of the actions that help to regulate and activate the CYP17A1 enzyme is serine phosphorylation.

Phosphatidylserine (PS) is a phospholipid nutrient that is found in high amounts in tissues with high energy requirements, such as the growing fetus, placenta, and reproductive organs. PS modulates receptors and enzymes among other things. Supplementation with PS has been shown to help attenuate cortisol levels due to its importance in the regulation of CYP17A1.[67] Research also shows that CYP17A1 affects 17OH-pregnenolone more than 17OH-progesterone.[68]

DHEA and dehydroepiandrosterone sulfate (DHEA-S) are produced in the zona reticularis. Huge amounts of DHEA-S are secreted by the fetal adrenal glands. It is converted into estrogen by the placenta before entering the maternal bloodstream. The fetal adrenal gland is nearly the size of the kidney at birth and produces more steroid hormones during fetal growth than during any time in adulthood. All the enzymes required for the fetal adrenal glands to produce DHEA and DHEA-S are found as early as 30 days gestation. CYP17A1 is the primary enzyme required for this large amount of DHEA production. DHEA and DHEA-S not only work as the precursors for estrogens produced via the placenta but they also help to balance cortisol levels in fetal maturation. In the placenta, the enzyme 17-beta-hydroxysteroid dehydrogenase (17β-HSD) converts the fetal DHEA-S to estetrol, estriol, estradiol, and estrone. These estrogens are going to be the key to all the physiological changes that occur maternally in preparation for childbirth. It's pretty awesome and my favorite topic in maternal functional medicine—the functional aspects of childbirth and the role nutrition plays. Don't worry, we'll touch on it.

This is a particularly important enzyme in pregnancy steroidogenesis for this reason. Vitamin A receptors are found on the same placental tissue, the endothelial cells lining the fetal compartment, that produce 17β-HSD, and research shows that vitamin A is important for enzyme activity in the placenta.[69]

The medulla is in the center of the gland. It contains specialized cells called chromaffin cells. These cells are your fight-or-flight response. Catecholamines such as norepinephrine and epinephrine are produced and secreted here in response to perceived and physical stress. These cells also produce enkephalins (natural pain killers), which are all particularly important in the natural labor process.

Steroidogenesis of female hormones is, well, complicated and varied based on cycles—information that, because we are primarily talking about pregnancy, may be a bit too much for this little book. But the understanding of production is important for our discussions.

The 3β-HSD enzyme is found not only in the mitochondria but also in the microsomes of the cells of both the ovaries and the placenta during pregnancy.

The ovary is complex, with multiple types of hormone-producing cells. The theca cells and the ovarian granulosa cells are the primary cells in steroidogenesis, and like the adrenal gland, specific cell types produce specific enzymes.

NUTRIENT HIGHLIGHT: VITAMIN E

Vitamin E is a complex group of multiple different fat-soluble vitamins. There are eight different forms: alpha-, beta-, gamma-, and delta-tocopherol, as well as alpha-, beta-, gamma-, and delta-tocotrienol. Of these, α-tocopherol is the only one that is recognized as an essential nutrient, but all forms do provide function in the body.

Like all fat-soluble vitamins, vitamin E needs fat to be absorbed. The fat type, though, makes a big difference. Polyunsaturated fats are extremely sensitive to heat and are prone to lipid peroxidation (rancidity). When diets are high in polyunsaturated fats, including our anti-inflammatory fish oils, we see an increase in the need for vitamin E. If this need is not met, we see an increase in vitamin E deficiency.[70]

It has been well-established that vitamin E affects the steroid hormones and reproductive health. Most research points to the role of vitamin E in its antioxidant capacity and its use in reducing oxidative stress in the cells. Research also shows that vitamin E deficiency has several negative effects on the female reproductive system, but the "how" behind these findings is still not well understood.

3β-HSD is essential to the production of progesterone from the corpus luteum during the luteal phase, as well as the corpus luteum and placenta during the first months of pregnancy. The mitochondria house vitamin B3-containing nicotinamide adenine dinucleotide (NAD) that works as a cofactor for 3β-HSD. During pregnancy, the expression of this enzyme is higher in the placenta and in the fetal adrenals.

An older study, done in 1975, found a correlation between vitamin E levels and steroid hormones. The study specifically highlighted the effects of vitamin E on the 3β-HSD enzyme. This was a rat study, and what they found was that the rats with vitamin E-deficient diets had significantly less 3β-HSD.[71]

NUTRIENT HIGHLIGHT: VITAMIN K

Vitamin K is a complicated little nutrient that comes in two dietary forms:
1. Vitamin K1 (phylloquinone): The form found in plants like parsley, kale, and spinach.
2. Vitamin K2 (menaquinone): The form found in animal products like organ meats, grass-fed butter, and pasture-raised eggs, and in fermented foods (bacteria, fermented . . . hint, hint).

K1 is the primary dietary source of vitamin K. K1 plays a role in the formation of blood clotting factors but has no other real function. Only 20 percent of vitamin K1 is absorbed from these sources, while a good portion of the remainder is fermented by gut bacteria to produce K2 or stored in the liver for future use.

The active form of vitamin K is the K2 form. K2 is also found in animal food sources and a portion of K1 is converted to K2 in the liver. Most of the K1, however, that is converted to K2 is converted by gut bacteria before absorption.

All vitamin K forms are similar in structure, with varying lengths in their side chains. K2 consists of a group of molecules with side chains between 4–14 units, hence their names: MK-4, MK-7, etc.
1. MK-4 is found, primarily, in meat, dairy, and eggs.
2. MK-7 is found, primarily, in fermented dairy and fermented soy production.

Vitamin K and Steroid Synthesis Regulation

Although research on vitamin K2 and its role in reproduction is still fledgling, connections between deficiency and poor fertility outcomes have been found.

A study done in 2006 on testosterone showed that vitamin K2 deficiency was associated with lower testosterone levels. What they found was that the expression of genes involved in the biosynthesis of cholesterol and steroid hormones was decreased in the vitamin K-deficient groups. The mRNA levels of CYP11A1 were positively correlated with the level of MK-4.[72]

This is a great step toward understanding the complex relationship fat-soluble vitamins and other nutrients have with the steroid hormones, especially as we see these nutrients being the most commonly under-consumed in the American diet. We see an abundance of clinical relations with nutrient insufficiencies and deficiencies and changes in reproductive ability. Understanding the chemical reasons behind why are still being explored with new studies coming out yearly. These connections can be transferred to the knowledge we have on the enzymatic and hormonal changes of pregnancy and the demand the body has for these nutrients.

Vitamin D and Steroid Synthesis Regulation

Prior to recent nutritional research history, the role of vitamin D in literature was limited to its function in calcium absorption and bone health. More and more studies have elucidated the connection between vitamin D and reproductive complications, including complications during pregnancy.

Vitamin D is essential for a healthy pregnancy and something we are going to bring up quite a bit throughout the rest of this book for various reasons. When you read about the actions of vitamin D, it is the calcitriol form they are talking about. This active form of vitamin D regulates the expression of the cytochrome P450 enzymes.[73]

A study done in 2014 analyzed the exact actions of vitamin D on the different enzymes in the steroidogenesis processes. Three key enzymes were found to be affected by calcitriol: CYP11A1, CYP17A1, and CYP21A2.

CYP11A1 and CYP17A1 mRNA levels were *upregulated* after vitamin D treatment, while CYP21A2 mRNA level was *suppressed* by the same treatment.

No significant changes were observed in the mRNA levels of CYP11B1, CYP11B2, or 3β-HSD.[74] Vitamin D also upregulated the enzymes that catalyze the conversion of DHEA to DHEA-S. Vitamin D also altered aromatase activity in the ovaries, testes, and placental cells.

NUTRIENT HIGHLIGHT: VITAMIN D

There are two dietary forms of vitamin D:

1. Ergocalciferol (D2) is synthesized in plants, yeasts, and fungi.

2. Cholecalciferol (D3) is synthesized in animals.

D3 is the form that we make in our skin when cholesterol meets ultraviolet rays and zinc-catalyzed enzyme reactions convert the cholesterol to 25-hydroxycalciferol (25(OH)D). This is taken to the liver to be converted to calcidiol, which is then taken to the kidneys to be converted to the steroid hormone 1α,25-dihydroxycholecalciferol (calcitriol).

Vitamin D is a fat-soluble vitamin, meaning that in the diet a fat must be present for the absorption of vitamin D to occur. So, when you tell the public to drink low-fat and fat-free milk that is fortified in vitamin D, you have done nothing to help them nutritionally but give them glorified sugar water. The absorption of the vitamin D from this source is limited by the amount of fat present, where the absorption of the dairy sugars is unlimited.

Many of the complications seen in pregnancy have a strong connection to vitamin D deficiency. Vitamin D deficiency is, currently, the most common nutritional deficiency found in the U.S. and thus could be a potential contributing factor to several different complications in the production and function of steroid hormones throughout gestation.

The maternal hormones, placental hormones, and fetal hormones are all connected in their dependence on each other for production. It is a beautiful cycle of hormone synthesis that is a delicate balance throughout pregnancy. This balance requires an understanding of the connected physiology as well as the nutrient involvement to fully use maternal functional medicine in treatment.

The placenta does not contain CYP17A1 and cannot create progesterone or estrogen without donated hormones from the mother and fetus. The fetus lacks the 3β-HSD enzyme and thus cannot make progesterone, so the placenta creates progesterone and provides it to the fetus. In return, the fetus provides the DHEA substrate of estrogen production to the placenta.

This complex interaction is the foundation of pregnancy support. Shifts in the natural balance of these hormones, their production, or their function are the base of maternal complications.

To me, vitamin D should be an essential component of standard prenatal blood work. Unlike many blood values for vitamins and minerals, serum 25-hydroxycalciferol, also known as 25-OH vitamin D or 25(OH)D, is considered a good evaluator of functional vitamin D in the body.

From my work with mothers in other countries, some systems are ahead of the curve and regularly run this preventative test because they understand from the research that the levels of vitamin D in pregnancy are linked to maternal complications.

Vitamin D Metabolism in Pregnancy

There is a noticeable difference in vitamin D metabolism in pregnancy. By 12 weeks gestation, calcitriol blood concentrations are twice what they were preconception. This rise continues to be two- to three-fold what they were prior to pregnancy.

In the non-pregnant mother this rise would be toxic, causing severe hypercalcemia throughout the body, but in pregnancy it is normal and necessary.[75] Research points to an "uncoupling" of calcium and vitamin D in pregnancy, with a shift in primary vitamin D function to be immunomodulating and steroid hormone regulating, among other things.

Yet, until recently, the medical community had a bit of a paranoia around supplementing vitamin D in pregnancy due to fear of fetal hypercalcemia, the only known side effect of vitamin D overdose. However, the fear of maternal vitamin D overdose causing hypercalcemia is based on outdated research.

A 2011 study set out to discover the dietary needs for vitamin D in pregnancy.[76] At the time, this was a bold study that countered all previously known measures of vitamin D in pregnancy. The researchers' goal was to raise and maintain serum 25(OH)D levels at a minimum of 32 ng/mL throughout pregnancy. What they found was that a dosage of 4,000 IU/day(d) safely maintained these levels. There was not a single adverse event during the trial that could be attributed to the dosage of vitamin D. This single study changed the course of how nutritional science viewed vitamin D in pregnancy. Several other studies followed and found that higher doses of vitamin D are not only safe but also reduce the risk of cesarean delivery,[77] reduce the risk of preterm birth,[78] decrease complications in pregnancy,[79] and decrease the incidence of gestational diabetes.[80]

Each of these studies used what would have been considered toxic doses of 4,000 IU/d on average. They each showed functional changes in serum vitamin D levels without becoming elevated. Based on these studies, many clinical nutrition researchers suggest that maintaining circulation levels of 25(OH)D of at least 40 ng/mL ensures maximum protection against maternal and infant complications.[81] In addition, to achieve these levels, dietary intake of vitamin D must be a minimum of 4,000 IU/d—significantly more than that the typically recommended 400–600 IU found in prescription prenatal vitamins or even the 1,000 IU/d found in most quality prenatal vitamins, meaning mothers need to be consuming vitamin D-rich foods daily and in high amounts.

Progesterone

There is an intricate balance between estrogen and progesterone throughout the menstrual cycle, both being produced by the same theca cells of the follicles at different rates before, during, and after ovulation. While estrogen stimulates tissue growth, progesterone gives it life.

Progesterone helps to increase vascular infiltration of the endometrial lining and facilitates a healthy placental attachment, which, when we look at how the maternal body functions and the importance of the placenta in this function, progesterone production at the beginning of pregnancy is crucial for pregnancy outcomes.

Production spikes sharply at the onset of conception and then stabilizes to a steady climb after the placenta has grown to a size capable of sustaining fetal life.

The surge of luteinizing hormone (LH) that causes ovulation also triggers a switch in the ratio of estrogen and progesterone to a higher amount of progesterone from the remaining corpus luteum. If no conception occurs that cycle, progesterone levels drop and menses occur. If there is successful conception, the newly formed embryo embeds into the endometrial lining and signals the corpus luteum to continue the production of progesterone in conjunction with the endometrial lining, thus sustaining the pregnancy.

The corpus luteum produces high amounts of progesterone until 7–9 weeks gestation and then slowly declines as the placenta takes over progesterone production around week ten. Throughout the rest of pregnancy progesterone production is controlled, chiefly, by the placenta. The rate of progesterone production throughout the remainder of the first trimester and the second trimester is stable, between 10–35 ng/mL in serum testing.

At the thirty-second week of gestation, there is a rise in progesterone production by the placenta, reaching a peak production at the end of pregnancy with serum levels of 100–300 ng/mL at term. The bulk of the progesterone produced by the placenta is pushed into the mother's bloodstream to affect the function of her body.

The ability of the corpus luteum to functionally produce progesterone is highly reliant on fat-soluble vitamins, specifically vitamin E and vitamin D—two vitamins that are highly deficient in the standard American diet, with greater than 90 percent of Americans not consuming adequate amounts. Receptors for these vitamins are found on the tissues that produce progesterone, and we see that deficiencies in these nutrients affectively downregulate the expression of the enzymes required for progesterone production.

Studies linking vitamin E and progesterone production go back nearly a century to the 1940s.[82] The connection between vitamin E and reproduction is well established and well known, but the inner workings of how are not quite elucidated.

Once the placenta is mature enough to take over hormone production, maternal LDL cholesterol enters the placental cells to be converted to progesterone. Unlike other steroid hormones during pregnancy, the growing baby gives nothing to aid in the production of progesterone. This is solely dependent on the mother's nutrient intake and cholesterol function.

Human chorionic gonadotropin (hCG), uterine and fetal cortisol, and progesterone suppress the actions of lymphocyte proliferation and actively prevent the mother's body from rejecting the placenta and fetus as they mature and grow in the first trimester.

As progesterone rises there is also a suppression of the calcium-calmodulin-myocin light chain kinase (MLCK) system that prevents contractions in the uterus to ensure that the embryo has a chance to embed and grow in the uterine lining without being expelled.

17OH-progesterone is transferred to the growing fetus to be the adrenal precursor for cortisol, aldosterone, and DHEA.

The additional rise in progesterone during the last trimester helps to balance the inflammatory effects that begin to occur during this time to prevent preterm labor. Higher levels of progesterone become a protective mechanism against rising levels of prostaglandins that begin the preparation for childbirth in the third trimester.

As the placenta begins to age toward the end of gestation, there is an increased production of corticotropin-releasing hormone (CRH). CRH increases the secretion of oxytocin and blocks the production of progesterone. As the progesterone levels go down, estrogen levels go up, and the effects of prostaglandins on the cervix are no longer regulated.

Estrogen

The placenta makes estrogens from the DHEA-S supplied from the fetal adrenal glands. Other sources of estrogens in pregnancy are the maternal adrenal glands and adipose tissues.

There are four types of estrogen (yep, four):

1. **Estrone (E1)** - The slow-acting estrogen that dominates after menopause.

2. **Estradiol (E2)** - The functional estrogen of female reproduction.

3. **Estriol (E3)** - The estrogen produced during pregnancy through conversion of fetal DHEA and DHEA-S by the placenta.

4. **Estetrol (E4)** - This estrogen is *only* produced in pregnancy by the fetal liver, transferred through the placenta, and no one talks about it. Seriously, we know it is there, but you don't find much research into its exact function or really any reference to its existence.

The functions of all the estrogens blend into each other a bit throughout pregnancy, with elevations in total estrogens and each estrogen being associated with similar processes. Each type of estrogen can bind with estrogen receptors (ERα and ERβ).

ERα receptors are found primarily on the endometrial tissues, breasts, ovaries, and placenta. ERβ receptors are found throughout the body in tissues, such as the bones, brain, lungs, heart, vascular systems, and kidneys. So, when we are talking about estrogen, we are talking about the cumulative effects of all the different forms of estrogen working together.

Of the four forms of estrogen, estradiol is the most potent and the most abundant during the reproductive years, while estriol is the weakest.

During the first few weeks of pregnancy, the corpus luteum is responsible for the production of estradiol. After the first trimester, like most other steroid hormones, the primary producer of estradiol and other estrogens is the placenta.

Estrone is produced by the maternal ovaries, adrenals, and peripheral tissues during the first six weeks of pregnancy. After the placenta has taken over steroid production, estrone levels increase steadily throughout pregnancy.

Estriol is first detectable in the maternal serum around nine weeks of gestation, around the time that the placenta begins to effectively transfer hormones and blood between the baby and the mother. The production increases steadily until 35 weeks when levels surge sharply as the increasing inflammation of pregnancy signals a final push in steroidogenesis and the cascade of processes that occur in preparation for childbirth.[83] A small amount is also produced in the fetal liver along with estetrol. While estriol is more pronounced in the maternal bloodstream, estetrol is more pronounced in the tissues of the baby.[84]

The rate of total estrogen production rises sharply throughout pregnancy and is the primary trigger for many of the biological changes that occur in the mother after the first trimester. The placenta lacks several important enzymes required to produce estrogen from progesterone, specifically CYP17A1 and 17β-HSD. Instead, it relies on DHEA-S from the fetal and maternal adrenal glands as a precursor to estrogen production. The CYP19A1-aromatase enzyme is used by the placenta to convert DHEA-S to estrogen.

Estrogen is a vasodilator, increasing blood flow to the growing placenta and baby. In pregnancy, we see dramatic increases in blood flow to the uterine tissues to transfer increasing amounts of oxygen-rich blood and nutrients to the growing baby and to keep the placenta functional. As estrogen levels increase, so does visible uterine blood flow.[85]

Binding of estrogen to the ERs in the vasculature increases the production of nitric oxide (NO), providing one mechanism to how estrogen increases blood flow to the uterus. Other estrogen-associated chemical changes that increase uterine blood flow include increased endothelial production of prostacyclin (PGI2), endothelial derived hyperpolarizing factor (EDHR), and carbon monoxide.[86] Of these, though, NO production has been shown to account for 79 percent of the increase in uterine blood flow, making it important for healthy placental function.

NO is synthesized from L-arginine, an amino acid found in meat and dairy. Arginine is not only the precursor of NO, but it also stimulates growth hormones, insulin, and other chemicals. Arginine is not an essential amino acid, meaning your body can also make some on its own from other amino acids.

Estrogen stimulates the synthesis of NO from arginine with the help of magnesium and riboflavin. Magnesium helps make healthy placentas, and deficiencies in early pregnancy may lead to lower uterine blood flow with weaker placental development. Weak placental development is associated with an increase in pregnancy-related complications. With an increasing number of women of reproductive age not consuming the minimum requirements for magnesium, this is an important nutrient to monitor throughout gestation.

Until about two-thirds through pregnancy, maternal cortisol is transferred from mom to baby via the placenta. From that point on, the baby can produce its own ACTH to stimulate cortisol formation.

What is the trigger of this change in the baby? Estrogen. As the estrogen levels rise, there is a threshold in which a specific amount of estrogen triggers the fetal pituitary to produce ACTH and thus adrenal cortisol.

A 1997 study from the University of Maryland at Baltimore elucidated the direct connection between elevations in estrogen and the trigger in the baby's pituitary. Using baboons, they blocked estrogen, specifically estradiol, in some and doubled estradiol in others. What they found was that by doubling estradiol halfway through pregnancy they could activate cortisol production in the developing fetus. When they blocked estradiol, the fetus never developed its cortisol production pathways.[87]

One of the researchers was quoted,

> *"Doubling the amount of estrogen also sped up the transformation of the stem cells of the placenta into mature cells whose structure and function is quite different . . . blocking estrogen resulted in miscarriage."*

Estrogens also work to regulate the production of progesterone in the placenta by regulating the availability of LDL for conversion to pregnenolone.

Fetal estrogen has a known role in the ovarian follicular maturity of female offspring during fetal development, meaning that estrogen is responsible for the growth and health of the follicles that develop in the female baby. These are the follicles that she will take with her into adulthood. This is an example of why maternal functional health is important for not only the mother and her child, but also the health of her possible future grandchildren and the fertility success of her daughter. It is interesting that fetal estrogens are responsible for this maturity and could be a potential function of fetal liver estetrol production. Cool fact: The fetal liver can take estradiol from maternal circulation and convert it to both estriol and estetrol.

Another super interesting finding is that estrogen plays a role in magnesium homeostasis by regulating the TPRM6 magnesium channels. This is extremely important in pregnancy as the demand for magnesium increases with the rise in estrogen levels. As these levels rise and magnesium is pushed more effectively to functional roles, we can see more symptoms of magnesium deficiency such as calf cramps and charley horses, typically starting during the weeks of gestation when estrogen levels rise sharply.

As labor comes closer, the high levels of estrogens stimulate many different processes necessary for delivery.

Now, this is exciting.

Rising levels of estrogens increase the expression of oxytocin receptors as well as prostaglandins in the cervix.

Estrogen influences the number of gap junctions between muscle cells in the uterus. Gap junctions are the gaps between the muscle cells that transport electrical impulses between cells. It is natural for there to be a growing number of these as the uterus expands and the gestation progresses. When active labor begins, these junctions and their electrical impulses will be used to create rhythmic contractions. (Hint: these actions need electrolytes.)

Estrogen stimulates the enzymes needed to convert essential fatty acids into prostaglandins. Lastly, estrogens affect collagen and hyaluronic acid (HA) production. We're going to talk a lot more about this in Chapter 12.

There is a beautiful balance between progesterone and estrogen functions throughout pregnancy. High levels of progesterone help to mitigate the labor-progressing effects of estrogen, allowing the increase in prostaglandins, changes in cervix structure, increased oxytocin production, and increased oxytocin receptor formation without causing active labor until the growing baby is fully mature. A hormonal signal that labor is imminent is the ratio of high estrogen and lower progesterone.

Testosterone

Testosterone is the androgen associated with male dominance, but it is also found in women and is important for certain characteristics and functions.

I would be remiss if I did not talk about it for a minute.

Maternal blood levels of testosterone increase by 70 percent in pregnancy. Wow!

Interestingly, the younger a mother is, the more testosterone she produces in pregnancy.[88] Unlike other steroid hormones in pregnancy, it doesn't seem as though this increase in testosterone affects the growing baby, as these increases are not seen in fetal circulation.[89]

The role of maternal testosterone is the least-researched hormone in maternal function. Most of the studies are linked to higher levels and conditions such as polycystic ovary syndrome (PCOS) and preeclampsia. The exact role of testosterone in supporting pregnancy outcomes is still up for debate.

DHEA-S

At this point, I think you fully understand that DHEA-S is produced by the baby's adrenal glands and that this androgen hormone is the precursor to estrogens produced by the placenta.

DHEA-S is the inactive transport form while DHEA is the active form. Both are produced in the adrenal glands, and DHEA-S is also converted to DHEA in the target cells around the body.

DHEA-S levels rise dramatically in the first trimester and then slowly decrease throughout the remainder of the pregnancy. The decrease in DHEA-S occurs in conjunction with the rise in estrogens, which makes sense when you know the physiology and that the majority of DHEA-S is used to make those elevated estrogen levels.

It has been speculated that the large surge in DHEA during the first trimester is essential for brain development. Several studies have been done connecting DHEA and DHEA-S with brain function, including neural tissue growth and cellular differentiation, showing that it works as a neuroprotectant.[90]

DHEA is neuroactive with actions at several neurotransmitter receptors, giving DHEA antidepressant effects.[91] This is important to remember when we are looking at things like prenatal depression and anxiety, which tend to coincide with a serum decrease in DHEA-S levels in maternal blood circulation.

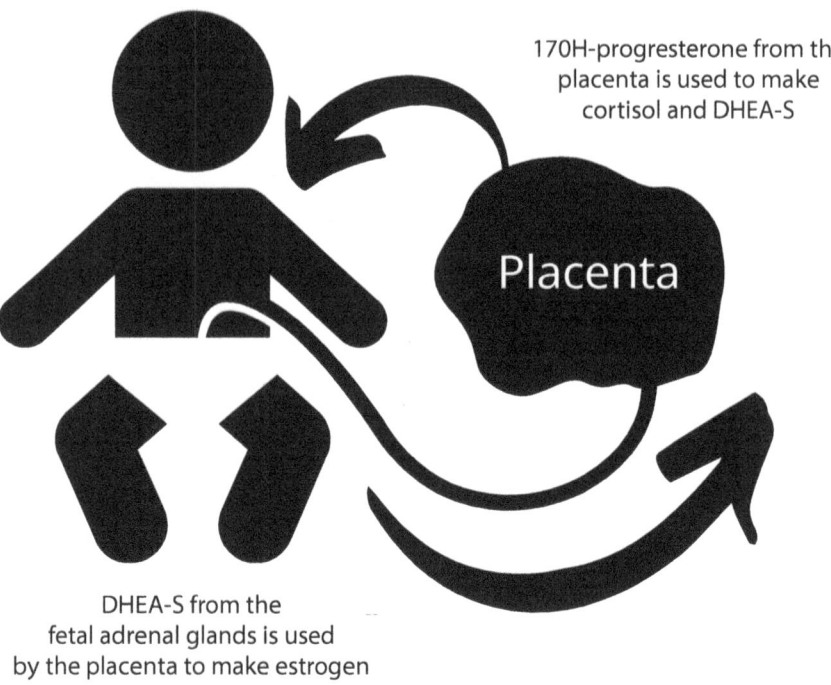

Figure 5: The relationship between the placenta and the fetus in the production of hormones.

The first- and second-trimester rise in DHEA may also have an immuno-modulating effect that helps to prevent rejection of the baby. Studies show that there is an inverse relationship between DHEA and serum levels of cytokines (inflammatory proteins).[92]

The fact that maternal circulation decreases during the later stages of gestation, while estrogen rises, is a clear, normal signal of the physiological changes that are occurring in preparation for childbirth. Childbirth is an inflammatory process, and the increase in cytokines at the tail end stimulates the actions of active labor.

Lastly, DHEA helps to balance the negative effects of cortisol.

Cortisol

In addition to DHEA and DHEA-S, the fetal adrenal glands produce copious amounts of cortisol. Cortisol is our stress hormone.

Corticotropin-releasing hormone (CRH) is a hypothalamic hormone, but during pregnancy, it is expressed by the placental and amniotic cells. From 16 weeks' gestation on, the placenta is the primary source of circulating CRH.[93]

Placental CRH stimulates the maternal pituitary to release ACTH and, in turn, adrenal cortisol production increases. As cortisol levels rise, the maternal expression of CRH decreases, while the rising cortisol levels increase the production of CRH in the baby and surrounding tissues. This fetal CRH then continues to drive maternal ACTH production, keeping cortisol levels elevated. This production of cortisol peaks during the third trimester with a three-fold increase.[94] This rise starts between 25 to 28 weeks gestation.

The primary role of cortisol during pregnancy is to help mature the growing baby. Specifically, the spike seen at the end of gestation is required for fetal lung maturity before delivery. This final hoorah of cortisol production not only helps get the baby ready for life outside the womb but can also give mom insomnia.

Insomnia in pregnancy is common, and I'm sure every mom reading this book who has mentioned that she can't sleep was told, "It's preparing you for when the baby gets here." That is not that comforting when the baby isn't here, and you really want to sleep.

Cortisol is our awake hormone. As the sun rises in the morning, the pituitary sends a flood of ACTH to the adrenal glands to, well, wake us up and give us a big boost of cortisol. This boost of cortisol is kind of like your cortisol reserve for the day. There is this large spike when we first wake up, and then we see it dropping throughout the day until we get to darkness and melatonin kicks in to help you sleep. This natural elevation in cortisol is important for survival.

When these natural levels increase due to changes in pregnancy physiology, some insomnia can be normal. Insomnia that is excessive is a sign of imbalance and dysfunction and should be differentiated to determine the cause.

Cortisol is more than your "stress" and "wakeful" hormone. Almost every cell in your body has a receptor for cortisol.

Cortisol functions:

- Regulates lipid, carbohydrate, and protein metabolism
- Regulates white blood cell production and function
- Promotes gastric secretions
- Regulates tissue healing post-injury
- Regulates bone formation
- Maintains normal blood pressure
- Regulates catecholamine production
- Affects sleep patterns
- Regulates thyroid production and function

During pregnancy, you can add to this list:

- Stimulates fetal maturation, specifically lung development
- Regulates placental and fetal CRH expression
- Regulates oxytocin expression
- Regulates prostaglandin expression

Magnesium helps to regulate cortisol[95] by modulating the hypothalamic-pituitary-adrenal (HPA) axis.[96] Magnesium deficiency is associated with an upregulation of CRH and ACTH. Experimental and clinical studies also suggest that fetal magnesium deficiency, secondary to maternal magnesium deficiency, and stress during critical developmental periods in gestation are involved in negative changes in fetal development, including sudden infant death syndrome.[97]

One of the functions of cortisol in the mother is to regulate her blood sugar levels. When blood sugars are too low, cortisol signals glycogenolysis, or a release of stored glucose, to raise blood sugars and keep them stable. Cortisol also makes fat and muscle cells resistant to insulin (part of the reason that women can experience calf cramps and charley horses during pregnancy at periods of high cortisol production).

The metabolic changes in pregnancy are partially stimulated and maintained by the increased secretion of cortisol by both the mother and the baby. When cortisol is elevated, blood sugars remain higher due to a boost in blood sugar-regulating functions. Too much cortisol or an imbalance between cortisol and progesterone and we can see blood sugar levels getting too high, causing conditions, such as gestational diabetes[98]

As cortisol levels change in pregnancy, so do serum total protein values. The higher cortisol is, the lower the total protein is. This is partly because cortisol binds to protein-based transport molecules. In fact, 90 percent of circulating cortisol is bound to proteins.[99] In turn, cortisol also triggers gluconeogenesis, the breakdown of proteins to make glucose in the liver, as well as lipolysis, to ensure an adequate supply of glucose. These are the catabolic functions seen in the third trimester.[100]

Balance is key. The interplay between the hormones is like a dance, each taking their turn, each stepping in time. If one steps out of place, there is dysfunction, and the dancers trip over themselves trying to maintain the movement.

Hormonal Interactions that Sustain Pregnancy

The production and function of each of these hormones is interconnected with the production and function of the others. The organs of the mother, the placenta, and the fetus each produces a slightly different combination of hormones and together they all work together to create a functional pregnancy and childbirth.

At the onset of pregnancy, the corpus luteum is the primary driver secreting large amounts of progesterone. At conception, the newly formed embryo begins to secrete hCG, which continues to stimulate the corpus luteum and the endometrial tissues to produce progesterone until the placenta has reached a mature size capable of taking over hormone production.

Once the placenta is well-established, it begins to produce 17OH-progesterone, which is transferred to the fetus to become cortisol and DHEA/DHEA-S. Rising levels of cortisol stimulate an increase in LDL cholesterol to fuel the increase in hormones and stimulate fetal growth. DHEA/DHEA-S is converted into estrogens that are used in the body to increase progesterone production, prostaglandins, and oxytocin receptor formation as well as to dilate blood vessels and increase blood flow to the baby.

As the placenta and baby grow, the production and actions of these hormones increase to affect other areas of the body. These processes are highly inflammatory and the demand for antioxidants—both innate and dietary—increases. At some point, there is a threshold in which the amount of inflammation is too much for the body, and oxytocin production from the pituitary signals labor.

When we are working in maternity functional medicine, knowing the changes in hormones, what they do, and how they affect the body at different phases of gestation are essential to proper diagnosis and treatment. These hormones dominate the changes of pregnancy. It is a lot of information, but as I dive into the different conditions and how we differentiate and treat them with functional medicine, these complex and deep connections become important.

Our steroid hormones are not the only hormones that affect and regulate the changes of pregnancy. Others such as growth hormones, insulin, and thyroid hormones interact with cells and influence the function of pregnancy.

CHAPTER 7

Thyroid Physiology

When you work in women's health, you have a love-hate relationship with the thyroid gland. With one in eight women having some form of thyroid disease, it's going to come up. The rate at which younger women are developing these conditions is rising. Understanding how the thyroid works in pregnancy may help women prevent complications associated with poor thyroid function and possibly help them prevent the onset of new thyroid disease during pregnancy or postpartum.

Let me introduce you to Kathy.

Kathy was referred to me by her midwife. Kathy had been trying to conceive for two years. She had a beautiful three-year-old daughter. She conceived her first pregnancy after one year of trying and had a healthy pregnancy and birth but struggled to breastfeed postpartum. Since the birth of her daughter, she had experienced three miscarriages at varying gestational ages but all within the first trimester. Her midwife was at a loss of why. They had run several medical tests and found nothing that would be a definitive cause of her miscarriages.

During our intake, I was reviewing her lab work. Her amazing midwife had done her due diligence and run a good number of labs before, during, and after her pregnancy losses. There was an interesting trend. Before her confirmed pregnancies, her thyroid-stimulating hormone (TSH) values were within normal ranges, but in her first-trimester blood work, it increased slightly, on average a jump from 1.5 mIU/L to greater than 2.5 mIU/L.

Now, when you look at standard TSH reference ranges, this is within normal ranges and wouldn't catch most practitioners' eyes. But, to me, that cued into a possible thyroid component to her miscarriages. You see, studies show that a TSH level greater than 2.5 mIU/L in the first trimester increases the risk of miscarriage.[101]

After doing some more digging, we found a combination of iodine deficiency and Hashimoto's thyroiditis, diagnosed with elevated thyroid peroxidase (TPO) antibodies. After treating her condition, she was able to conceive, carry her pregnancy, have a beautiful delivery, and breastfeed her baby.

Understanding thyroid physiology during pregnancy was key to identifying this hidden pattern of dysfunction.

How the Thyroid Works

If you are a functional medicine practitioner, much of this is going to be familiar. If not, this is going to be fun and important when addressing many of the conditions seen in pregnancy and postpartum.

The thyroid gland is located at the base of the neck, just below the Adam's apple. It has a right and left lobe, with an isthmus in the middle that holds the wings together, making it resemble a butterfly.

It also houses the four parathyroid glands that help to regulate calcium levels in the body.

The thyroid gland is an endocrine organ, which means it releases hormones in the body. It has the important job of regulating much of the metabolic processes we discussed in Chapter 5. In addition, it affects other endocrine hormones, such as the steroid hormones. Thyroid hormones affect every cell in the body.

Thyroid hormones stimulate metabolic processes by directly affecting the size and number of mitochondria within each cell, stimulating sodium-potassium channels, and increasing beta-adrenergic (β-adrenergic) receptors in tissues.

Thyroid hormones are made from the binding of the amino acid tyrosine to iodine molecules. Thyroid hormones include the following:

- Thyroxine (T4)
- Triiodothyronine (T3)

	Thyroid Hormone Production	
A	Active Transport	This is the transport of iodine to the follicular cells in the thyroid. This is controlled by the sodium-iodine symporter (NIS). The ability of the thyroid gland to accumulate iodine is crucial to the formation of thyroid hormones. The numbers (4 and 3) in T4 and T3, respectively, represent the number of iodine molecules present on the hormones. NIS is a protein found in the thyroid cells that transports iodine. TSH stimulates this protein to increase iodine accumulation in the thyroid follicular cells. This process is heavily influenced by magnesium status. A 2020 study showed that magnesium helps to balance the uptake of iodine into the follicular cells, especially in cases of iodine-deficient hypothyroidism.[102] An interesting fact about NIS is that it is also found in cells outside of the thyroid gland, most notably the mammary glands, where its job is to transport iodine into breast milk for the breastfeeding infant's own thyroid health.
T	Thyroglobulin	This is a large protein that is rich in tyrosine. Tyrosine is an amino acid that makes up the "T" component of T4 and T3. Thyroglobulin is formed in the follicular ribosomes and stored in vesicles.
E	Exocytosis	Thyroglobulin is excreted into the colloid with iodine. There, it awaits the TSH signal to be synthesized into thyroid hormone.

Table 4: Mnemonic for remembering the steps in thyroid hormone production.

	Thyroid Hormone Production	
I	Iodination	Iodine in the colloid is activated by thyroid peroxidase (TPO) enzymes. The TPO enzyme production is stimulated by the actions of TSH on the thyroid cells. Iodine binds to the tyrosine amino acid components of the thyroglobulin, forming monoiodotyrosine (MIT) and diiodotyrosine (DIT). For TPO to do its job, it needs calcium and iron cofactors. The action of making thyroid hormone is highly oxidative, and the need for antioxidants, such as selenium, is crucial to preventing oxidative stress in the thyroid gland during the hormone-making process.
C	Coupling	MIT and DIT join to make triiodothyronine (T3), while the coupling of DIT and DIT makes tetraiodothyronine (T4/Thyroxine).
E	Endocytosis	Newly formed thyroid hormones are taken up into the follicles of the epithelial cells again. These hormones are not "free" and are attached in a larger protein group. The breaking apart of this larger molecule gives us our free T4 and T3 that enters circulation.

Table 4: Mnemonic for remembering the steps in thyroid hormone production.

There are other thyroid molecules that contain iodine, but these are considered inert or at least don't serve a function we know about yet. Ninety percent of the hormones produced by the thyroid gland are inactive T4, with 10 percent being the active T3 form. The bulk of cellular T3 comes from the removal of an iodine molecule within the target tissues.

At a microscopic level, the thyroid gland is amazing.

The cells responsible for producing thyroid hormones are called epithelial cells. These cells create rings called follicles, and at the center of these follicles is a pool of thyroglobulin and iodine called the colloid. The production of thyroid hormone is unlike the production of any other hormone in the endocrine system.

This process is stimulated by the secretion of thyroid-stimulating hormone (TSH) from the anterior pituitary gland. TSH binds to receptors on the epithelial cells of the thyroid, stimulating the formation of thyroid hormones. High concentrations of TSH increase the rate of thyroid hormone formation and secretion, while lower concentrations of TSH slow the rate of thyroid hormone formation and secretion.

The concentration of TSH is regulated by a negative feedback mechanism. Thyroid-releasing hormone (TRH) from the hypothalamus regulates the expression of TSH from the anterior pituitary. As the levels of circulating thyroid hormones increase, there is an inhibition of the production of both TRH and TSH. If there are low-circulating thyroid hormones, there is an increase in the production of TRH and TSH, stimulating an increase in thyroid hormone production to keep the system balanced.

The thyroid hormones are bound to transport proteins in the bloodstream and brought to target tissues. Once inside these tissues, the hormones bind to receptors, which enable them to stimulate DNA gene expression, inhibiting or activating the sequences required.

Making thyroid hormones is not as simple as the stimulation of the thyroid gland by TSH. There are six steps to the hormone-producing process. A hiccup in any of these steps and we can see issues in the production and later function of these hormones in the body. Once in circulation with its transport proteins, the thyroid hormones can act on the cells.

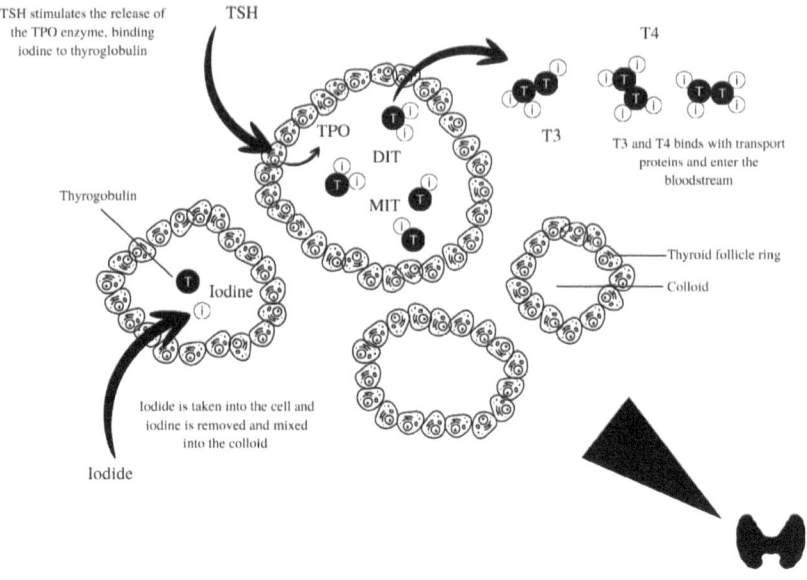

Figure 6: The production of thyroid hormones.

Thyroid Hormone Activation

Thyroid hormones are transported throughout the body by thyroid-binding globulin (TBG) and albumin proteins. TBG is a transport protein that is produced by the liver. The production of TBG is increased with higher levels of estrogen. During phases of increased estrogen production, like in pregnancy, we see a higher demand for thyroid hormones.

After inactive T4 enters the cells, it needs to be activated so it can bind to the receptors and do its job. Deiodinase enzymes remove an iodine molecule from the T4 structure to create active T3. Deiodinases are selenium-containing enzymes that require zinc to catalyze the removal of iodine and the cofactors B2 and B3. Deficiencies in zinc or selenium can affect the ability of the body to remove iodine from T4 and create active thyroid hormones.[103]

Once T3 is formed, it can bind to its receptor and do its job. There are currently four known types of thyroid receptors in the body: α1, α2, β1, β2. These different receptors have different patterns of expression based on where they are located and the developmental age. The beta receptors increase significantly during the fetal growth periods and right after birth. The upregulation of these receptors is crucial for the brain development of babies.

All thyroid receptors need zinc to function. Without zinc, T3 cannot activate the receptor and thus no action is performed.[104] This is the reason you will see women taking synthetic hormone medications and still presenting with hypothyroid symptoms. You can give all the synthetic thyroid hormone you want, but if that hormone cannot bind to the receptor it cannot function. All the medication has done is raise levels of circulating thyroid hormones; it has not changed the actual function and really hasn't corrected the disease.

An example of this in research is a study on hair loss associated with hypothyroidism. The study found that hair loss symptoms did not improve with the supplementation of thyroid hormones in medication form unless zinc was also supplemented. A Catch-22 is that thyroid hormones are required for zinc absorption, so with low thyroid hormones, we also see lower zinc levels, perpetuating and exasperating the condition.[105]

This is functional medicine at work. Understanding the link between receptor function and zinc deficiency is key to proper treatment success.

The Iodine Debate

Iodine is a trace dietary element whose sole purpose is to be the precursor for thyroid hormones, at least that we know. Yet newer research points to a protective mechanism of iodine against cancer in other tissues of the body.

It is found in high amounts in the oceans, including foods from the oceans, and in some soils around the world. There are iodine "dead zones" where we see little to no iodine in soil content. These areas are growing as poor crop rotation, management, and erosion strip the soils of the iodine they contain.

This influences the iodine content of the foods grown in these regions as well, leading them to be iodine deficient. One of these "dead zones" is the Midwest region of America, where most of our crops are grown.

The actual form found in foods and nature is iodide. Iodide is the ionic state of iodine. It is, basically, a salt compound formed when iodine bonds to another element, such as potassium or sodium. This potassium- or sodium-bound iodide is transported to the thyroid gland follicles via NIS. It is in the follicle that iodide is oxidized into iodine.

NUTRIENT HIGHLIGHT: SELENIUM

Selenium is a trace mineral essential to human life. It is the foundation of over a dozen known selenoproteins that affect reproduction, thyroid function, DNA synthesis, and immune function and serves as an antioxidant for regulating oxidative stress.

Selenium is found in two forms: organic and inorganic.

1. Organic - Selenomethionine and Selenocysteine
2. Inorganic - Selenate and Selenite

Although all forms of selenium seem to be readily absorbed, their retention and function in the body seem to differ.[106]

Much of the function of selenium is as the component of enzymes. TPO is one such enzyme but so is glutathione peroxidase, a potent antioxidant that protects the liver, thyroid, and other organs from oxidative damage.

Selenium content is higher in the thyroid than any other organ in the body. It is partly due to its important role in the structure of TPO enzymes but also because the process of making thyroid hormones is highly oxidative and leaves behind free radicals that increase the risk of oxidative stress in the thyroid gland. Glutathione peroxidase protects the thyroid from this oxidative stress.

Studies show that selenium supplementation, specifically in the selenomethionine form, improves thyroid markers.[107]

While most of the iodine is found trapped in the thyroid, there is still a small percentage found in mammary glands, eye and gastric mucosa, salivary glands, and the cervix. The role that these iodine molecules play is still unclear,[108] but newer studies link iodine to decreased rates of cancer in these organ systems.[109]

So, how much iodine is too much?

Honestly, it's debatable.

There are two very conflicting schools of thought on dietary iodine intake and supplementation dosage—both sides with research to support their theories.

From the early 1900s to the mid-1950s, high doses of iodide solutions were used to treat a variety of health conditions. This changed when a 1948 study pointed to high doses of iodine in the development of certain thyroid diseases.[110]

After the fear of iodine toxicity took hold, daily recommended intakes were lowered, with the current recommended upper limit being no more than 1mg/day. Over the course of the next few decades, changes were made in food fortification and grain preservation that removed iodine from the food systems.

A kink in the iodine toxicity theory was a comparative analysis of iodine intake in countries such as Japan as well as newer studies. Japan has the highest iodide intake in the world. It is estimated that the average Japanese woman consumes up to three times the general safe limit of 1 mg daily[111], most of this in seaweed and seafood. Interestingly, these seemingly excessively high levels seem to have no suppressive function on the thyroid.[112] I find this interesting since I just love looking to cultural traditions in food consumption and nutrient profiles. Japan has a low rate of autoimmune thyroiditis as well,[113] which also adds to the puzzle, as studies show that a high intake of supplemental iodine can trigger autoimmune thyroiditis.[114]

The studies linking high intake of iodine to increasing rates of autoimmune thyroiditis list an increase in the iodination of thyroglobulin and the resulting oxidative stress as the trigger for immune system reactions.

If we take a second to look at the role that selenium and zinc play in modulating these actions in the thyroid and the fact that dietary intake via seafoods in Japan is rich in both selenium and zinc versus more modern western countries—where the rate of autoimmune thyroiditis is higher—then we may have a dietary component that increases the risk of iodine-induced autoimmune thyroid disease, and it's not the increased intake of iodine but the deficiency in the supporting minerals. It would also be remiss of me to not note that food sources of nutrients are complex, with a range of supporting nutrients and phytochemicals that we do not fully understand. Supplementation with isolated nutrients, in many studies, has been shown to have undesired effects.

In 1998, Dr. Guy E. Abraham, a former professor of obstetrics, gynecology, and endocrinology at the UCLA School of Medicine, founded the Iodine Project. He proposes that much of the controversy over iodine intake had to do with poorly performed early studies on iodine intake. In Dr. Abraham's preface to Dr. David Brownstein's book *Iodine: Why You Need It, Why You Can't Live Without It,* he stated:

> *"Of all the elements known so far to be essential for human health, iodine is the most misunderstood and the most feared. Yet, iodine is the safest of all the essential trace elements, being the only one that can be administered safely for long periods of time to large numbers of patients in daily amounts as high as 100,000 times the RDA. However, this safety record only applies to inorganic, nonradioactive forms of iodine. Some organic iodine containing drugs are extremely toxic and prescribed by physicians. The severe side effects of these drugs are blamed on inorganic iodine although studies have clearly demonstrated that it is the whole molecule that is toxic, not the iodine released from it."*

What we see in the studies seems to be a "U" shaped pattern in the effects of iodine on thyroid function. Too little and we have poor thyroid function, too much and we overburden the system. Currently, the World Health Organization (WHO) and the U.S. Institute of Medicine recommend a higher iodine intake of 220–250 μg/day in pregnant women.

Just like everything we drive home in functional medicine, there is a complicated and intricate design of systematic balance that must be attuned with each process in the body. It is all connected and dependent on a broad range of nutrients.

Environmental Halogens and Thyroid Hormones

Iodine is an element on the periodic table that falls into the category of halogens or halides. Who remembers basic chemistry? This group of elements includes chlorine, fluorine, bromine, and iodine.

Interestingly, we see that each of these elements can affect thyroid function, and they are found in nearly every aspect of our lives.

Prior to the 1950s, iodide was used in the storage of grains to keep them from spoiling. After the Wolff study, bromide replaced iodide in grain storage methods (we don't want those grains sprouting in storage). Bromide is commonly used in pesticides, and residues of this compound are found throughout our grains, dried fruits, nuts, and seeds.[115] Bromide can replace iodide in the thyroid, and thus replace the iodine molecule in the formation of thyroid hormones with bromine.[116][117] Studies also show that increased intake of bromides causes the body to excrete higher amounts of iodine through the urine.[118]

Chlorine is naturally found in the body and makes up a component of stomach acid, hydrochloric acid (HCl). Both chlorine and bromine are used to disinfect swimming pools and drinking water and are found in bleach. Theoretically, intakes of chlorine could affect thyroid health, but there are no definitive studies linking chlorine to lower thyroid function.

Fluoride is toxic, but despite its toxicity, it is found in our water, toothpaste, dental care, vitamin supplements, and baby formulas. Unlike chloride, studies do link excess fluoride intake with decreased thyroid function. A 2018 study found that the fluoride found in drinking water had a negative effect on all thyroid values. The study concluded that a water filtration system should be implemented to remove fluoride.[119]

Other studies have shown that people living in areas with water fluoridation are at a higher risk of developing hypothyroidism than those living in areas without water fluoridation.[120]

Halogens are all around us—in our drinking water, food, agriculture, plastics, and other toxic compounds. The studies clearly point to a connection, and when we begin to factor this into the big thyroid puzzle, it becomes a bit clearer why western countries have higher rates of thyroid disorders.

Thyroid Antibodies – Autoimmune Disease in Pregnancy

Autoimmune conditions, like all diseases, are on the rise. An estimated five percent of the general population has some form of autoimmune thyroid disease.[121] The most common autoimmune disease affecting women is autoimmune hypothyroidism, a.k.a., Hashimoto's disease, accounting for nearly 90 percent of all hypothyroid cases.

The research on autoimmune thyroid disease really is fledgling, with studies only beginning to be published in 2005, and, there is still so much we do not know about this common diagnosis.

What we do know is that autoimmune thyroid disease results from a combination of genetic and environmental factors, coupled with poor dietary intake and lifestyle choices that weaken the immune system, increase its sensitivity, and decrease its ability to distinguish between antigen proteins and thyroid proteins.

These thyroid proteins are the enzymes and components of thyroid hormone production and function. When we have an autoimmune thyroid presentation, we must shift our treatments to not only supporting the production and function of the thyroid and its hormones but also to reducing the triggers and immune responses to foreign proteins to control the immune reactions. This is a complex idea that requires its own book and, luckily, many amazing practitioners have written them. Izabella Wentz's book *Hashimoto's Thyroiditis: Lifestyle Interventions for Finding and Treating the Root Cause* is a great reference.

Thyroglobulin is the protein base of the thyroid hormones. Some cases of autoimmune thyroid disease involve antithyroglobulin antibodies that attack and destroy thyroglobulin proteins. This antibody is found in both Graves' disease and Hashimoto's disease. Often, women with this antibody have a difficult time regulating their thyroid medications.

The thyroid peroxidase enzyme is the key to thyroid hormone production and the primary target of autoimmune antibodies in thyroid disease. The destruction of this enzyme means that iodine cannot be activated and bound to the tyrosine protein to form thyroid hormones, decreasing thyroid hormone output, increasing TSH, and causing hypothyroidism.

Like other proteins in the thyroid hormone-producing process, we can see autoimmune antibodies associated with NIS destruction. It has been documented that many with Hashimoto's thyroiditis also have autoantibodies to the NIS protein affecting iodine transport and uptake into the cells. This is not an antibody typically tested for in hypothyroid patients, but maybe it should be.

Recent studies have shown a correlation between low levels of vitamin D and an increase in thyroid antibodies.[122] Most immune cells express vitamin D receptors, including antigen-presenting cells.[123] These cells mediate the immune response by processing and presenting antigens for T-cell activation. Vitamin D in these cells seems to neutralize overactive presentation and decrease the cytokine expression by these cells.[124] Basically, it increases our immune tolerance so we do not actively trigger proteins we really should not.

Autoimmune thyroid disease, even in the absence of overt thyroid disease, is associated with an increased risk of pregnancy complications, including recurrent miscarriage, preterm delivery, growth restriction, and others.

The idea that thyroid antibodies could be associated with miscarriage was first discussed in 1990 after a study identified thyroid autoimmune antibodies as a marker for pregnancies at risk of miscarriage.[125] Since then, other studies have confirmed this idea. Interestingly, this association is present even if TSH values are normal at conception.[126] We also have studies that show that treatment of hypothyroidism with levothyroxine to normalize TSH values does not decrease the rate of miscarriage in Hashimoto's patients.[127]

In pregnancy, identifying an autoimmune disease can make the difference in maternity care. Knowing each of the autoantibodies in autoimmune thyroid disease and using the elaborate info I've already given you, you can support these women successfully throughout pregnancy.

Testing is key. As you saw in the studies, normal TSH values are not indicative of thyroid health, and autoimmune presentations can be hiding under normal lab values.

Conventional medicine doesn't typically run antibody levels because the standard method of treatment is the same: Supplement the deficient thyroid hormone and make the thyroid blood panel look pretty.

From a functional medicine perspective, knowing the autoimmune factors can help define a treatment plan that specifies the deficient enzyme or protein, address nutritional components known to reduce autoimmune load, identify and remove triggers, and, in turn, increase thyroid function.

Thyroid Hormones in Pregnancy

The extreme metabolic, hormonal, and physiological changes that occur during pregnancy result in modifications in thyroid hormone production and function.

Total thyroid hormone significantly increases during the first half of pregnancy. During this phase, the fetus is reliant on thyroid hormones from the mother. Between 6–12 weeks gestation, there is a sharp rise in thyroid hormones. From there, they rise more slowly, peaking at 20 weeks.[128] After this point, the baby can produce its own thyroid hormones for body function.

Both alpha and beta receptors are present on the placenta during gestation, and the placenta expresses several types of deiodinase enzymes. The placenta produces a large amount of the type III deiodinase that makes reverse T3. Therefore, you will see higher serum reverse T3 values in pregnancy thyroid labs.[129] Remember, this process requires a significant amount of selenium and zinc.

The placenta and the maternal thyroid have a wonderful and complicated relationship. In early gestation, as thyroid hormones rise, the placenta and the fetus mature and grow. Elevated levels of human chorionic gonadotropin (hCG) from the placenta stimulates an increase in thyroid hormones. Without adequate thyroid hormones, we get weak and poorly formed placentas that are at a higher risk for placental-related complications in pregnancy.

Throughout gestation, different phases of physiological change create unique demands on thyroid hormones. These periods of increased and decreased thyroid function mark some of the symptoms and complications seen in pregnancy. Understanding the interactions between the metabolic shifts, hormonal changes, and nutritional demands gives us a foundation for applying functional medicine in maternity care.

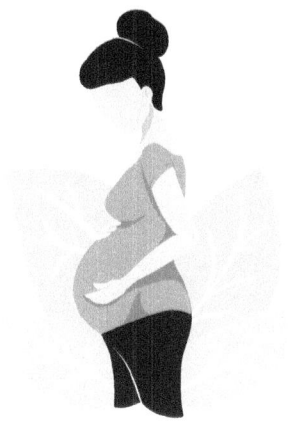

Part Three

Applying Nutrition and Functional Medicine to Maternity Healthcare

"First, they ignore you, then they laugh at you, then they fight you, then you win."

- Nicholas Klein

Nausea in pregnancy • Anemia in pregnancy •
Depression and anxiety • Gestational hypertension •
Functional childbirth • Why method of birth matters

Chapter 8

Nausea In Pregnancy

When I was pregnant with my second daughter, I thought it would be as smooth as my first. In my first pregnancy, I felt amazing, better than I had pre-pregnancy, with boundless energy and a positive mood. I was that quintessential glowing pregnant woman. I loved everything about it. I couldn't wait to be pregnant again.

Then came my second pregnancy, two years after my first. I knew I was pregnant as I walked through a mall with my sister. We took a turn down to the food court to grab lunch and we walked past a Boston Market. The smell of the rotisserie chicken (something I genuinely like) triggered immediate nausea. There was no stopping it, and I ran to a trash can and vomited. Thus began my second pregnancy and unrelenting nausea (and heartburn).

I was sick my whole first trimester. Now, in relation to many of my patients, it wasn't bad, but it was there, and it was something new that I had not experienced with my first pregnancy. I was sick morning and night.

"Morning sickness" does not do pregnancy nausea justice. For many women, like myself, these symptoms were not isolated to the morning and occurred at varying times throughout the day and night. I would wake up and be sick until I ate breakfast, but eating breakfast was hard since nothing sounded good. I lived off carbs. I hate to admit it, but my go-to breakfast was a brownie. Seriously. I jokingly refer to my second daughter as my "brownie baby" because I, literally, ate an entire pan of brownies every week while pregnant with her. I do not recommend this, and this is one of those "do as I say, not as I do" moments.

I would feel decent until a few hours after lunch and it would hit again, typically around three to five o'clock in the afternoon. If I didn't get a snack in, I was done for, and no amount of food or water would help. My nausea stopped just before the end of my first trimester—just in time for the heartburn to kick in.

Nearly all women will experience some element of nausea during their first trimester of pregnancy, 70–80 percent. Interestingly, the rates of nausea in pregnancy are more common in western countries, and there are some theories as to why. Of the women who experience nausea in the first trimester, 3 percent may develop a condition called hyperemesis gravidarum (HG), a severe form of nausea and vomiting that is more likely genetic in nature.

The pathogenesis of nausea in pregnancy is still considered unknown. The reality is, there are multiple causes and a combination of causes that make up a variety of different presentations and patterns.

- Metabolic factors
- Hormonal factors
- Helicobacter pylori (H. pylori)
- Nutritional deficiencies
- Genetics

Understanding and differentiating the presentation is important for accurately diagnosing and providing support for these women. The function of these factors helps us identify specific patterns of symptoms and increase treatment success.

I'm about to show how everything I discussed in Part Two rolls into this single aspect of maternity health—from metabolic factors to hormonal and nutritional factors. Therefore, I've started my discussion on applying maternity functional medicine here. It's not just that it is seen as the first and most prominent group of symptoms associated with pregnancy, but because in this one example, we can see the complexity of maternity care and the amazing power of functional medicine in applied treatment.

As I break down each condition, you'll see that treating these common complaints isn't a set protocol of supplements and treatments. It's the differentiation of the possible causes of the conditions. It is up to you to determine the mechanisms of action for each presenting pattern you see in the clinic and to correctly choose supplements and dietary and lifestyle treatments that best suit the individual. Generic protocols don't work.

Therefore, what you will not see in the remainder of this book are generic protocols. I am giving you the tools you need to understand the foundation of these conditions and to begin breaking down the conditions into different patterns of dysfunction. Treatment always requires considering other factors such as other medical conditions, injuries, sensitivities, illness history, and all the beauty and experiences of life that make us individuals.

Metabolic Factors

We have already touched on the changes in glucose metabolism that occur in the early months of pregnancy. All women have an increased demand for insulin during the first trimester. With the increase in insulin production, it is easier for a new mother to have her blood sugar drop too low, causing mild or severe hypoglycemia.

If you've been pregnant and experienced nausea, you'll remember how important small and frequent meals were to management.

The typical presentation for nausea associated with lower blood sugar may look like nausea that is worse in the morning before eating and is better after, strong cravings, and nausea better with starchy carbohydrates. Nausea can continue into the second trimester, depending on the severity of insulin production and the rate at which the pancreas is able to return to a stable state.

An increase in insulin production is a normal part of maternal physiology during pregnancy, but a large increase in insulin is a sign of dysfunction. A sharp increase in insulin production, up to 15-fold those of pre-pregnancy, is more likely to occur in those who have had insulin dysregulation issues prior to pregnancy, such as those with type 1 and type 2 diabetes, insulin resistance, and PCOS.

To strengthen the connection between nausea and vomiting in pregnancy and the connection to insulin production, a 2013 study found that infants born to women who experienced HG had 20 percent lower insulin sensitivity, higher fasting insulin, 22 percent higher baseline values of cortisol, and were at an increased risk of developing type 2 diabetes.[130] In addition, daughters of mothers who experience severe blood sugar swings associated with nausea tend to be more likely to have the same issues in their own pregnancies.

Vitamin B1 (thiamine) is a B vitamin seldom discussed but is crucial for glucose metabolism. It aids in the regulation of blood sugar within every cell of the body, with a strong emphasis on brain development and health.

Glucose requires thiamine for metabolism.

During the first trimester, the demand for both glucose and thiamine intensifies as the cellular growth of the fetus and placenta increases rapidly. We see in women with long or severe nausea an increase in thiamine insufficiency and deficiency. It could be connected to a decreased nutritional intake, but it could also be due to the rate at which sugar is metabolized in the system and the increased demand for thiamine for maternal function.

Insulin is produced by the beta cells in the islets of Langerhans of the pancreas. Alpha cells in the islets of Langerhans produce another chemical called glucagon. Glucagon works to balance the effects of insulin. In the first trimester of pregnancy, while insulin production goes up, glucagon production remains the same as it was pre-pregnancy. It is not until 16–18 weeks gestation that the production of glucagon rises, thus lowering the hypoglycemic effects of elevated insulin production. This is one reason that you will see patients with persistent nausea that continues well past the first trimester.

Vitamin D is an important nutrient in the regulation of insulin production from beta cells, yet research is not 100 percent sure how. The beta cells themselves contain vitamin D-specific receptors and express the enzyme 1-α-hydroxylase to convert 25(OH)D. Significant correlations have been found between decreased vitamin D and glucagon levels. In addition, 1,25(OH)2D directly activates the transcription of the insulin receptor gene and enhances the ability of insulin to transport glucose throughout the body. Vitamin D has been shown to influence the effects on insulin secretion and insulin sensitivity. Because of this connection and studies showing lower levels of vitamin D in patients with HG, there is some speculation that vitamin D may play a crucial role in the development of HG in some cases, but there are no definitive studies.

Hormonal Factors

Most of you have heard that nausea in pregnancy happens because of elevated hormones that occur in the first trimester, right? How many of you have stopped to ask *how*?

Human chorionic gonadotropin (hCG) is the hormone of pregnancy. When a woman takes a pregnancy test, this is the hormone that they are testing for. HCG production has long been associated with increased symptoms of nausea in early pregnancy.

Shortly after conception, the trophoblast cells that surround the embryo begin to secrete hCG. These are the cells that will eventually become the placenta. HCG stimulates the corpus luteum to continue to produce progesterone to maintain pregnancy. Once the placenta has matured, it increases production of steroid hormones while hCG production decreases and plateaus around 20 weeks.

Research has found an association between hCG and nausea in that there are higher blood values of hCG in those with increased severity of nausea. So, yes, the more nausea a woman has, typically, the more hCG we can find in her blood. Whether hCG is the primary cause of nausea and how higher levels of hCG cause nausea are still being elucidated. The fact that hCG is higher in those with more severe nausea seems to be more of an association than a cause because other conditions with elevated hCG levels, such as choriocarcinoma, do not cause an increase in nausea symptoms. In addition, it does not account for the cases in which nausea continues past the gestation age in which hCG naturally decreases. We'll come back to this.

Progesterone is another hormone that has also been linked with higher rates of nausea in pregnancy. Elevating hCG from the placenta signals the corpus luteum to continue to produce large amounts of progesterone to sustain pregnancy. So, with higher hCG levels, you find higher progesterone levels. Again, this seems more of an association because women given supplemental progesterone do not have an increase in nausea symptoms. Even when we compare birth control use, progesterone-only containing birth control types are less associated with nausea than estrogen.

Nausea is, however, highly associated with several conditions associated with elevations in estrogen, such as higher body mass index (BMI),[131] and is also a common side effect of estrogen-based medications. Although there are studies that show associations with elevated levels of estradiol and severity of nausea, these are still only correlations. There is, though, more of a connection with conditions related to elevated estradiol and nausea than hCG and progesterone.

A retrospective survey done in 1983 showed an increased likelihood of nausea in pregnancy among women who had used estrogen-based oral contraceptive before conception, which could add support to the theory that nausea in pregnancy is more associated with rises in estrogen than other pregnancy hormones.[132] But it could also lend to the theory of nutritional deficiency, as birth control is known to deplete certain vitamins and minerals in the body after long-term use.

We also must consider that the estrogen elevations in the first trimester have a functional role in the maturation of the placenta and the growing fetus. Estrogen is known to increase insulin sensitivity in tissues, and it is supposed to increase insulin sensitivity in the tissues of both the mother and fetus to increase fat stores for the mother and maturation for the placenta and fetus.

Based on the information we have, estrogen alone cannot be solely connected to increased rates of nausea.

So, if hCG, progesterone, and estrogen alone cannot be decisively linked with pregnancy nausea, what other pregnancy hormones do we have?

The thyroid. Its hormones and their functions are often under-discussed in pregnancy.

During the first months of pregnancy, the thyroid gland becomes highly stimulated by hCG, progesterone, and estrogen. See a connection already? In addition, increasing levels of thyroid hormone stimulate increased levels of hCG and progesterone as the placenta increases in size and maturity.

hCG is remarkably analogous to TSH in structure, and during early pregnancy, it binds to the TSH receptors on the thyroid gland to stimulate an increased production of thyroid hormones. In a normal pregnancy, TSH levels drop slightly and free triiodothyronine (T3) and thyroxine (T4) levels rise as hCG levels increase.

Unlike TSH, hCG is not regulated by a negative feedback mechanism that helps prevent an overload of thyroid hormone in the cells. Instead, the placenta produces a specific type of deiodinase (remember that zinc-dependent enzyme?) that helps to deactivate and clear surplus thyroid hormone. As the levels of maternal thyroid hormones rise, there is an upregulation in these chemicals. The inert metabolites of T4 and reverse T3 increase and are a possible trigger of increased nausea. But why?

Higher levels of hCG can overstimulate the thyroid, causing a temporary hyperthyroid presentation called gestational transient thyrotoxicosis (GTT). GTT has been found in two-thirds of women suffering from HG.[133] There are multiple variants of hCG, and there are some theories that a specific variant is more stimulating on the thyroid and more likely to cause the

GTT condition. As hCG encourages this hyperthyroid presentation, there are also more of the thyroid hormone metabolites produced by the placenta.

Based on this knowledge that hCG affects thyroid function, basically hijacking the mother's thyroid to deliver thyroid hormone to the growing fetus, biology professor Scott Forbes published a research paper in the *Journal of Evolution and Human Behavior* that suggests that the connection between this temporary hyperthyroid function and nausea is an iodine-regulating mechanism to ensure proper fetal development.[134]

Iodine is the key nutrient for thyroid hormones. The numerical component of T4 and T3 indicate the number of iodine molecules attached to a tyrosine protein. The shunting of unneeded thyroid hormone by the placenta and induction of vomiting may be a regulatory mechanism to decrease iodine intake to help regulate thyroid hormone production. This may also explain why in conditions such as choriocarcinoma, hCG levels do not induce nausea and vomiting. There is no placenta and no production of placental chemicals to deactivate elevated thyroid hormone. The opposite condition, hypothyroidism, can be seen associated with lower iodine levels, a higher risk of miscarriage, and an absence of nausea symptoms.

So, pregnancy nausea may be a regulatory mechanism for iodine intake. It is interesting that we do not see as many cases of pregnancy nausea in areas with iodine deficiency. Pregnancy nausea is more common in western countries and urban populations where iodine intake may be higher through food fortification and supplementation and the exposure of halogens is greater.[135]

Bacterial Dysbiosis – The Case of H. Pylori

H. pylori is a type of bacteria that colonizes the stomach. It is one of only a few bacteria species capable of thriving in the highly acidic conditions of the stomach. It has been associated with stomach conditions such as ulcers, gastroesophageal reflux disease (GERD), and other gastric upset presentations. The bacteria infect the cells that line the stomach and weaken the ability of the duodenum to protect itself against stomach acid.

In 2000, Puerto Rican researchers identified a link between H. pylori and nausea in pregnancy. Blood tests from this study found H. pylori infection in 89 percent of women experiencing nausea during pregnancy and only 7 percent of women who were not experiencing nausea.[136]

This seems like a highly significant finding. Yet we also need to keep in mind that H. Pylori is one of the most common bacterial infections in the world. Some research points to a symbiotic relationship with H. pylori that only becomes pathogenic in conditions of stress and a weakened immune system, hence the stronger connection between stress and ulcers versus H. pylori and ulcers.

When H. pylori was first discovered as a cause of ulcer formation in 1983, it made big waves in the medical communities, which long held that stress was the cause of ulcers. They were both right. H. pylori is associated with the formation of ulcers and the increase in gastritis—yes. But this doesn't account for the 15 percent of ulcers with no known bacterial cause or the patients with a positive H. pylori diagnosis with no digestive symptoms. Only 10 percent of the people infected with H. pylori get ulcers even though H. pylori is seen in 85 percent of ulcer cases.

When we think of stress, we tend to think only of perceived stress or emotional stress. Perceived stress is our view of the world, demands, responsibilities, fears, and emotions. But there are two other categories of stress that we should also be discussing: endogenous and exogenous.

Endogenous stress is physical stress. Cortisol is our primary stress hormone, and its job is to keep you alive in times that require an increase in the neurotransmitters and hormones of fight or flight. That is not all cortisol does. It is also responsible for gastric output, TSH production, immune responses, and so much more. Endogenous stress is inflammation in the body. This can be caused by injury, oxidative stress, and pregnancy.

Exogenous stress is like endogenous in that it is stress associated with inflammation. This inflammation, though, is caused by external sources, such as viral and bacterial infections, pesticides, and environmental chemicals. These, too, will raise cortisol levels and increase stress in the body.

Stress affects H. pylori.

Not all stress is negative. Acute, normal stress reactions have been shown to increase immune health and overall body function. Long-term stress, however, can have a significant negative impact on the body. Chronic stress has been discovered to be an underlying cause of many common diseases and conditions, including gastritis.

It is this long-term stress response that is associated with an increased expression of H. pylori pathogenesis.

In a stress reaction, we have different phases.

During a stressful response, whether emotional, endogenous, or exogenous, there is the release of corticotropin-releasing hormone (CRH) from the hypothalamus, which stimulates the pituitary to release ACTH. ACTH then travels to the adrenal glands to stimulate the release of corticosteroids. Glucocorticoids are a specific type of corticosteroids that are highly effective at reducing inflammation and suppressing our immune system. During early pregnancy, there is a rise in these specific corticosteroids. Glucocorticoids rise in early pregnancy to help regulate the processes required for successful embryo implantation as well as the initial phase of fetal and placental growth by stimulating the secretion of hCG.

We have now come full circle.

Higher amounts of stress hormones increase the secretion of hCG. In fact, studies show that supplementation with corticosteroid medications can increase hCG production 10-fold.[137]

So how does this affect H. pylori?

As the glucocorticoids rise, there is a suppression in immune responses. When this happens, the natural mechanisms that keep a homeostatic relationship with H. pylori fail, allowing the bacteria to become more pathogenic in nature, creating gastritis.

Anxiety is the physical manifestation of stress. Although there are no studies linking stress, anxiety, and morning sickness, we do see the correlation between stress, anxiety, nausea, and gastritis in other conditions, such as ulcer formation.

You will not be able to lower the natural stress responses of pregnancy nor would you want to. You can, however, regulate the emotional stressors and work on removing other endogenous and exogenous causes of stress.

Nutritional Factors

When you explore the research surrounding nutrition and pregnancy nausea, you'll notice that most studies are done on the nutrients that are depleted due to nausea, not connections between preexisting nutritional insufficiencies and deficiencies with the development of pregnancy nausea.

I've already mentioned a few individual nutrients that if insufficient or deficient can affect the natural processes of the first trimester, such as vitamin D and thiamine regarding proper glucose metabolism and iodine in the regulation of thyroid hormones. These deficiencies could predispose a woman to issues with nausea. I've got a few more particularly important nutritional connections that are highly associated with an increase in pregnancy nausea symptoms that we should touch on. One, especially, is going to seem familiar: vitamin B6 (pyridoxine).

B6 has been known to have antiemetic effects since the 1940s. There are multiple forms of B6 in blood circulation and knowing which form was the most effective in treating nausea and vomiting had been a bit of a mystery until a newer study pointed to the pyridoxal-5-phosphate (P5P) form of B6 as being associated with a decrease in nausea and vomiting symptoms.

A study done in 2014 and published in the *Journal of Clinical Pharmacology* found a correlation between levels of P5P and a decrease in nausea and vomiting symptoms. The results came after an analysis of 283 pregnant women experiencing nausea symptoms. The participants were randomized to receive a vitamin B6 medication in the form of pyridoxine hydrochloride (pyridoxine HCl) or a placebo for 14 days. The effectiveness of the treatment was assessed by the Pregnancy-Unique Quantification of Emesis (PUQE) scoring system. Blood samples were taken at days 0, 4, 8, and 14 to measure the values of the different vitamin B6 forms: pyridoxal, pyridoxine, and P5P.[138]

Among the women in the group receiving the supplemental pyridoxine HCl, PUQE scores consistently improved over the 14 days. When they broke down the blood samples, the values of pyridoxal and pyridoxine remained constant and low, while the blood values of P5P increased in association with the antiemetic effects.

How cool is that?

From this study, we can deduct that pyridoxine and pyridoxal were preforms of the P5P and that the P5P form was the form with the therapeutic effects. Based on these findings, treatment with the P5P form may be more beneficial than the pyridoxine HCl form typically found in supplementation, especially for those women who may have genetic conditions that limit their ability to convert pyridoxine to P5P or who are insufficient in nutrients needed for conversion to happen.

So how does P5P help with nausea?

During pregnancy, there is an increased demand for the enzyme tryptophan dioxygenase (TDO), which requires B6 as a cofactor. TDO is important in the tryptophan pathway that creates NAD, a vitamin B3-dependent compound needed for cellular metabolism and steroid hormone synthesis (more on this in Chapter 10).

To work as a cofactor for the TDO enzyme, vitamin B6 must first be converted into its active form. Dysfunction of the TDO enzyme pathway and a disruption in the NAD metabolic pathway is one of the known mechanisms of insulin resistance. In addition, P5P deficiency impairs insulin secretion.

B6 activation requires vitamin B2 and magnesium.[139] Zinc is necessary for the transport of B6 through the body and across cell membranes. Lower zinc and B6 levels are seen in pregnancy nausea patients.

Outside of pregnancy, hyperthyroidism has been shown to be a cause of lower levels of vitamin B6, and we now know that the mother's body in the first trimester becomes synthetically hyperthyroid thanks to rising hCG levels. Demand for zinc increases during the first trimester as the demand for thyroid hormone increases.

Zinc is an enzyme catalyst for deiodinase, which converts inactive T4 to active T3. It is also required for the placenta to produce several chemicals required for normal pregnancy function, including the deiodinase for thyroid hormone clearance. There are several different types of deiodinases and all of them need zinc. If zinc is low, B6 is low. Deficiencies in both zinc and B6 have been associated with increased severity of nausea.

Interestingly, the only medication approved to treat nausea and vomiting in pregnancy is a combination of pyridoxine and doxylamine/Unisom. But, unless the cause is related to issues associated with a B6 or zinc deficiency, this medication may not give any relief. Differentiation and understanding function, as always, is the key to successful treatment.

In the clinic, we find that P5P supplements work significantly better for nausea management, and they work even better when given with a small amount of zinc. Knowing what you know now, you get why.

Magnesium is another nutrient that is highly associated with increased severity of nausea in pregnancy. As progesterone levels increase, so does the demand for magnesium. As blood sugars drop, so does magnesium. Not only is magnesium one of the most important nutrients for maternal health throughout pregnancy, but it is also one of the most commonly insufficient and deficient nutrients in the maternal diet.

Magnesium levels are closely related to shifts in cortisol, progesterone, and estrogen. Cortisol is the primary hormone that helps to regulate blood sugar levels. As we've already discussed, in the early stages of pregnancy, there is a shift in insulin production and a tendency toward hypoglycemia. When blood sugar drops, cortisol rises. When cortisol rises, so does the demand for magnesium. Cortisol has a lovely diurnal pattern throughout the day. As cortisol drops, in response to decreases in blood sugar, we see a specific pattern of nausea dysfunction, which can be treated by regulating magnesium levels.

Afternoon fatigue with hypoglycemia is common in this pattern as are symptoms that are worse in the afternoons and evenings and better with sleep. And often there is constipation and poor gut motility as well. Research studies on the role of and use of magnesium in pregnancy nausea are pretty much nonexistent.

Genetics

Clinical experience and research both show us that severe nausea in pregnancy runs in families. This familial relationship points to a genetic predisposition.

A study done in 2018 identified genes associated with hyperemesis gravidarum. The genes, growth differentiation factor 15 (GDF-15) and insulin-like growth factor binding protein 7 (IGFBP7), play important roles in the development of the placenta as well as appetite.[140]

Another 2018 study found a direct correlation between elevations in GDF-15 and nausea and vomiting in the second trimester.[141]

GDF-15 is a stress response cytokine or inflammatory protein. Outside of pregnancy, elevations in this protein are shown to be associated with type 2 diabetes and insulin resistance. It is now being used as a marker for impaired fasting glucose.

IGFBP7, too, has been associated with insulin resistance and an increased risk of metabolic syndrome[142]. This protein is a binding protein that increases and decreases binding of insulin growth factors to their receptors.

These genetic cases are specific to HG, a severe form of nausea in pregnancy that can result in hospitalization, severe dehydration, malnutrition, and, in extreme cases, pregnancy loss.

This is a vastly different condition than other forms of nausea in pregnancy. Although some of the factors mentioned—hormones, hypoglycemia, nutrition, and H. pylori—may still play into symptoms, this seems to be more of a genetic condition that affects glucose metabolism and function. The research on this topic is new and exciting, and I look forward to reading and learning more about it as it unfolds.

Keep in mind that the evidence that there is a genetic predisposition does not mean that the symptoms cannot be managed. Though they may be prone to the condition and have symptoms regardless of the grasp of function, we can still help these women manage their symptoms by lessening severity, reducing the need for medical intervention, reducing the risk of nutritional deficiencies seen in women with severe nausea, and reducing their risk of other pregnancy complications that seem to be higher in these women, such as preeclampsia.

IV nutrition therapy is often a tool utilized with great success by women with HG. Most medical management of HG focuses on rehydration, which can give women acute symptom relief and increase electrolytes but misses the big nutritional picture. Severe nutritional deficiencies are seen in these women and the addition of IV nutrients to hydration methods, is essential for preventing complications with their pregnancies and in their babies' growth.

Ginger Versus Peppermint: Which Is Best for Nausea Symptoms?

Differentiation is key to the effectiveness of any treatment plan but is especially so in the use of herbal therapies.

In TCM, diseases are classified into multiple pattern types. Pregnancy nausea, for example, can be associated with more than five different patterns of dysfunction. Each pattern requires a slightly different approach to treatment. Conventional medicine, too, as we see from the breakdown of pregnancy nausea, also has differentiated patterns of diagnosis that should affect the method of treatment prescribed. Whether we are looking at disease from a TCM or conventional perspective, differentiation is the key to treatment.

There is no one cause of any disease in the human body. Studying and understanding how the body functions and interacts—not just how an individual organ system works—helps in the differentiation of disease progression and symptoms.

In comes ginger and peppermint. These are prime examples of the importance of differentiating symptoms in treatment. Many of you have heard of, personally used, or prescribed ginger for pregnancy nausea.

How many of you had negative results?

This is because you did not differentiate the symptoms and the pattern presentation was not indicative of the use of this herb. Peppermint would have been a better choice, most likely.

Ginger has a long history of use in gastric issues, such as nausea and poor gut motility. In fact, the treatment of many gastrointestinal conditions, such as small intestine bacterial overgrowth (SIBO), uses ginger to increase gut motility to prevent bacterial colonization in the small intestine during and post-antibiotic treatments. Ginger is energetically hot in nature. It increases gastric emptying and reduces nausea by affecting serotonin signaling along the vagal nerve.

Peppermint is the opposite of ginger in that it is cooling and works differently in the body. While ginger increases movement through the gut and affects serotonin signaling, peppermint works as a muscle relaxant and numbing agent in the stomach and intestines. In fact, studies show that peppermint is as good at relaxing gut spasming as antispasmodic drugs.[143]

Now, if you were to give a woman with poor gut motility a peppermint solution to treat her nausea, that only relaxes the gut further, you may cause more nausea symptoms. In turn, if you were to give a woman with a spastic gut more ginger that stimulates movement, you would also cause a worsening of symptoms. Therefore, when we look at the research that does not differentiate patterns in treatment, we see a mix of success and failure in nausea treatment with herbal management and probably other treatments, such as medication therapy that includes pyridoxine and doxylamine. The pattern was not differentiated, and thus accurate treatment was not given.

There is no one cause of nausea and vomiting in pregnancy, but there are several possible connections that need to be addressed with any mother experiencing symptoms severe enough to affect her daily life. It is not just a symptom of pregnancy but a dynamic condition that should be monitored so it does not cause nutritional deficiencies that can affect the future pregnancy. Many factors play into the development, severity, and duration of nausea in pregnancy.

Understanding the maternal function and how nutrition plays a role is important in proper diagnosis and treatment regardless of the limiting research linking treatment approaches. Maternal function in pregnancy is an area of research that is lacking, and great advances are still needed.

Knowing what I know now, I believe my nausea was metabolic and nutritional. With my first pregnancy, I had taken my diet very seriously and lived what Dr. Price wrote. Once my daughter was born, I was preoccupied with being a new mom and I let my own nutrition slip. I am prone to low blood pressure and hypoglycemia by nature, and a combination of nutritional deficiencies from a less-than-adequate diet (I *may* have been on a brownie kick), genetic predisposition to hypoglycemia, and the use of birth control between my pregnancies predisposed me to a specific presentation of nausea in pregnancy.

Chapter 9

Anemia In Pregnancy

In my practice, the diagnosis and management of anemia in pregnancy are all too common. Each case is completely different as to why the mother ended up becoming anemic and the treatment varies. Take Sam for example.

Sam was referred to me by her midwife. She had been struggling with anemia throughout her entire pregnancy. She had had low hemoglobin at the beginning of pregnancy, and it had followed her throughout. She had been taking a high-dose iron supplement since she was 12 weeks pregnant, and her numbers had not changed. In fact, they had gotten worse. She was aiming for a homebirth, but the local homebirth midwives have a hemoglobin cutoff of 11.0 grams(g)/deciliter(dL).

In her first trimester, she had been 10.6 g/dL—so, borderline. Her midwife was confident that some extra iron would get her levels up. They didn't. By 32 weeks, her hemoglobin had dropped to 9.3 g/dL. Why? Because she wasn't iron deficient; she was B vitamin deficient.

She came to see me at 32 weeks gestation. She was experiencing extreme fatigue, so much so that she just didn't want to get out of bed. She had also been diagnosed with depression and was having carpal tunnel symptoms. She had been extremely nauseous in her first trimester and had been living off crackers, potatoes, and carbohydrates. She still didn't have the greatest appetite and ate mostly bland and nutrient-poor foods, such as chicken nuggets, mashed potatoes, and mac and cheese.

I looked at her old labs and her most recent. Her hemoglobin levels had continued to decline even though she was taking 40 mg of iron per day, prescribed by her midwife. What was interesting was that her mean corpuscular volume (MCV) was going *up*.

Unlike many other blood cell values that change throughout pregnancy, MCV should remain constant and unchanged. This rise in MCV was an indicator of vitamin B issues. Instead of increasing her iron, as her midwife suggested, we supported her iron intake with IV B vitamins and oral active form B vitamins and, of course, changed her diet.

We ran another CBC at 35 weeks and her hemoglobin had increased from 9.3 g/dL to 10.8 g/dL. We were on the right track. At 37 weeks, her hemoglobin had risen to 11.9 g/dL—just high enough for her amazing home birth.

Gestational anemia continues to be a condition seen commonly throughout pregnancy. Anemia is defined as a deficiency of red blood cells or hemoglobin. NHANES reported that 18 percent of pregnant women were iron deficient, while only 5.4 percent were anemic.[144]

Anemia should be taken seriously. When a mother is anemic, she is unable to supply the required oxygen to both herself and her baby. It is typically a sign of several nutritional deficiencies that should be addressed. Anemia is associated with low birth weight, poor placental functioning, increased rates of hypertension and preeclampsia, and maternal mortality.

The primary cause of anemia is malnutrition of the nutrients needed for proper blood cell formation and function. Certain habits and events can increase the risk of anemia in pregnancy:

- Multiples
- Subsequent pregnancies
- Morning sickness
- Younger mothers
- Anemia prior to pregnancy
- Poor diet
- Vegan diet
- Antacid medications
- Oxidative stress and inflammation

Depending on the individual woman, the nutritional cause may be one of many different nutrients required for blood cell formation and function and is not limited to iron deficiency.

Birth of a Red Blood Cell

Erythropoiesis is the fancy term for red blood cell (erythrocyte) formation. The production of red blood cells happens in the marrow of the bones and is triggered by a hormone produced in the kidneys when blood oxygen levels are low, erythropoietin. The gestation and birth of a mature red blood cell takes about seven days. (Did you like that analogy? Nerd humor.) These red blood cells then live for 100 to 120 days.

In the fetus, blood cell formation begins in the yolk sac. From two to five months' gestation, the fetus makes red blood cells from liver and spleen stem cells, and then from five months on the baby produces red blood cells from bone marrow just like its mother.

Each red blood cell starts out as a stem cell called a hemocytoblast. These cells are the base for both red and white blood cells, but for now, let's stick to red. There are multiple steps to becoming a red blood cell.

First, hemocytoblast becomes erythroblasts. This stage is highly governed by erythropoietin, which signals the differentiation of the stem cell to become a red blood cell through genetic modifications. The DNA transcription that differentiates what the hemocytoblast will become is dependent on genetic acetylation and methylation; it is not just for fetal programming. Remember, this is reliant on several vitamins in the diet: folate, choline, B2, B5, and B12.

Erythroblasts still resemble all other cells in the body by having organelles like the nucleus that houses DNA. As the erythroblasts mature into reticulocytes, they lose their organelles, including the nucleus and the plasma membrane. Red blood cells are unique in the fact that they do not contain a nucleus. Without these structural changes, red blood cells could not take on their concave shape. These changes require a breakdown of chromatin and increased acetylation.[145] This process is dependent on the vitamin B5-containing acetyl-CoA.

There is always a balance, and methylation is pivotal to preventing excess acetylation that will cause apoptosis. Therefore, you see B9 and B12 being crucial to the proper formation of red blood cells. Deficiencies in B12 are associated with a specific type of anemia due to an increase in apoptosis. In mild cases of B9 and B12 deficiency, you see an increase in misshapen red blood cells, not enough to cause full-on death and anemia but enough that they are malformed and not functioning well.[146]

Reticulocytes are also called immature red blood cells. They have now become baby red blood cells, and these cells are released into the bloodstream to mature. Maturation takes about three days.

The hallmark of what makes a red blood cell able to do its job is the formation and function of the hemoglobin unit. Heme is produced by the mitochondria of the red blood cell before it reaches the reticulocyte phase. Heme consists of an iron ferrous molecule surrounded by a ring of four pyrrole molecules. These rings are linked by methane bridges. This heme compound is then surrounded by a globin protein that protects the iron.

The process for making a hemoglobin starts with a glycine (an amino acid) and a succinyl coenzyme A (succinyl-CoA), from the Krebs cycle. B6 is the coenzyme for the reaction that starts the initial step in hemoglobin formation, which is the formation of the pyrrole rings. These rings are highly dependent on both B6 and zinc.

Iron accumulates in immature red blood cells early in the developmental process. It is stored in the cell as ferritin until hemoglobin synthesis begins. Increasing iron levels signal the synthesis of globin by ribosomes in the cells. Vitamin C levels have been linked to the absorption of iron into the cells.

Once hemoglobin is formed and the red blood cell is matured, it is functional and able to travel through the bloodstream, carrying oxygen throughout the body.

In Pregnancy We Double

The second trimester is marked by the need for the mother to double her blood volume to support the increasing needs of her baby. From the second trimester through the third, there is a 50 percent increase in plasma volume and a 35 percent or more increase in red blood cells.

The increase in plasma and the increase in red blood cells are governed by two different processes. There is little change in the first trimester, with a rise that plateaus around 30 weeks and peaks at 34–36 weeks. The largest rise in plasma occurs between the first half of the second trimester and the mid-third trimester.[147] The plasma volume change is associated with the size of the growing baby. The larger the baby, the more plasma.[148]

The rise in plasma is greater than the rise in red blood cells, so a dip in some red blood cell measurements is considered normal in later gestation. What shouldn't change is the mean corpuscular volume (MCV) and mean corpuscular hemoglobin concentration (MCHC).

Plasma carries waste products, water, electrolytes, enzymes, sugars, fats, proteins, and nutrients throughout the body. The rise in plasma helps to regulate blood pressure and water retention for kidney function. This increase is highly regulated by estrogen and aldosterone.

More blood and blood volume means a healthier mom and baby.

Shifts in Iron Metabolism

Throughout gestation, like in all aspects of metabolism, there are shifts in the absorption and use of iron throughout the pregnant body. Different phases of gestation are characterized by different patterns in iron regulation.

Unlike many other minerals, iron isn't excreted when excess is consumed. It accumulates in the system. Because of this unique feature, iron metabolism is tightly controlled.

There are three hormones that regulate iron in the body:

1. Erythropoietin - produced in response to low blood oxygen levels.

2. Erythroferrone - produced in response to anemic stress.

3. Hepcidin - produced in response to iron stores, low blood oxygen levels, and systemic inflammation.

NUTRIENT HIGHLIGHT: IRON

Iron is a dietary mineral. It is best known for its requirement in red blood cell production and function, but it also makes up another protein complex called myoglobin. It is also a component of several enzymes in the body, specifically the cytochrome P450 (CYP) enzymes required for steroidogenesis.

Dietary iron comes in two forms:

1. Heme - Iron bound to protoporphyrin IX. This form is found in blood and muscle, so in the diet it is found in meat.

2. Nonheme - This is the elemental form of iron that is found in many different food sources as well as supplements.

Heme iron is considered the most absorbable form because it is not affected by antinutrients, such as phytates or oxalates. In pregnancy, the placenta favors heme iron. The gut easily absorbs this form of iron, with the system transporting it whole to the placenta where it readily accepts and shuttles this form directly to the baby for accumulation.[149]

Nonheme iron, which is found in both animal foods and plant-based foods, is less absorbed because it is influenced by several other factors, such as phytates and oxalates.

On average, heme iron is about 15–35 percent absorbed, while nonheme absorption ranges from 2–20 percent, based on the food source and cooking methods used.[150]

Nonheme iron is notoriously difficult to absorb.

Of these three hormones, hepcidin has been linked the most to the regulation of iron absorption and metabolic changes in pregnancy. Hepcidin inhibits iron absorption and helps to regulate the amount of iron in the system to prevent overdose. When ferritin levels are high, so is hepcidin.

This increase in hepcidin binds to iron transport proteins and prevents their ability to bring iron through the gut or into target cells. When iron stores are low, hepcidin is low, increasing the expression of iron transport proteins and increasing the absorption of iron through the gut and into the cells for storage.

Iron absorption drops at the beginning of pregnancy due to an increase in hepcidin production. The loss of menses and the preconception diet should have set a mother up for this drop with adequate iron absorption and ferritin storage. The mother is living off the red blood cells she had in circulation and her ferritin reserves more than the iron she is consuming at this phase of gestation.

Iron absorption increases again at 24 weeks, after a normal anemic phase signals the release of stored iron, decreasing ferritin in the cells, decreasing hepcidin, and increasing absorption. Now, there is a significant reduction in hepcidin production from 24 weeks to 40 weeks to signal a significant increase in iron absorption in the system. The mechanism behind this is considered unknown. Mothers with adequate ferritin and iron values at birth will still have decreased hepcidin levels.[151] Many of the hormonal and inflammatory features that would naturally raise hepcidin levels are present during this time—inflammation and elevated progesterone—yet levels stay low.

A 2012 study found that estrogen regulates hepcidin through genetic expression of the hormone in hepatic cells.[152] Several studies have since found that increased estradiol is linked to lower levels of hepcidin.

Testosterone has also been shown to decrease hepcidin and correct anemia when administered to female anemic mice.[153] Could one of the reasons we see a 70 percent increase in testosterone production in pregnancy be partly due to the need to reduce hepcidin and increase the ability of the body to absorb iron? Who knows?

Heme transport proteins are found throughout the placenta, and much of the iron absorbed in the third trimester is transported directly to the placenta for transport to the fetus. Throughout pregnancy, the baby needs to accumulate approximately 300 mg of iron before birth. Most of this iron is accumulated in the last trimester of gestation. During this time, the baby is absorbing 5–8 mg of iron per day from the mother.[154]

The need for iron throughout pregnancy cannot be fully supplied by the diet and is heavily reliant on the iron stores a mother has prior to pregnancy[155] in addition to the amount of iron she is able to accumulate before the point in which the fetal demands take over.

During the second trimester, when a mother is doubling her blood volume and increasing her ferritin stores, she is doing so in preparation for the third trimester and the increased demand in iron that her baby will put on the system. If she is unable to prepare correctly and increase her iron reserves, she will be unable to keep up with the iron demands in the third trimester. The 5–8 mg per day that the baby will take from the mother's reserves and her diet leave her with little else. We also see that in the third trimester iron transport favors the placenta over maternal needs, making it difficult, if not impossible, to raise maternal ferritin levels at a certain point in gestation.

A better preventative measure would be to increase dietary iron and iron supplements in the months prior to conception to improve iron stores as well as the crucial periods before iron transfer favors fetal accumulation. In addition, assessing ferritin levels at the beginning of pregnancy can be a biomarker for anemia later in pregnancy and as an assessment of maternal iron metabolic function. In anemia, as in most other conditions, prevention is easier than treatment.

Inflammation and Iron Deficiency

For some women, no amount of iron supplementation is going to raise their iron levels. Inflammation, such as in the form of oxidative stress, chronic pain, or environmental chemical absorption can cause a rise in the hepcidin hormone, reducing iron absorption in the gut regardless of systemic iron levels. This is often seen when ferritin levels are high and/or normal but serum iron is low.

Inflammatory cytokines have been shown to increase hepcidin production from the liver, decrease red blood cell life spans, and decrease red blood cell production in the bone marrow—making a perfect recipe for functional anemia.[156]

One form of inflammation seen in many conditions in pregnancy that seems to connect to anemia is oxidative stress. When cells are under oxidative stress conditions, we can see apoptosis. When cells die, they release their ferritin into the bloodstream, increasing serum ferritin values. At the same time, we see oxidative stress-mediated destruction of red blood cells.[157] This connection is seen in cases of preeclampsia, where we find correlations between oxidative stress markers, iron status, and vascular function.[158]

For women who do exhibit higher oxidative stress patterns, decreasing inflammation is key to improving blood values and preventing complications.

A Cultural Approach to Oxalates

Oxalate is the biggest stealer of iron in foods, yet oxalates are highest in the foods we often think of as being the best sources of plant-based iron, such as green leafy veggies like spinach. Anyone who has worked with me knows how much I dislike raw spinach and many other raw greens, especially in pregnancy, simply due to their high levels of oxalates.

Oxalates are also known as oxalic acid. This compound is naturally produced in our bodies and found in plants. A little serves a purpose because it binds minerals—good and bad—and helps to clear them out through the urine. Too much and we see stone formation in the kidneys as well as mineral deficiencies throughout the diet and the body.

Have you ever looked at cultures that eat food sources that are high in oxalates? There is almost always a universal preparation method used in each of these cultures: blanching.

In Korean cuisine, we have banchan, which are these little veggie and meat side dishes that are served at each meal. One that you almost always see on a Korean table is a simple seasoned spinach salad. This salad is not raw but a blanched spinach that has been drained, cooled, and seasoned. Other cultures that use spinach also incorporate similar practices. Think saag in Indian cuisine and spanakopita in Greek cooking. Each of these spinach preparations requires the step of blanching the spinach before use. Why?

Yay science! Thanks to studies that have investigated how cooking methods affect the percentage of oxalates in foods, and we now know that boiling/blanching removes a significant amount of oxalate from the spinach and other oxalate-rich veggies. Nearly 90 percent of the oxalates in these plants were removed through boiling.[159] The oxalates remained in the water and to remove oxalates you need to dump the water.

My grandmother used to say that the bitter taste that spinach gave your mouth was a sign it was no good. Only when it was cooked was it good for you. Seems those crazy cultural approaches to food preparation were onto something.

Other greens that are high in oxalates are beet greens, chard, turnip greens, etc. I have a rule of thumb at my house to be safe. If the leaf is a big, dark green leaf, we cook it. If it's smaller and lighter, we don't. In all things in nutrition, it's about balance. By cooking the big greens that are rich in iron, calcium, magnesium, and other helpful minerals, we can be sure to maximize absorption. Then, by leaving the smaller leaves that are rich in vitamin E, vitamin C, B vitamins, and other heat-sensitive nutrients, we can maximize our overall nutrient density.

Anemia Is More than Just an Iron Deficiency

A study of young pregnant women found that 25 percent were anemic in the third trimester and of those women only 6.1 percent had iron-deficiency anemia.[160] In another study that followed healthy women who were carrying multiples, they found anemia was evident in 45 percent of the women at delivery, but only 18 percent had iron deficiency anemia—leaving us to postulate that other nutritional components are associated with anemia in these other cases.

Nutritional deficiencies that affect the absorption or the formation of red blood cells can easily be a contributing factor to anemia presentations.

Zinc-deficiency anemia is more common in pregnancy than studies suggest. The balance between copper and zinc is fickle, and as the copper levels naturally rise throughout pregnancy, we see lower levels of zinc and, if levels get too low, we see insufficiency and deficiency symptoms. Zinc is found in the structure of the enzymes required for iron absorption and hemoglobin formation. A 2009 study found that zinc supplementation improved all parameters of anemia.[161]

There is a 10–20-fold increase in folate requirements, and a two-fold increase in the need for B12 during pregnancy.[162] Deficiencies in these nutrients not only affect methylation for fetal programming and placental health but also affects the formation of red blood cells.

Folate deficiency in early pregnancy is a predictor of anemia in later gestation. One study of 502 women found 97.5 percent of them had inadequate dietary folate intake at their early gestation visit. Eighteen percent of these women presented with anemia. Of these women, 43.4 percent were anemic in the postnatal period. This study found a direct relationship between first-visit folate levels and the development of anemia in pregnancy.[163]

B12 deficiency is associated with a special type of anemia called pernicious anemia. For the body to absorb B12, we need intrinsic factor, which is produced by the parietal cells of the gut with stomach acid. Pregnant women with heartburn who take antacid medications are more likely to have a B12 insufficiency or deficiency and could have anemia presentations associated with poor red blood cell formation due to B12. This is another nutritional deficiency intricately connected to anemia, preeclampsia, and HELLP syndrome. Many of the symptoms of B12 deficiency mimic HELLP syndrome.[164] (For more information on the HELLP syndrome, see chapter 11.)

NUTRIENT HIGHLIGHT: VITAMIN B12 (COBALAMIN) AND COBALT

Vitamin B12 is a term used for a group of vitamins, called cobalamins, that contain cobalt. There are two forms of B12 used in the body: methylcobalamin and 5-deoxyadenosylcobalamin.

Like many other dietary nutrients, B12 is bound to proteins in the diet. In the gut, the mixture of HCl, digestive enzymes, and bacterial fermentation breaks these bonds. This free B12 binds with intrinsic factor, a glycoprotein that is secreted with stomach acid, and is absorbed through the small intestines. There is a limit on how much B12 can be absorbed at a single sitting. Only about 50–60 percent of a 1 mcg dose of B12 is absorbed, and the amount of B12 absorbed is rate limited by the amount of intrinsic factor produced. It is estimated that your body will absorb 10 mcg of a 500 mcg dose; overdosing like this is considered safe because your body will flush what it does not use. Now, this is in healthy people who are producing adequate amounts of intrinsic factor, HCl, and digestive enzymes and have a healthy microbiome. People taking proton pump inhibitors and certain other medications cannot absorb their B12 regardless of the form they are taking.

B12 is a primary cofactor in several different enzymatic functions throughout the body, not just methylation pathways. B12 is also important for cellular metabolism, neurotransmitter formation, and the health of the myelin sheaths that surround nerves.

A little sidenote on cobalt. No one talks about this mineral, but it is considered an essential trace mineral. Cobalt in the diet is converted to B12 by gut bacteria, so having a healthy gut is important for fermentation and formation of some of the B12 in the body.

HELLP syndrome is another complication of gestational hypertension and preeclampsia.

It stands for:

> H – Hemolysis
> E L – Elevated Liver enzymes
> L P – Low Platelets

Other nutritional factors seem to be more associated with other systemic causes of anemia, such as inflammation and oxidative stress.

Several studies have indicated a correlation between vitamin D status and anemia, specifically hemoglobin concentrations.[165] Studies seem to point to this connection being greater in cases associated with inflammation, and because vitamin D plays a role in immune regulation, that the correlation is due to this action.

Other studies seem to indicate that taking vitamin A with iron supplements is more effective than taking iron supplements alone in improving anemia yet with an unknown mechanism of action.[166]

Something interesting in these studies is that there was no measure taken to assess for inflammatory markers as a cause of anemia in patients. It is plausible that the improvements in anemia were due to addressing the inflammation through vitamin A antioxidant functions and had nothing to do with iron use in the body. It is also important to note that the demand for vitamin A increases in the third trimester, as we'll discuss in Chapter 12.

When you really look at the data, iron deficiency seems to be a relatively small portion of gestational anemia cases. Yet conventional medicine has a standardized one-size-fits-all approach to treatment. If we standardize our care to only include iron deficiency as a cause of anemia, we will be missing many women desperate to improve their blood chemistry, their health, and their pregnancies. Understanding the different nutrients involved in the formation of red blood cells and the regulation of other factors known to be associated with anemia can help with the differentiation of anemia types.

Anemia in the Vegan Diet

Anemia is more common in plant-based diets—fact! I know many of you reading this right now are yelling, "You can meet all your nutritional requirements with a vegan diet." Yes, you can, but it is hard and requires a focused diet.

You can get defensive, or you can get educated.

I find many women consuming a vegan diet are eating higher intakes of breads and carbs with lower-than-adequate actual plants. These women need help and support just like the women I see who are eating a high-carb, low-fat standard American diet.

I do not believe it is my job to change someone's dietary philosophy. In my practice, I work with many different women with many different cultural and philosophical beliefs on diet. I am never going to tell people who choose, for whatever reason, to avoid a certain food that they cannot have a healthy pregnancy if they don't consume that food.

What I am going to tell them is the truth. What science shows us is that they are more prone to being deficient, so they can focus on the foods within their philosophical beliefs to fulfill the needs that may not be met. For vegans, B12, vitamin D, calcium, and iron are the nutrients that are the most commonly deficient and the hardest to get in this type of diet.[167] This is a fact. It does not mean that a plant-based diet cannot fulfill the requirements; it just means it is harder in a select few nutrients and often requires extra supplementation.

Here is a quick look at this from a different perspective.

In the third trimester, a mother needs to consume >9 mg of iron per day to fulfill both her needs and her baby's. Depending on the type of iron-rich foods the vegan mother is consuming, and in what preparation form, may determine her ability to meet this demand. Three ounces of spinach has 2.5 mg of iron (give or take). Locked up with oxalates in the raw spinach form, say, in a smoothie, a mother may get 2 percent of this, or 0.05 mg of iron. If she prepared it correctly by boiling and draining her spinach before use, she may get a max of 0.875 mg per serving. Next, take lentils. These little guys are great because they are lower in both oxalates and phytates, and they contain a good amount of iron: 6.5 mg. Knowing that in the best of conditions the most absorption we see with iron is 35 percent of intake, 1 cup of cooked lentils would provide 2.3 mg. To meet the daily requirements, she would need to consume just under five cups of lentils per day.

Now, it isn't just vegan moms who struggle dietarily to meet the demands of iron in pregnancy. Studies show that in the third trimester no woman can compensate for the demand of iron dietarily. The iron in the third trimester is dependent on the iron stores from the first and second trimester. Keeping up with fetal iron demands in the third trimester on a vegan diet is harder, typically requiring supplements. If you understand the unique needs of these women, and instead of shaming them into eating meat, you support their beliefs by helping them choose better quality foods and better preparation techniques, they can have amazing pregnancies where they feel supported, listened to, respected, and empowered. (My doula days are kicking in . . . empower the mothers!)

I had a patient years ago that came into my office during her pregnancy. Before I could even start talking, she aggressively told me she was plant-based and would not go paleo. I chuckled a bit and asked her why she thought I was going to tell her to eat paleo. She told me that every nutritionist and functional medicine practitioner she had seen before her pregnancy had told her she needed to eat meat and that her vegan diet was not healthy. I gave her my normal spiel about how I don't care what food sources she gets her nutrients from, just so long as she gets the nutrients she needs.

We looked at her diet, made some tiny tweaks, but all in all, she was doing better than the women I see consuming a standard American diet, which is the worst of the extreme diets—and it is an extreme diet. She had a beautiful pregnancy, a beautiful birth, and a beautiful postpartum. She later told me I should advertise that I'm a vegan-friendly functional medicine practitioner because they don't seem to exist. I never did. I don't want to fall into any one school of thought on nutrition and diet mostly because I don't think any one school is right, and if I did, I could not support all the women I see.

Lost Mothers

The American College of Obstetrics and Gynecologist currently recommends iron supplementation during pregnancy to prevent anemia.[168] Even though systematic reviews show that iron supplementation does not have a positive effect on maternal iron status, and the evidence showing that routine high-dose iron supplementation improves maternal outcomes is inconsistent.[169]

With the understanding that iron metabolism changes throughout pregnancy, and that standard anemia testing often doesn't occur until after 28 weeks gestation, there may be a smaller window of opportunity in which we can affect maternal iron levels with iron supplementation. After this point, the supplementation of iron is less to the benefit of the mother and more to ensure that the baby receives the required reserves of iron before delivery.

The conventional treatment of anemia is to increase iron supplementation only. I've wondered, knowing what I know and now what you know, if that has really been for the benefit of the mother or more to support the iron requirements of the baby in the third trimester.

If the system were designed to genuinely care for mothers and treat their anemia to support their overall health, function, and birth outcomes, why would the system not address all aspects of anemia support and sooner than the third trimester? Instead, the focus seems to be directed to only supporting the iron requirements of the growing baby.

Preparing for preparing. The work that goes into supporting maternal health regarding anemia prevention occurs before the shift in iron metabolism and in addressing the many other nutritional components associated with the proper formation and function of red blood cells.

A Case of Anemia

Colleen was a fertility client of mine who had struggled with unexplained infertility and recurrent miscarriages after the birth of two previous children. She came to see me after she had lost a pregnancy at 13 weeks per the recommendation of her midwife. After addressing some underlying conditions, she became pregnant nine months after we started our functional medicine and acupuncture treatments.

In her first trimester, she had nausea but did not want to treat it as it gave her comfort, especially as she reached 13 weeks when she had experienced her previous miscarriage that ended in a traumatic dilation and curettage (D&C) with severe blood loss. She had multiple ultrasounds to confirm pregnancy and fetal health, and all looked good. We did some work on second trimester nutrition, and I gave her some generic tips on what foods to include during this phase of gestation.

Our next meeting was at 24 weeks when she came in saying she felt better at this phase in gestation than she had in any of her previous pregnancies. She was experiencing mild fatigue but chalked it up to being a mom of two children, one autistic, and being pregnant. She said the fatigue wasn't stopping her from doing daily activities.

At 28 weeks, things "shifted," in her words. She had been feeling as though she was a bit fatigued but nothing that seemed abnormal for her life, and now it was like she had been hit by a truck. She was exhausted, but not normal fatigue—exhaustion like she couldn't get out of bed and felt she had to sit down after the slightest exertion. No amount of extra sleep or self-care seemed to make a difference. We decided to run some blood work.

We did a basic CBC, serum iron, and ferritin. Her red blood count (RBC) was well within the normal range for her gestation of pregnancy, but all her other values showed anemia. She had been able to build her red blood cells, but they were weak. Her hemoglobin was 10.2 g/dL, iron was 56 mcg/dL, and her ferritin was 8 ng/mL—functionally and clinically anemic. Specifically, iron-deficiency anemia. Now, I don't believe that iron-deficiency anemia stands alone, so we worked on building her blood (hopefully quickly) with iron supplements as well as B vitamins. The hope was that we were not too late to make changes in her values.

Her next set of labs were done two weeks later. We had a small success. Her hemoglobin had popped up to 11.1 g/dL, just over the cusp of what a mama needs, but her ferritin had not shifted. She was obviously getting the additional iron and using it to make red blood cells, but she was not storing it. More labs. This time, a comprehensive metabolic panel.

It's amazing what these standard labs can tell you.

Zinc is required for so many processes in iron metabolism and *storage*. For iron to be stored within the cells, we need zinc. Zinc is also important for the formation of alkaline phosphatase. This is a liver enzyme that has a placental form that is produced in high amounts in pregnancy. Naturally, there is an increase in alkaline phosphatase in pregnancy, with levels being nearly double pre-pregnancy levels by the third trimester. This enzyme contains zinc, and zinc deficiency can cause lower than functional values of alkaline phosphatase. Her levels were low for gestation at 57 U/L. This single measure indicated a possible zinc component. Zinc is also required for protein metabolism. Some decrease in total protein is 100 percent normal in pregnancy, but her levels were low for gestational norms at 5.4 g/dL.

I started to suspect that zinc deficiency may be playing a role in her anemia as well. We increased her dietary zinc and gave her a supplement. Within a week she was feeling better, less exhausted, and able to get up in the mornings. We went off her symptoms and continued with treatment as she was feeling better. Another round of testing was done at 34 weeks to confirm our hopes that her anemia had been corrected.

Her hemoglobin had remained steady at 11.1 g/dL, but her ferritin had jumped up to 18 ng/mL, just over the anemia border. In addition, her other values such as her proteins and alkaline phosphatase had also increased and were within our normal, functional ranges.

Colleen went on to have a beautiful, natural birth with no complications.

This is an example of how looking at the complete anemia pattern and running the right labs at the right time is important for accurate treatment. In this case, there was a combination of other factors in addition to poor iron intake. Her untreated morning sickness in the first trimester had prevented her from eating an adequate volume of foods to increase iron reserves. She had been able to function fine, with only mild fatigue, until she hit the shift in iron metabolism that required her to work off her ferritin stores in addition to her diet. It was at this point that her diet was unable to keep up with the increasing demands of her baby.

Her case encouraged me to test my mamas earlier in pregnancy for ferritin levels. Knowing these levels earlier can help with building these iron stores and prevent the associated risk of anemia later in pregnancy.

Chapter 10

Depression and Anxiety

For every 100 Americans, 34 show signs of depression and anxiety, but few will be treated or seek help due to the stigma around mental health. Thirteen percent of pregnant women will experience some form of depression during their pregnancy, with even more experiencing subclinical depression that never gets diagnosed correctly.[170] Higher rates are seen in lower-income communities and urban areas, which are the communities that are at the highest risk of nutritional deficiencies, poorer healthcare, and increased stress and trauma.

Subclinical depression is often underdiagnosed because symptoms can be confused with the common complaints of pregnancy—fatigue, poor appetite, and insomnia. As you now know, these common pregnancy complaints are signs of underlying dysfunction, and depression is just another symptom.

Many women are reluctant to tell their providers about their symptoms for fear of the prescription of medications they are looking to avoid during pregnancy or the stigma that comes with a mental health diagnosis. The rate of antidepressant use in the United States has increased nearly 400 percent over the last two decades.

Some women show symptoms and ask for help but are dismissed, such was the case for Meghan Markle. You would expect someone in her station to have access to the best maternity and prenatal care money could afford, yet she was left in the dark with her requests for help. Her brave interview with Oprah will hopefully open more conversations on these feelings that many women experience during pregnancy.

There are strong connections between prenatal depression and anxiety and complications in maternal and fetal health, often because the underlying mechanisms and nutritional components are the same. Depression and anxiety being just another symptom of systemic imbalance, which makes this a condition that should be properly differentiated and correctly treated for not just the mother's emotional experience, but for the health of both her and her child.

Depression and anxiety are often dismissed as emotional components of pregnancy and less related to physical conditions in the body. Yet research points to the idea of these conditions being more than our perception of the world around us but being associated with physical inflammation, changes in hormonal patterns, and nutritional factors. This is not to say that the trauma and emotional experiences a woman has will not affect her mental health, but that these physical conditions can lower her threshold for emotional stimuli and that there is significantly more to these conditions.

Getting to Know the Nervous System

The nervous system is a complex network of cells.

The nervous system is divided into the central nervous system (CNS) and peripheral nervous systems (PNS). The CNS constitutes the brain and spinal cord. This is the core and controller of the PNS. The PNS includes all the portions that are outside of the brain and spinal cord. They relay messages from the periphery and send messages to the periphery to perform functions. There is also the enteric nervous system (ENS) of the gut that can function without the brain, but that's another topic for another day.

The PNS is further divided into the somatic nervous system (SNS) and the autonomic nervous system (ANS). Somatic nerves control our voluntary movements, while the autonomic nerves control our involuntary movements and system functions.

Of course, to make it more fun, the ANS is further divided into the sympathetic and parasympathetic nervous systems. These are the systems that we are assessing when we are discussing depression and anxiety conditions.

The sympathetic nervous system controls our fight-or-flight responses. Think of it as the nitrous oxide system (NOS) in a racing car. The sympathetic nervous system is action.

The parasympathetic nervous system controls rest and digest functions when there is no threat. This is the cruise control set at the speed limit as well as the brakes. The parasympathetic system is regenerative.

Neurons don't actually touch. There is a gap between the nerves called a synapse, where neurotransmitters transmit messages to the next nerve. Within the synapse, you find receptors for neurotransmitters and neurotransmitter transporters. Neurotransmitters are released through vesicles that burst when calcium enters the synapse. These neurotransmitters then elicit the desired effect. Most neurons only contain a few types of neurotransmitters, each packaged in their own vesicles.

The first neurotransmitter, acetylcholine, was discovered in 1921. Since then, dozens of others have been discovered. These neurotransmitters have been the foundation of research behind mental health conditions, such as depression, anxiety, schizophrenia, ADHD, and more.

Neurotransmitters are chemical messengers that regulate physical and emotional processes in the body, facilitating the communication needed between the cells of the brain and cells of the body. Neurotransmitters travel between the synapses of neurons and activate signals that travel between the cells.

The regulation of neurotransmitter release, receptor formation and function, as well as reuptake is governed by hormones and the amount of neurotransmitter available.

Neurotransmitter Life Cycle	
Synthesis	Proteins are enzymatically converted into neurotransmitters.
Packaging	Neurotransmitters are packaged into small fluid-filled bubbles called vesicles.
Release	Calcium floods the neuron, causing vesicles to tear open, releasing neurotransmitters into the synapse.
Interactions	The neurotransmitter travels across the synapse and attaches to a receptor, causing either a firing of the nerve or an inhibition.
Reuptake	Neurotransmitters are returned to the original cell and recycled into vesicles for reuse.
Death	In each reaction, some neurotransmitters are lost or scavenged.

Table 5: There is a life cycle to neurotransmitters that includes birth and death in a series of six steps.

Brain and nervous system cells are like electrical wires in the body, sending messages through electrical impulses and neurotransmitter signaling. These wires are coated in a waxy substance called myelin. Like the plastic that coats electrical wires, this myelin helps to keep the signals and electricity traveling down the wire and not sparking out into the world. Just like an electrical wire with a damaged plastic coating, damage to the myelin can cause electrical impulses to jump and shock the system, *literally*.

In the brain, we have gray matter and white matter. Gray matter contains numerous cell bodies and a few myelinated nerves, while white matter contains few cell bodies and numerous myelinated nerves. Myelin is crucial to how neurons function.

Can Cholesterol Be Too Low?

Just like everything in the body, there is a functional range for cholesterol. Too much and we have issues, too little and we still have issues. I can't tell you how many people I've seen with low cholesterol. Cholesterol in pregnancy is crucial, yet it is not part of routine blood work in maternity care.

Lower cholesterol levels have been found in both prenatal and postpartum depressed mothers, with lower levels correlating with increased severity of symptoms.[171] Studies on rats given cholesterol-lowering medications showed an increase in depressive symptoms, and in humans, lower cholesterol is associated with a higher rate of suicide.[172] Why?

One explanation is that lower blood cholesterol levels equal lower brain cholesterol levels, which alter brain and neurotransmitter function. Studies also show that cholesterol-lowering medications affect brain function, increasing the probability of this correlation.[173]

Cholesterol and neurotransmitters go hand in hand, literally. Cholesterol affects the receptors for neurotransmitters, and without enough cholesterol in the brain, these receptors cannot function correctly. Some receptors are upregulated and some are downregulated, causing patterns of dysfunction.

Myelin is cool stuff. It is composed of cholesterol, and deficiencies in cholesterol mean weaker myelin sheaths. Twenty-five percent of total body cholesterol is found in the myelin.[174] The integrity of the myelin is a component in the progression of depression symptoms.[175]

I know we're talking maternal depression and anxiety, but a sidenote: Cholesterol levels rise in pregnancy for several reasons, not just as the base for the steroid hormones. It also comprises the fetal myelin sheath formation. Lower maternal cholesterol levels are associated with not only maternal depression and anxiety but also fetal growth issues.

So contrary to the standard American guidelines of consuming less cholesterol, eat those eggs ladies.

Nutrition in the Tryptophan Pathway

Tryptophan is an essential amino acid that is the base for the formation of pregnancy neurotransmitters: serotonin, melatonin, and dimethyltryptamine (DMT) as well as the nicotinamide adenine dinucleotide (NAD).

Serotonin (5-HT) is the primary neurotransmitter that is produced from the amino acid tryptophan. It not only affects mood but also plays a crucial role in gut motility. Ninety-five percent of serotonin is produced in the gut, in the ENS. The enzymes that help to synthesize serotonin from tryptophan requires an array of nutrients to do so: iron,[176] calcium[177], B9[178], magnesium[179], B6[180], B3[181], vitamin D[182], zinc[183], and vitamin C[184]. A deficiency in every one of these nutrients has been linked to depression.

Melatonin is produced by the pineal gland and works to regulate circadian rhythms of sleep and wakefulness in ratio with cortisol. These two have an inverse relationship—when one is up, the other is down. Melatonin is synthesized from serotonin in two steps that require a B5-containing acetyl-CoA as well as SAMe—the two primary acetylation and methylation compounds.

Rising levels of cortisol and cytokines have compounding effects on nearly all systems of maternal physiology as well as fetal growth. As these levels rise, there is an increase in the production of two enzymes, indoleamine 2,3 dioxygenase (IDO) and tryptophan dioxygenase (TDO), that shuttle tryptophan toward the kynurenine pathway. We touched on the TDO enzyme and B6 in Chapter 8.

Tryptophan is degraded through the kynurenine pathway, with the end products of this process being quinolinic acid, NAD, and picolinic acid.

The two enzymes IDO and TDO catalyze the first reactions that degrade tryptophan into kynurenine. IDO is activated by increased levels of cytokines in the cells, like those found with oxidative stress, while TDO is activated by cortisol.

As tryptophan gets shuttled to the degradation pathway, we get less tryptophan being converted into serotonin or melatonin, but we get an increase in the production of NAD.

NAD is the cofactor for many of the enzymes required for pregnancy function such as metabolism and steroid hormone production. As we see increases in the pregnancy cortisol levels, we see an increase in the need for NAD as both maternal and fetal metabolism increases at specific times in gestation as well as the need to produce more steroid hormones.

The precursor to NAD is quinolinic acid, which is a neurotoxin that if not degraded to NAD can cause neurological conditions and increased neurological stress. Certain patterns of depression are associated with a heightened activation of this tryptophan pathway that leaves less serotonin and more quinolinic acid. For quinolinic acid to become NAD, we need adequate amounts of magnesium, and for kynurenine to become picolinic acid, we need B6. In fact, if there is adequate B6 and magnesium, quinolinic acid is correctly degraded into NAD.[185]

As shifts in the tryptophan pathway favor the side that synthesizes NAD during pregnancy, this can lead to lower levels of serotonin and melatonin if the dietary needs for tryptophan or cofactors are not met.

During the transitional point of labor, we see an increase in the production of both melatonin[186] and DMT. These two neurotransmitters help to induce a hypnotic state often seen in women who are birthing naturally.[187] (See Figure 7.)

Picolinic acid is a chelator in the body, but it also helps to negate the negative effects of quinolinic acid. Studies show that it has antiviral properties as well.

This rise in the kynurenine pathway activation has a combination of effects that include immunomodulation, NAD production, and mechanisms that have not been elucidated. But like all mechanisms in the body during pregnancy, there is a natural rise in these inflammatory and almost toxic compounds that must be balanced by the natural counterbalancing chemicals. The nutritional components are crucial to this balancing act that must occur for a functional pregnancy.

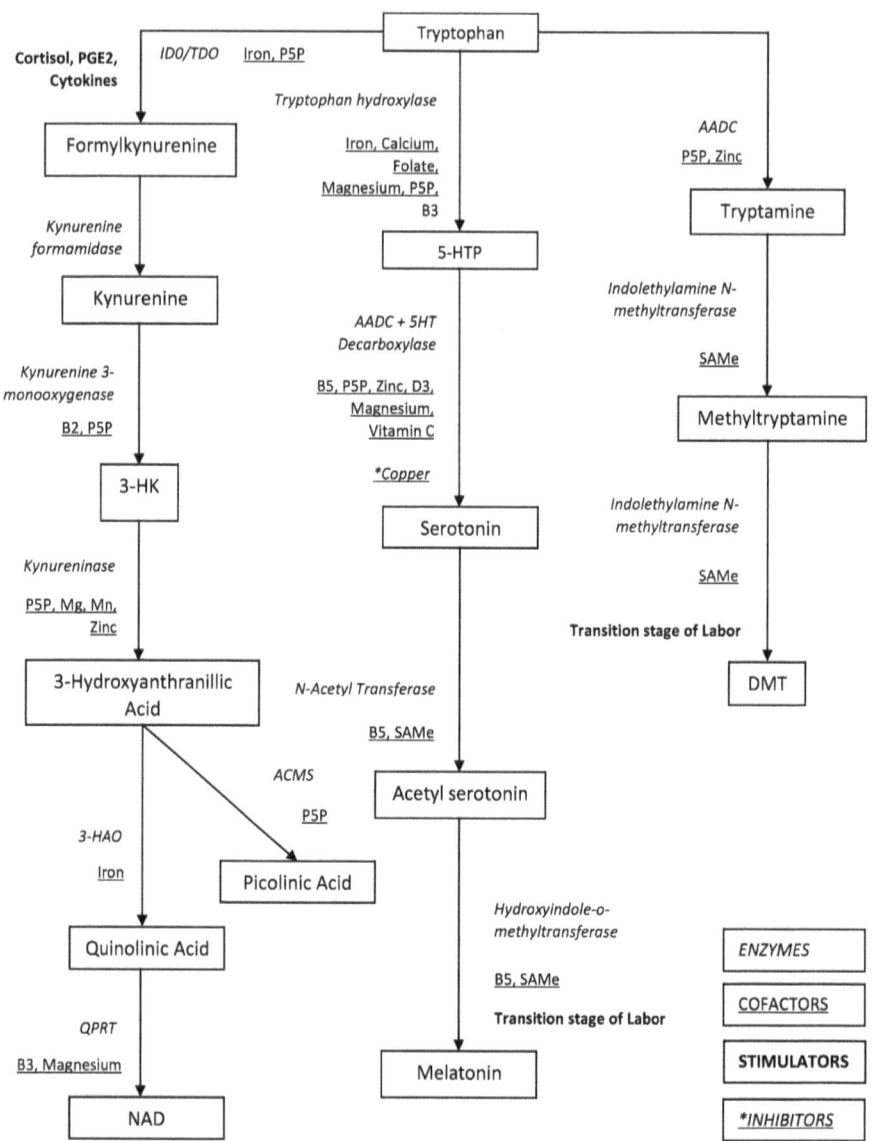

Figure 7: Tryptophan pathway.

Understanding these natural and unnatural shifts in neurotransmitter function can help diagnose the mechanisms of action behind the presentations of depression.

Nutrition in the Tyrosine Pathway

Tyrosine is a nonessential amino acid, meaning the body makes it from other essential amino acids, primarily phenylalanine. Fifty percent of all dietary phenylalanine is used to make tyrosine. Tyrosine can be and is consumed in the diet as well. The neurotransmitters produced in this pathway are called catecholamines. The enzymes that synthesize dopamine, norepinephrine, and epinephrine from tyrosine require the same nutrients that are required for the synthesis of serotonin in the tryptophan pathways. Deficiencies in these nutrients are also associated with conditions related to catecholamine dysfunction as well.

Dopamine is an important neurotransmitter for motivation. It encourages movement of the muscles and emotional responses. Vitamin B6 in the P5P form is required for the enzymatic steps that synthesize dopamine from tyrosine.

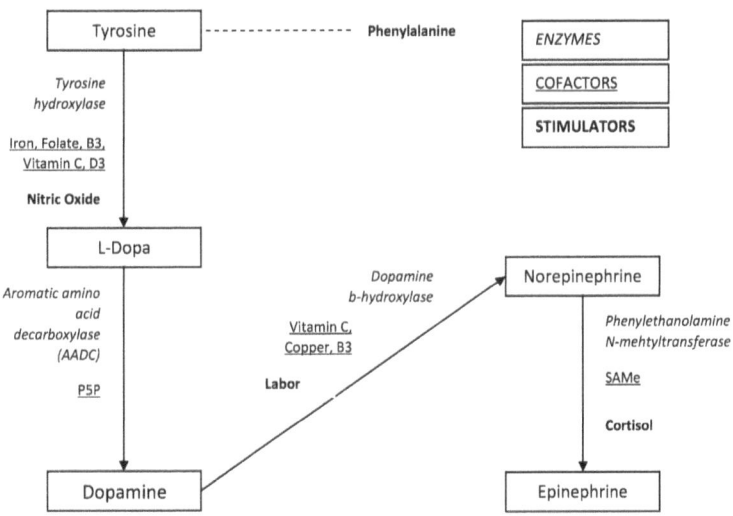

Figure 8: Catecholamine pathway.

Norepinephrine is produced by the neurons as a neurotransmitter and the adrenals as a stress hormone. Norepinephrine increases alertness, energy, memory, and focus. This is the primary neurotransmitter of the sympathetic nervous system. A balanced amount of norepinephrine is necessary for the function of our body. Nearly every organ system requires norepinephrine for its actions. Norepinephrine is produced in steady and constant low-grade levels. Epinephrine, on the other hand, is like souped-up norepinephrine that is released only in times of stress.

Epinephrine is methylated norepinephrine. SAMe donates a methyl group to norepinephrine to create the increased response of fight or flight in response to elevated cortisol levels.

Nutrient Power

The idea that nutrition plays a role in the symptoms of depression and anxiety are only slightly known and used in treatment. Yet some of the symptoms of common nutritional deficiencies include the symptoms of depression and anxiety, fatigue, weakness, lack of motivation, changes in heart rate, and overall feelings of being unwell. Some women know their emotional triggers or scenarios that elicit these symptoms. Others can't identify a cause.

I'm prone to anxiety. I joke that I'm like a mouse. I have a high resting heart rate. I'm constantly on the move. I don't know how to sit still. I am high fight or flight. If I stop moving, I notice it. If I keep going, I'm good. Social situations are my trigger. I get overwhelmed with people very quickly and don't love being the center of attention.

So, I wrote a book to get me more attention. Smart.

I know my natural predisposition, or my constitution as we call it in TCM, and know where I personally need to focus my nutrition and self-care to manage who I am as a person. Part of this is knowing which nutrients I tend to be lower in because my constitution leans that way. I am a biochemical individual and care for myself and my health is determined by how I treat this unique presentation.

Each of us has a unique biochemical constitution that influences our personality, sensitivities, propensity to disease, and overall function. Think of the possibilities in genetic combinations that can occur during development and the influence that epigenetics has on these genetic expressions, and you have the recipe for the creation of individuals where no two can ever be alike. The same diets, supplements, medications, and lifestyles will not work for everyone. In treatment, you must look at each individual person and her or his unique biochemical code.

These differences make the Recommended Dietary Allowance (RDA) for nutrients seem irrelevant for many people who, due to genetics, may need many times these amounts for overall body function, and others who may need significantly less.

For centuries, TCM has looked at all conditions as not a single disease, but a group of different patterns that results in similar symptomatology. Depression and anxiety are no different. There are multiple patterns in TCM theory that are connected to the different types of depression and anxiety presentations.

Nutrient Power: Heal Your Biochemistry and Heal Your Brain is a book written by Dr. William Walsh. After working with tens of thousands of patients, he developed a biochemical nutrition approach to mental health conditions.

In his studies, he determined four different subtypes of depression presentations based on nutrient and biochemistry involvement. He did, with modern science, what traditional Chinese practitioners had done with observations: created different versions of the same disease that required different treatment methods. By treating each group differently and not giving them the same treatment approach, he increased his treatment success. He treated them as biochemically unique individuals, not a disease name.

The power nutrition has on mental health is underrated but vital to the care of pregnant women who cannot use many of the prescription medications used to manage these conditions. Nutrients compose the base for the formation and function of all neurotransmitters. Proteins, vitamins, minerals, antioxidants, and phytochemicals are needed for these processes to work and are supplied by the diet.

Depression as a Sign of Inflammation

In the case of Meghan Markle, there was real-life pressure and emotional stress that was a contributing factor, but for some women, they don't know why they feel this way, leading us to a more systemic cause of dysfunction and not a reaction to perceived stress.

Once you begin to understand the dynamics of the body and our reactions to oxidative and physical stressors, the more you begin to visualize depression as a physical manifestation of inflammation. Metabolic imbalances, genetics, infections, toxic chemicals, and changes in the hormones due to pregnancy can increase the imbalance in neurotransmitter function.

It is normal for cortisol to rise in pregnancy; it has a job to do. If a mother is predisposed to sensitivity to cortisol rises and drops prior to pregnancy or is suffering from nutritional deficiencies that deplete the nervous system, then she is prime for depression and anxiety in pregnancy and postpartum.

We focus so much on the rising of cortisol and the implications, but what about the deficiency of cortisol? Cortisol has several jobs to do and if there is not enough to get the job done the body will go into a sleepy state to induce regeneration.

The parasympathetic nervous system has the important job of making us rest. When we are sleeping, the parasympathetic nervous system regenerates our cortisol, serotonin, and dopamine. This can be during sleep, meditation, relaxation, and just overall resting.

Stress is more than just our perception of the world around us. The hormone cortisol has numerous jobs in the body, and one of those is the reduction of inflammation. Inflammation can be caused by several factors, such as spinal injuries, chronic pain, oxidative stress from poor diet, and toxic buildup in the body. We also see it with parasite infections, viral infections, and, of course, pregnancy.

Oxidative stress is one of the most common connecting factors between diseases in pregnancy. Nearly every condition associated with negative outcomes has a link to cellular oxidation somewhere. This is a form of stress and inflammation that affects cortisol and causes a dysfunction in the sympathetic and parasympathetic states. When the inflammation is high, the body must shut down to heal this damage. To clean out the cells, they must sleep. Oxidative stress has been shown to play a significant role in the pathogenesis of depression and should always be considered with mothers experiencing depression.[188]

During an acute stress response, cortisol increases catecholamine production and, in turn, increases the genetic expression of transporters that vacuum up serotonin from the synapses to allow for fight-or-flight responses. When the acute reaction is over, a period of depression occurs to signal regeneration of cortisol and neurotransmitters. Cortisol levels that are chronic or adrenals that cannot regenerate enough cortisol to function elicit a more chronic depressive state.

Being depressed and fatigued is the body's signal that something is wrong and that a regenerative phase is required to promote the production of cortisol and other neurotransmitters as well as clean out cellular damage and debris.

If depression is persisting in pregnancy, assessing a patient's stress levels is imperative to treatment. Identifying emotional and physical causes of stress will make a difference in treatment approaches.

Anxiety Is the Physical Manifestation of Stress

When there is a threat, and the body feels stressed, there is a spike in cortisol that wakes up the sympathetic nervous system to either fight or run away. This is normal and natural. After an acute stressful experience, the natural response is to induce a parasympathetic response to, well, regenerate the cortisol and dopamine that was just used in the fight-or-flight process.

A natural balance of systems is in place to help us survive stressful scenarios but also regenerate and restore the body afterward. When we get chronic stress—too much of the sympathetic responses and too little of the parasympathetic responses—we can see the presentation of anxiety as the body is in a constant state of fight-or-flight and a state of depression where the body is in a constant state of recovery.

Symptoms such as palpitations, agitation, changes in breathing patterns, gut pain and motility changes, nausea, and the feeling of fear are signs of stress in the body.

Catecholamines change little throughout pregnancy even though there is an increase in cortisol production. Only in cases of oxidative stress or true stress reactions do we see an increase in these neurotransmitters and hormones.[189] If catecholamines do rise during pregnancy, this can be a marker for preterm labor and has been associated with uterine and placental infections.[190] Because of this, I take the acute onset of anxiety in pregnancy very seriously with the target of finding the cause of inflammation or stress triggers.

During childbirth, though, we see a substantial rise in these neurotransmitters and hormones. Between week 37 and the onset of labor, the increase of cortisol and epinephrine is nearly 500 percent and norepinephrine 50 percent.[191] That's huge and really hammers home the physical and mental stress a mother goes through during childbirth and the amazing cascade of mechanisms in place to help her manage these changes. Interestingly, when an epidural is used, there is a moderate decrease in catecholamines but not cortisol. More on this in Chapter 13.

Pregnancy Depression & Anxiety and DHEA

The effects of cortisol in the progression of depression have been well studied. The connection between DHEA and anxiety is new. A 2020 study found that women with depression during pregnancy had lower levels of DHEA, flattened DHEA diurnal variability, and smaller DHEA to cortisol ratios.[192]

Another 2020 study found similar results with elevations in cortisol and lower levels of DHEA in women with pregnancy anxiety.[193]

DHEA not only helps to mitigate the negative effects of cortisol, but it also works as a neuroprotectant on its own. Studies show that DHEA helps to regulate emotional processing and reduces emotion reactivity, specifically in the amygdala and hippocampus. These regions of the brain regulate our fear and anger, and DHEA reduces these emotions in patients.[194]

What this means for maternity care is unknown because there are no studies on the use of DHEA supplementation during pregnancy and no data on safety and effectiveness in treating pregnancy symptoms. But since the studies are new, I thought it would be good to add them in to keep the idea in the back of your mind; I know it is in the back of mine.

Assessing Depression and Anxiety in Pregnancy

Regardless of the continued advances in research supporting the different patterns and causes of depression and anxiety, these conditions are more commonly treated as a single presentation with the primary cause being low serotonin, which is why most women diagnosed with mental health conditions are given the same treatment, a selective serotonin reuptake inhibitor (SSRI) medication.

While these medications may help a portion of these women feel better, it neglects a large population that does not fall into the simplified category of low serotonin, nor does it elucidate the cause and address the mechanisms behind the symptoms.

Treating women from a functional medicine standpoint, understanding the changes that occur during pregnancy and the effect on neurotransmitters becomes crucial to truly helping women reduce the risk of mental health conditions during and after pregnancy. Determining the underlying cause of the symptoms is always of utmost importance to proper treatment.

In pregnancy, we are limited by time in our ability to treat these conditions. Outside of pregnancy, nutrient-based treatments can take months to change neurotransmitter function and improve depression and anxiety symptoms. In pregnancy, we see a quicker turnaround once the mechanism is discovered.

When assessing depression and anxiety in pregnancy, it is important to consider other factors, such as anemia, nutritional deficiencies, oxidative stress, infection, trauma, and fear.

Some of the functional lab testing you would use in patients outside of pregnancy becomes useless in pregnancy. So often we are using educated deduction to assess and treat these conditions with nutritional and functional support.

Chapter 11

Gestational Hypertension

Many of you reading this book are not physicians. There is a growing number of women choosing to have unattended births. This means they are planning to deliver at home with no midwifery or other support. It is possible that these women, if experiencing symptoms associated with emergency complications, may seek out help from other professionals.

As maternity functional medicine practitioners, our goal is to set up a mother for pregnancy success from the beginning to help prevent the possibility of these conditions before they start. If symptoms arise, we must do our best to slow the progression and reduce the risk of complications, *not* diagnose, and treat without medical supervision. It is not your role or responsibility to become the primary care providers for these women, unless you are a physician.

For example, differentiating gestational hypertension from the life-threatening preeclampsia, eclampsia, and HELLP syndrome is something that should always be guided with the collaboration of trained medical professionals that can monitor and make medical decisions when needed.

Gestational hypertension and preeclampsia often get lumped into the same category. These conditions can have a multitude of causes and pathologies. These pathologies are poorly understood, with multiple theories being proposed but no single cause determined.

Hypertensive conditions are the third-leading cause of maternal death in the United States, just behind hemorrhage and stroke.[195] The CDC states that hypertension in pregnancy is a preventable and treatable condition.[196]

Throughout this chapter, we will discuss the complex presentations of gestational hypertension and possible etiologies. Because of the nature of the condition, for many women, treatment becomes management. As you will see, some of the causes occur before pregnancy even begins and complete regression is not an option. Management of symptoms becomes the primary goal. With proper differentiation and treatment, women can have great success in management, allowing them to continue with a healthy pregnancy and natural delivery.

Categories of Hypertension	
Chronic Hypertension	Hypertension prior to pregnancy.
Gestational Hypertension	A pregnant woman has hypertension without protein in the urine or other organ involvement, and symptoms were not experienced prior to pregnancy.
Preeclampsia/Eclampsia	A serious condition where a woman may have had normal blood pressure throughout pregnancy and has had a sudden increase with other associated symptoms and protein in her urine.
Preeclampsia Superimposed on Chronic Hypertension	A woman who had hypertension prior to pregnancy and during pregnancy develops proteinuria.

Table 6: Categories of hypertension in pregnancy.

Diet and Hypertension

The idea that diet influences the onset of hypertension is a huge component of the functional medicine approach to chronic disease. Outside of pregnancy, hypertension remains one of the most commonly diagnosed conditions in the United States. According to the CDC, nearly half of all Americans have some form of hypertension, with only 25 percent of those diagnosed having it managed and under control.[197]

The primary causes of hypertension are diet and lifestyle choices. Therefore, it is considered a preventable chronic disease. Dietary patterns that we see being highly associated with an increase in the presentation of hypertension are, well, the standard American diet: diets that are high in sodium, specifically, from processed foods and less associated with table salt, high in processed fats, excess in calories, and low in vegetable intake.[198]

A 2019 Danish study compared seven dietary patterns to assess diets that increased and decreased the risk of hypertension in pregnant women. Of the seven, only two had a measurable effect on hypertension symptoms: a seafood- and vegetable-based diet and the western diet. The seafood and vegetable diet was characterized by a high consumption of, well, seafood and vegetables and was inversely related to the development of hypertension in pregnancy. The western diet was characterized by high consumption of potatoes, white bread, a variety of meats, and low vegetable intake and was related to the development of hypertension in pregnancy. They concluded that the western diet created an increased likelihood of developing hypertension in pregnancy.[199]

Other studies have shown vegan and vegetarian diets also seem to protect against the risk of gestational hypertension.[200] But these benefits are less associated with the reduction of animal and meat products and more associated with the increased intake of vegetables that are rich in nutrients, fibers, antioxidants, and phytonutrients.

A mother who does not have chronic hypertension before the onset of pregnancy may have had a predisposition to the condition due to these dietary influences, and the increased demand on her body triggered an increase in blood pressure. Other factors can influence the onset of non-preeclamptic hypertension. These include pretty much anything that can cause a decrease in the ability of the cardiovascular system to function properly or a decrease in the availability of nutrients and oxygen needed to grow a baby and nourish a mother's tissues.

Anemia and Hypertension

Studies show that women with severe and uncorrected anemia have a 3.6 times higher risk of developing gestational hypertension and preeclampsia.[201]

The question becomes does anemia cause hypertension, or does the same mechanism that is causing hypertension, such as oxidative stress, also cause anemia?

It is probably both.

Hemolysis is the destruction of red blood cells due to inflammation and oxidative stress. It is one of the hallmark symptoms of HELLP syndrome, a serious complication and association of symptoms in gestational hypertension and preeclamptic presentations. Elevated markers of oxidative stress and hypoxia are seen in cases of hemolysis and HELLP syndrome.[202]

Outside of this specific and severe presentation, we also see that gestational hypertension can be secondary to true anemia due to malnutrition or disease. A study done in Africa looked at the increase in anemia in women who had experienced malaria and their increased risk of developing gestational hypertension. They determined that the severe anemia, caused by malaria, was the primary driver of gestational hypertension in these women.[203]

We don't really get a lot of malaria here in America, but we do see malnutrition anemia from vitamin and mineral deficiencies, and we see many people living at altitude, like where I practice in Colorado. Altitude is directly associated with increased gestational hypertension and preeclampsia.[204]

Oxygenation of the placenta, the mother, and the fetus becomes greater as gestation goes on. If there is anemia due to poor red blood cell formation, then the job is harder, the body becomes stressed in its efforts to increase oxygenation and, thus, increases blood pressure. Living at altitude with less oxygen in the air means women tend to need more red blood cells than women living at sea level to provide the necessary oxygen requirements.

Hypoxia and anemia in early gestation have also been associated with poor placental development, poor mitochondrial function and, in turn, a greater risk of developing placental dysfunction and related conditions.

In treatment, when anemia is present, we go backwards to diagnose the cause of the anemia and treat it accordingly. If the mother has reached the third trimester, changing her blood counts may be difficult to do. Prevention of hypertension associated with anemia begins in the weeks where the body is working to double blood volume in preparation for the demands of the next phase of pregnancy.

Electrolyte Balance and Dehydration

Pregnant women all around the world know how hard it is to maintain hydration in pregnancy. Depending on where you live, it may be harder due to things like elevation and air moisture. With my local patients here in Colorado, maintaining hydration is harder than for those who live in more tropical and sea-level locations.

As the plasma levels begin to double, the increased need for hydration becomes daunting. Add in the amniotic fluid and its replacement and we are looking at a lot of water.

The amniotic fluid begins to surround the embryo at four weeks gestation. Ninety-nine percent of amniotic fluid is water and electrolytes. The amount of amniotic fluid grows with the growing baby: 20 mL at seven weeks, 800 ml by 34 weeks, and 600 ml by the end of pregnancy. There is a dip at term as the placenta begins to age. Each of these volumes is replaced every three hours. No wonder women feel as though they are unable to keep up and why dehydration is a real thing.

We've all heard of electrolytes, but what do you really know about them other than they help when you have tight muscles?

Electrolytes are substances that carry an electrical charge when dissolved in water. In nutrition, these are minerals. Minerals are either positively charged or negatively charged and categorized as cations or anions.

The electrolytes found in the body include sodium, potassium, calcium, chloride, magnesium, phosphate, and bicarbonate.

These electrolytes dance a beautiful ballet throughout the body, keeping balance in and out of the cells and regulating nerve impulses, muscle contracture, cardiac function, body pH, and cellular hydration.

We also need to consider the increased need for these electrolytes, not just for hydration but enzymatic function throughout the body. Certain minerals are more commonly depleted because of this increase, thus causing imbalances. We also see that the hormonal changes in pregnancy speed up the loss of minerals, such as potassium and magnesium through the kidneys, and retention of sodium and water.

Dehydration occurs when the body loses more water and electrolytes than it can take in, and pregnancy is a perfect example of mechanisms that increase the propensity for dehydration. Imbalances in the electrolytes are more common in pregnancy than typically discussed.

We know that conditions associated with nausea and vomiting can cause imbalances in electrolyte ratios. So, it would seem rational to expect that women who have suffered from severe pregnancy nausea will have more issues with electrolyte imbalance. Women who experience HG are more likely to have placental dysfunction, hypertension, and preeclampsia[205], specifically if the symptoms persist into the second trimester.

Most studies on electrolytes and blood pressure focus on the balance of potassium and sodium solely. Reductions in blood pressure are seen when there is a reduction of sodium chloride in the diet but also an increase in potassium, magnesium, and calcium.[206]

The current pregnancy RDA for potassium is 4,700 mg/day. According to the NHANES survey, the average American woman is only getting 2,100–2,300 mg of potassium per day, half what she needs in pregnancy. Yet potassium gets little recognition in pregnancy. It's not typically added to prenatal vitamins because it doesn't play a role in fetal growth. Its only known function is as an electrolyte, but it is a key electrolyte that balances sodium in the cells, helping to regulate water movement for nerve function. It's pretty important in cardiovascular and muscle health.

Calf cramps have long been associated with a potassium deficiency. Studies show that potassium supplementation lowers hypertension in elevated sodium conditions.[207] An association between sodium and potassium imbalances has been identified in some patterns of gestational hypertension.[208]

We also see significantly lower magnesium levels in gestational hypertensive patients.[209] The demand for magnesium grows exponentially from 28 weeks of gestation through childbirth. Unlike potassium, magnesium isn't just an electrolyte; it is responsible for the formation and function of over 300 enzymes in the body, regulates calcium channels, increases nitric oxide production, and is crucial for the cascade of maternal physiological changes that occur in preparation for childbirth.

Magnesium is also essential to the sodium-potassium movement in and out of the cells, and studies show a direct relationship between magnesium deficiency and electrolyte imbalances.[210] This imbalance can create the presence of edema in the pregnant mother. Fluid can get into the tissues, but it can't get out, not without magnesium. This, accompanied by calf cramps and charley horses, is a clear indication of an electrolyte imbalance that requires correcting.

Magnesium deficiency has been implicated in several pregnancy complications with no definitive studies saying it helps treat any single condition. What studies show is a general "better pregnancy" when magnesium is sufficient. A 2017 randomized control trial (RCT) study found that magnesium supplementation reduces the probability of multiple pregnancy complications.[211]

Another article in the journal *Nutrition Reviews* highlights that magnesium deficiency is prevalent in women of reproductive age in both developed and underdeveloped countries. The need for magnesium increases throughout pregnancy and a majority of women are not meeting this increased need.[212]

Magnesium deficiency as well as other nutritional deficiencies have been linked to gestational hypertension and other pregnancy complications. The mechanisms behind preeclampsia differ from gestational hypertension. Preeclampsia is a multi-system disease that is characterized by placental dysfunction and a few associated nutritional deficiencies.

Nutritional Associations to Preeclampsia

When you look at the studies, literally every nutrient known to man is somehow associated with an increased risk of preeclampsia. The consensus seems to be that diet and nutrition play a role in the prevention of preeclampsia.[213]

Vitamin D supplementation has been shown to reduce the risk of recurrent preeclampsia.[214] Vitamin D modifies the early pregnancy transcription of genes associated with placental implantation and immune regulation. It also regulates the genetic transcription of endothelial growth factor.[215] Preeclampsia is more common in women living at altitude, and so is vitamin D deficiency.[216]

Latitude also plays into vitamin D deficiency and preeclampsia risk. Studies of people living above the 37th parallel show that they do not get enough vitamin D through sun exposure alone and need more dietary vitamin D.[217]

Riboflavin-Vitamin B2 is also highly associated with an increased risk in preeclampsia.[218] The mechanism of action is primarily through the production of B2-containing enzymes needed for mitochondrial function and NO release, causing both oxidative stress and increased vasoconstriction. Symptoms of B2 deficiency can mimic other nutrient deficiencies and so it can be hard to diagnose—anemia, dry/cracked lips/nose/mouth, and a magenta-red tongue (for all you TCM practitioners out there that always look at tongues).

Even though several vitamins and minerals have been found to be deficient in those with preeclampsia, studies do not consistently find the use of supplementation during acute preeclampsia effective in preventing the progression of the disease. Too little too late.

Calcium is the exception.

Calcium supplementation in pregnancies at a higher risk for preeclampsia has been shown to reduce the risk of hypertension and preeclampsia[219] as well as reduce the maternal mortality risk due to preeclampsia.[220]

The lack of evidence in nutrition therapy surrounding acute preeclamptic presentations is possibly because the nutritional deficiencies associated with the progression of preeclampsia occurred in the preconception and early placental developmental phases. Once a placenta is matured, you cannot reverse poorly formed vascular development or the associated oxidative stress damage. You cannot reverse damage. All you can do is support the system, improve function as best you can, and attempt to delay the onset of severe complications as long as possible.

If you genuinely want to use diet and nutrition to help prevent preeclampsia, you must work backward. You must go back to the beginning—literally the beginning of this book when I talked about preconception nutrition. What a mother and father bring to the pregnancy will influence the development of the placenta.

Epigenetics, Placental Development, and Preeclampsia Risk

Scientists who've studied the "why" behind preeclampsia have racked their brains in trying to find an underlying cause to the condition since the early 1900s. In the 1960s, studies linked placental vascular dysfunction to preeclampsia. Other theories have surfaced, with most being refuted. Changes in liver function, kidney function, and placental vascular structure are all found in varying amounts in preeclamptic presentations, with placental dysfunction seeming to be the root.

In the early weeks of gestation, the placenta and uterus create a spiral of blood vessels. This process is stimulated by hormones, immune responses,

DNA methylation, and vascular function and is reliant on matrix metalloproteinases (MMPs). MMPs consist of zinc and calcium. The completion of this arterial spiralling occurs at 20 weeks gestation. Because the initial stages of placenta development can occur before a mother even knows she is pregnant, the prevention of preeclampsia and hypertension begins in preconception, with proper maternal nutritional intake to create a healthy connection, but it also continues through the 20th week of pregnancy.

Preeclampsia and placental issues were once theorized to be caused by a deficiency in the B complex. Recent studies have linked elevated homocysteine, low B9, and low B12 as increased risk factors for preeclampsia.[221] In addition, polymorphism C677T MTHFR SNP is associated with an increased risk of developing preeclampsia.[222]

Epigenetics in the progression of preeclampsia is also gaining more ground.

Numerous studies link gene alterations in placental development to the pathology of preeclampsia.[223] These genetic changes have an influence on the structure of the placenta but also the production of enzymes needed for oxygen signaling that is associated with increases in placental oxidative stress. This oxidative stress then increases the aging and degeneration of the placenta, increasing dysfunction.

Maternal Vascular Changes in Preeclampsia

Preeclamptic women seem to present with weak vascular function. Blood vessels of preeclamptic women show signs of oxidative stress, inflammation, damage, poor tone, and reduced dilation responses.[224]

There is also an increase in glomerular endothelial swelling in the kidneys. This is associated with a deficiency in the endothelial growth hormone they need to function in pregnancy.[225] The genetic transcription of this hormone is regulated by vitamin D, and it is produced by the placenta. Thus, a poorly functioning placenta causes the kidneys to "leak" protein. This change in kidney function can continue for months postpartum, which is one of the reasons there is a continued risk of eclamptic presentations after delivery. Delivery is not the cure for preeclampsia; it helps, but it doesn't mean complications cannot occur.

In a normal and functional pregnancy, nitric oxide (NO) rises in pregnancy to help regulate the flow of blood through the body, thanks partially to rising estrogen levels.[226] Estrogen signals the breakdown of the amino acid arginine in the formation of NO with the help of magnesium. NO regulates vascular tone and blood flow; it is also an antioxidant in lipid peroxidation reactions. Oxidative stress is highly associated with the presentation of preeclampsia. Interestingly, epithelial cells taken from preeclamptic women show that these women produce less NO.[227] Studies have also shown that blocking NO production induced preeclampsia-like symptoms.[228]

Prostacyclin (PGI2) is a prostaglandin (more about prostaglandins in the next chapter). These prostaglandins increase in healthy pregnancies, but in preeclamptic pregnancies, they decrease.[229] [230] Prostacyclin has vasodilatory properties that when deficient could contribute to poor maternal vascular function. Prostacyclin increases with EPA consumption, not DHA.

Thromboxane A2 (TXA2) is a vasoconstrictor and platelet aggregator that is necessary for childbirth, but elevations in early pregnancy can cause vascular constriction and poor function. Maternal blood levels of thromboxane A2 are higher in pregnant women presenting with preeclampsia.[231] These compounds are produced in the placenta and may signal a placental dysfunction due to poor genetic methylation or a decrease in the dietary consumption of docosahexaenoic acid (DHA). In studies on preeclamptic women with elevated thromboxane A2, there was an increase in the expression of thromboxane synthase due to reduced DNA methylation and, thus, a connection to B9 and B12 deficiencies with preeclampsia.

Oxidative Stress in Hypertension and Preeclampsia

Oxidative stress comes up in nearly every section of this book. Its association with all forms of gestational hypertension is undisputable. At a cellular level, this seemingly simple process of balance between reactive oxygen species and the antioxidants that neutralize them is the primary driver of hypertensive and preeclamptic conditions.

Studies on hemolysis changes in pregnancy show oxidative stress affects the placental functions and increases the release of fetal hemoglobin into maternal circulation.[232] Unbound hemoglobin is toxic and causes many of the complications seen in the progression of preeclampsia.

First, the iron-rich hemoglobin binds to NO and reduces its availability for vasodilation, which causes vasoconstriction and increases the pressure needed to push blood through the system.

Second, the iron-rich hemoglobin spontaneously produces reactive oxygen species, specifically superoxide, that increase vascular oxidative stress.

Lastly, these iron-rich proteins increase immune inflammatory responses that include increased neutrophil and cytokine production.

Sidenote: We can see increased serum hemoglobin in preeclamptic women: >14.5 g/dL increases the likelihood of preeclamptic conditions associated with maternal serum fetal hemoglobin leakage and is an indicator of placental damage.

Addressing the oxidative stress components has become a new target for prevention and acute treatment of preeclampsia.

Vitamin E is known for its lipid oxidation inhibition—the same oxidation typically seen in preeclampsia. There is also a decrease in both vitamin C and vitamin E in preeclamptic patients. Studies assessing vitamin C and vitamin E in the treatment of preeclampsia have traditionally used low doses of these supplements and found no correlation in their effectiveness—1,000 mg vitamin C and 400 IU of vitamin E.[233] These studies were also short-term, considering that gestation has a time limitation.

Studies outside of pregnancy that focus on supplementation to reduce oxidative stress use significantly higher dosages and significantly longer treatment times. These studies hint at a threshold of vitamin E supplementation (outside of pregnancy) that must be hit before oxidative stress markers are reduced. Statistically significant reductions were not seen until 1,600 IU/day and 3,200 IU/day, with the maximum suppression occurring at 16 weeks from the start of trials.[234] Studies at this dosage found no clinical toxicity, even at the 3,200 IU/day dose. A comprehensive review of all published safety observations for vitamin E supplementation in clinical trials concluded that vitamin E supplements up to 1,600 IU/day were safe for most adults.

No studies have been done to this effect in pregnancy, but we know that oxidative stress and increasing inflammation in the system requires an increase in the amount of dietary and innate antioxidants.

The deficiency of other antioxidant nutrients, such as coenzyme Q10, zinc, and manganese has also been associated with increased oxidative stress and poor maternal outcomes.[235]

Manganese is a trace mineral rarely discussed in nutrition, especially prenatal nutrition. Studies show it has a protective effect against oxidative stress, especially in cases of iron-associated oxidation, such as the release of fetal hemoglobin cardiovascular inflammation. Manganese is a cofactor for an antioxidant called superoxide dismutase (SOD).

Superoxide Dismutase Enzyme Families	
Copper/Zinc SOD	Uses copper for a catalyst and zinc for structure
Manganese/Iron SOD	Uses either manganese or iron as cofactors
Nickel SOD	Exceedingly rare and uses nickel

Table 7: There are multiple families of SOD enzymes, based on their metal cofactor.

Although the manganese-iron SOD family can use either metal as a cofactor, there are differences in how the enzymes function, depending on the cofactor used. Manganese SODs will readily bind to iron, yet iron inactivates the enzyme.[236] What's worse is that these enzymes then increase oxidation in the body.[237]

This iron replacement is rare but occurs with mitochondrial damage, such as in the cases of oxidative stress to the placental trophoblast cells that allows for fetal hemoglobin dumping.

Limited studies have been done on manganese in pregnancy, but several studies have linked manganese deficiency in the progression of hypertension outside of pregnancy, specifically, in the increase of systolic blood pressure.[238]

A new study, published in 2020, may possibly be bridging the gap among manganese deficiency, oxidative stress, and preeclampsia risk. This study was led by researchers at Johns Hopkins Bloomberg School of Public Health. It was an analysis of data from more than 1,300 women who were followed throughout their pregnancies. The analysis found significantly lower levels of manganese in early pregnancy increased the likelihood of the development of both gestational hypertension and preeclampsia. This is the first paper linking manganese to preeclampsia.[239]

These same researchers had previously found that red blood cell manganese, measured shortly after delivery, was lower in women who had been diagnosed with preeclampsia.[240]

This connection between SOD and preeclampsia is not new, though, just the connection to manganese. It has been recommended in the past that SOD serum values be used as a biomarker for predicting preeclampsia.[241]

Manganese SOD enzyme activity has been shown to decrease with age.[242] This could be a contributing factor to the increased risk of preeclampsia in older mothers.

As we age, the body produces fewer SOD antioxidants. Results obtained from comparative reverse-transcription-polymerase chain reaction (RT-PCR) analysis found that coding for the copper-zinc and manganese SOD enzymes significantly decreased, specifically in women equal to or older than 38 years of age[243], which resulted in lower measurable levels of these enzymes in the bloodstream and an increase in oxidative stress.

The rate of gestational hypertension is skyrocketing in all age groups but especially in older mothers. And the age at which the average mother becomes pregnant for the first time is going up. As much as we all try to stay healthy and keep our bodies young as much as we can, there is no denying that we all age. As we age, oxidative stress increases in our bodies.

Studies on dietary consumption and preeclampsia development found the most protective dietary mechanism was the consumption of fruits and vegetables during pregnancy. Now if you remember, we have 80 percent of the American population not meeting the minimum daily requirements for fruit and vegetable intake. The consumption of fruits and vegetables is more than nutrient density. These foods are high in phytochemicals and antioxidants that have a protective effect against inflammation and oxidative stress.[244]

Mitochondria, CoQ10, and Preeclampsia

Mitochondria are found in all cells, including the placental trophoblast cells. Remember the Krebs cycle? The production of energy through the cycle is imperative for proper placental function. The malfunctioning of these cells leads to oxidative stress and the cascade of reactions that can lead to multi-organ disease and poor pregnancy outcomes, not just preeclampsia.

Coenzyme Q10 (CoQ10) is not only a cellular antioxidant but is required for enzymes in the Krebs cycle to function. More and more studies point to the true etiology of preeclampsia being placental dysfunction and, specifically, beginning with abnormal mitochondrial function in the trophoblast cells.[245]

Only a few studies have investigated CoQ10 in pregnancy. These studies show that levels of CoQ10 rise slowly throughout pregnancy. A 2003 study found a marked decrease in CoQ10 in women with preeclampsia.[246] The theory is that increasing oxidative stress "consumes" the CoQ10, decreasing mitochondrial function. Interestingly, this difference is more prominent in women living at altitude than women living at sea level.[247]

As we age, CoQ10 declines in tissues. Longevity and oxidative stress are closely related, and whether the deficiency of CoQ10 causes oxidative stress and aging, or if the oxidative stress and aging cause a CoQ10 deficiency, is still not known. Either way, it happens, and it influences older mothers.

Studies on preeclampsia risk and age consistently show an increase in risk with advanced age, particularly in women over the age of 35.[248]

Because of the connection among mitochondrial function, age, and fertility, CoQ10 has been well publicized and researched. In the application of CoQ10 to age-related maternal conditions, little research has been done. One study did find that supplementation with 200 mg of CoQ10 reduced the risk of preeclampsia in at-risk women.[249]

Know Your Scope

Preeclampsia occurs in one in 25 pregnancies in the United States. In severe cases, this condition can progress to maternal seizures. This is called eclampsia and is obviously a serious condition.

Knowing the symptoms that distinguish hypertension from preeclampsia is crucial when working with pregnant patients. Preeclampsia is life-threatening, and if you are working with a pregnant mother who is showing signs of preeclampsia, it is crucial that she receives the correct and immediate care she needs.

Symptoms of preeclampsia include hypertension, pitting edema, sudden weight gain, headaches, and vision changes.

When assessing your patients for conditions associated with hypertension, even when they are being supervised by a physician, you need to know these symptoms and be able to refer them back to medical or emergency care if these arise.

As much as I want every mother I meet to have a functional and natural birth experience, for some this is not to be, and it is why we need to respect the role that physicians play in maternity care and understand that this is the situation that needs this sort of intervention.

Chapter 12

Functional Childbirth

This, people, is the end game, the *pièce de résistance* so to speak. Everything I've discussed up to this point culminates into this final act of maternity. The birth of the child.

This is my absolute favorite topic in maternity functional medicine and the primary driver behind everything I've strived to learn and do in my practice. The idea that nutrition plays a role in how a mother's body will function during labor is practically unheard of.

If you look up nutrition for natural labor, you'll find article after article titled, "What to eat during labor," "Evidence on eating and drinking during labor," and "Best foods for labor." But nowhere is there an article that describes nutrition as it applies to the beautiful function of childbirth.

This intricate balance of hormones and connections that built upon each other throughout the course of gestation, to end in a triumphant finale that relies heavily on a nutrient-dense mother to proceed functionally, is never discussed. Not even within the functional medicine and natural health communities. It's like this information doesn't exist. I promise you it does, and I am beside myself with enthusiasm to be the one to share it with you.

These are the theories and studies I use in my practice to help women achieve their maternity and childbirth functional health goals. Note, though, that the amount of information it would take to fully address and unveil the magic of this progression would take a separate book (wink). In this chapter, my goal is to introduce you to the idea that we have an influence over the progression of birth and the functionality of birth through nutrition.

Old Discoveries, New Applications

The idea that a mother's nutrition influences childbirth progression and function is not new. In fact, it was one of the primary connections that Dr. Weston Price made nearly 100 years ago.

His book was filled with stories of cultural shifts from traditional lifestyles to life on reservations and rationed food or the "civilization" of communities and the effects this had on the ability of women to birth naturally. He found that within a few generations there was a stark difference in a woman's ability to birth without medical intervention. The closer a traditional group lived to civilized society and the more they relied on modern foods, the less functional their births were.

Dr. Price writes:

> *"Among primitive races living in a primitive state childbirth was a very simple and rapid process, accompanied by little fear or apprehension; whereas, in the modernized descendants, even in the first and second generations of those individuals born to parents after they had adopted the foods of modern white civilizations, serious trouble was often experienced....*
>
> *"One of the outstanding changes which I have found takes place in the primitive races at their point of contact with our modern civilization is a decrease in the ease and efficiency of the birth process. When I visited the Six Nation Reservation at Brantford, Ontario, I was told by the physician in charge that a change of this kind had occurred during the period of his administration, which had covered twenty-eight years and that the hospital was now used largely to care for young Indian women during abnormal childbirth."* [250]

Like most of what Dr. Price and his colleagues discussed all those years ago, the connection between nutrition and childbirth has been forgotten to medicalized approaches to care and management. These old discoveries are poised to take a new stance in maternity care. The idea that a mother's diet influences her childbirth experience is novel in our generation but, if applied correctly, could save mothers and help them achieve their birth goals.

A Quick Look at Labor Physiology

The onset and progression of labor is measured and described by the frequency and strength of contractions, the cervical effacement, the cervical dilation, and the position of the baby. But there is so much more to this beautiful process—so much that is never explained or discussed.

No two women go into labor in the same way. Even the same woman can have vastly different birthing experiences. This makes it difficult to put together a flowchart of birth. Instead, I discuss the mechanisms of action, possibilities, and end results (birth).

Before a mother goes into active labor, there can be a period of pre-labor. During this time, the mother may be aware or unaware of changes in her body. Mild contractions—horribly termed "false labor"—can occur. Like a marathoner training for the big race, a mother's body is training for the big event. The weeks leading up to the active labor are crucial for preparing the body for labor and delivery with more than just exercising the uterus.

These contractions are typically mild and can go unnoticed by the mother, or they can be bothersome. There are a couple of factors that control these early labor contractions.

As the placenta begins to age, it produces higher amounts of corticotropin-releasing hormone (CRH). Toward the end of pregnancy, as the placenta nears the end of its functional life, this production increases drastically. This CRH rise signals the mother's body that it is the end of gestation. Oxytocin production is stimulated in small amounts, which then begins to affect the uterus, causing mild early labor contractions.

At the same time, estrogen levels increase, which stimulates the increase of oxytocin receptors in the fundus of the uterus.[251]

In the early stages of pre-labor, there are mild progressive changes occurring. As the small amounts of oxytocin affect the uterus, causing the pre-labor contractions, there is irritation—a normal part of the labor process—that occurs in the uterus. Oxytocin stimulates the production of prostaglandins and cytokines, which cause localized inflammation. This is good inflammation, as it signals a multitude of reactions necessary for labor and delivery.

Premature labor is different from pre-labor. Premature labor is the start of labor prior to full gestational age. There are many causes of premature labor: infection, inflammation, trauma, and nutritional deficiencies. All these underlying issues can create an inflammatory environment that triggers labor before the baby or mother are ready.

As the progesterone levels begin to drop and estrogen begins to rise, this stimulates an increase in oxytocin receptors as well as prostaglandin receptors. As the number of receptors increase, so does the effect of the oxytocin, causing more and stronger contractions that signal the beginning of active labor. At the same time, the amount of CRH secreted by the placenta is at its peak, stimulating more oxytocin from the pituitary. (See Figure 9.)

This oxytocin not only stimulates uterine contractions but stimulates the prostaglandin production needed for cervical ripening.

Research points to the role of the baby in signaling the onset of labor. As the baby reaches full developmental age and the lungs become fully developed, a protein is secreted from the baby's lungs. This protein reacts with macrophages and creates inflammation that irritates the endometrial lining of the uterus. This inflammation stimulates the production of prostaglandins, cytokines, and oxytocin.

Estrogen stimulates cervical ripening as well as the production of relaxin, which keeps the ligaments and muscles loose and flexible, allowing the pelvis to widen—all leading to the end goal of the natural vaginal birth of a healthy baby.

Functional Childbirth

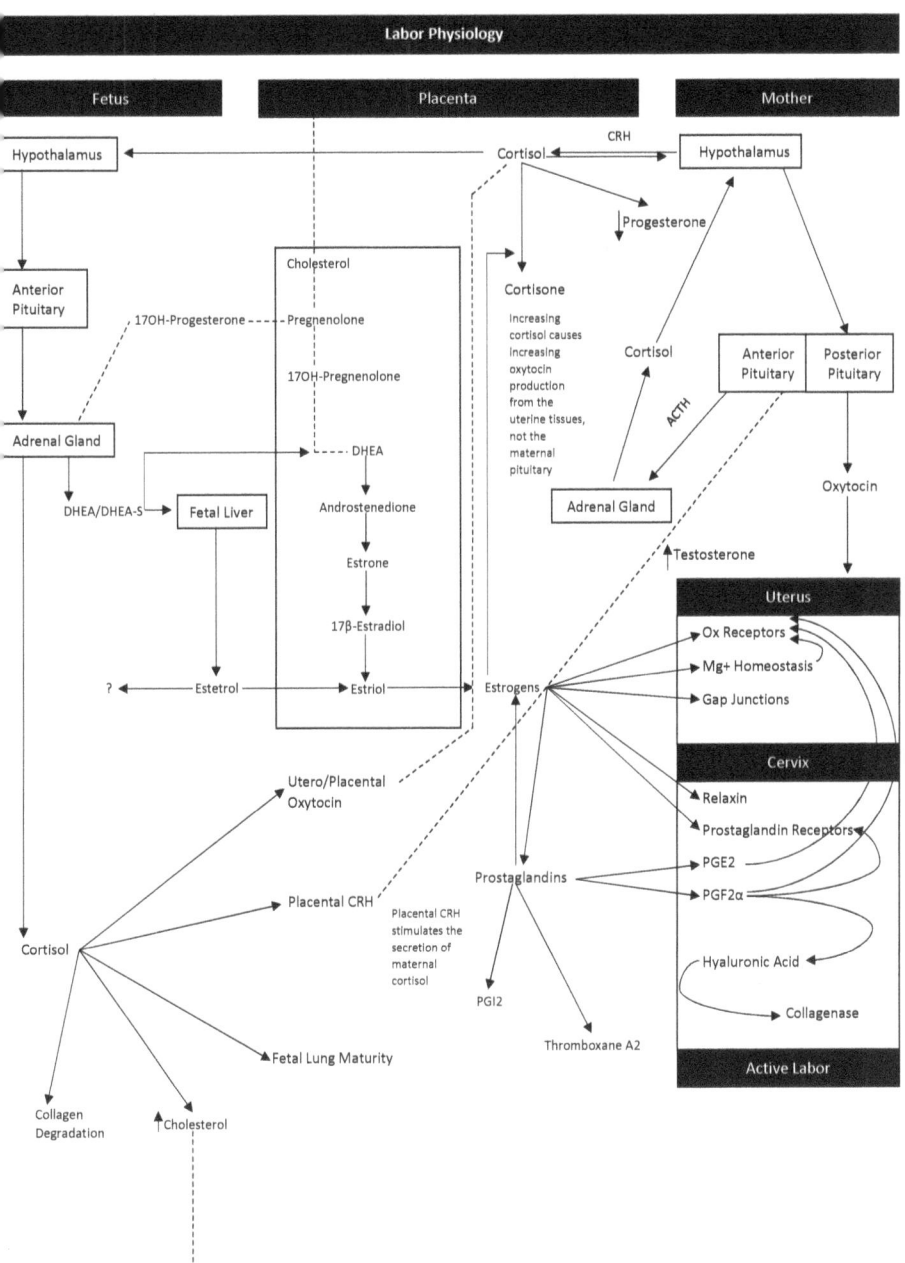

Figure 9: Chemical changes in the baby, mother, and placenta all contribute to the onset of labor. Without each of these steps working correctly, there can be hiccups in the initial activation of labor.

All the interactions and connections we have discussed before this point have led us to the progression of childbirth. Knowing how the hormones work to facilitate birth will help you help women facilitate a natural and functional birth. Addressing the different components that lead to labor starts all the way back at 28 weeks gestation with changes in the structure of the cervix that allows for effacement during active labor.

The Wonderful, Amazing Cervix

Oxytocin causes contractions, but before those contractions can push the baby out, the cervix must open. To do so, the cervix must first ripen and efface. The process of cervical ripening is, in my opinion, the most important component of a successful labor and delivery; if it's not soft, it cannot stretch with the contractions and there will be no or slow dilation.

The cervix is a magical piece of tissue; I find the actions and changes that the cervix goes through during pregnancy and childbirth significantly more fascinating than the uterus. More importantly, I find the lack of respect and knowledge for the cervix even more so.

Why have we neglected this tissue for the more prominent uterus?

The cervix is the door between two worlds. If the door cannot open, the baby cannot pass. If the cervix cannot soften and efface, then no amount of uterine contracting will deliver a baby.

Even research supports this.

In 2011, a systematic review was done to assess the evidence supporting the use of each method of induction.[252] The review concluded that cervical ripening agents were more effective than synthetic oxytocin in successful vaginal birth within 24 hours with fewer cesarean deliveries. Why? Because they unlocked the door.

This systematic review was one of the driving factors in the changes we've seen in induction protocols.

When I had my first baby in 2008, Pitocin was all the rage. The documentary *The Business of Being Born* focused heavily on the excessive use of this medication in controlling birth, with increasing rates of cesarean delivery and complications as a result. Since then, the new induction protocol is to first ripen the cervix if it is deemed unfavorable, meaning it cannot open successfully if contractions are initiated with the use of Pitocin. This change alone has helped reduce induction complications that use to be seen with Pitocin-only induction.

The cervix is a fibrous chunk of tissue that is a bit of a mystery. Because it can disrupt normal pregnancy to study the human cervix, little is known about its true structure and function during this period of life. Most of what we know about the cervix comes from studies done in the 1940s.

Crazy, right?

The cervix is 80–90 percent collagen. The rest is a blend of stromal extracellular matrix (ECM), fluid, proteins, and elastin fibers.[253] The conventional school of thought, until recently, was that the cervix was a passive organ in parturition. (That's a fancy word for labor. Anyone have *Fancy Nancy* kids?)

Collagen Types	
Type I	Accounts for 90 percent of the collagen in the body and is made of densely packed fibers that provide structure to skin, bones, tendons, cartilage, connective tissue, and teeth.
Type II	Found in the elastin cartilage that protects your joints.
Type III	Protects the structure of muscles, organs, and arteries.
Type IV	Helps with filtration and is a component of skin.

Table 8: There are 16 collagen types. Only four are regularly discussed.

The collagen of the cervix is two-thirds Type I and one-third Type III.[254]

This little chunk of collagen goes through a complete remodeling process that is stimulated by the production of prostaglandins, cortisol, estrogen, and who knows what else. However you put it, this door and its remodeling processes throughout pregnancy are the missing links to a functional childbirth.

Collagen Remodeling

Cervical collagen remodeling is well-known but not well-understood. It is the progressive change that occurs in the cervix through pregnancy in preparation for labor. Remodeling is divided into phases.

The first thing that must occur in the progression of natural labor is softening. This is the initial change in the cervical structure that constitutes the restructuring of the cervical collagen fibers.

At the onset of pregnancy, the purpose of the cervix is to tighten up its collagen fiber matrix to prevent this new life from, basically, falling out and to prevent nasties like bacteria, viruses, and yeasts from getting in. The fibers of the cervix create an interwoven tangle of fibers knotted and cinched together. This structural tightening of the cervix maintains throughout the first and second trimester.

The cervical collagen then starts to change structure, untying the knots that held the cervix closed, changing the fibers from resembling a bird's nest to a series of rows and columns with space that can be filled with fluid.[255]

Little has been known about what and how this trigger starts, but a new study published in 2020 is shedding light on the role cortisol, progesterone, and estrogen play in this restructuring process.[256]

At the beginning of gestation as progesterone levels rise, there is an increase in the expression of Type I collagen that helps to maintain the structure of the cervix, giving it that woven, knotted look. This is important as the other steps in cervical remodeling begin to make changes. This additional rise in progesterone throughout pregnancy helps to maintain the proper structure and slowly change the cervix so that the cervix does not soften, ripen, or dilate too early in pregnancy as cortisol and estrogen prepare for childbirth.[257]

If you remember from Chapter 6, cortisol levels begin to slowly rise at 16 weeks gestation, making a sharp turn at around 25–28 weeks and peaking in the last month of pregnancy.

Phases of Cervical Remodeling		
Softening	Slow progression	Increased progesterone function Increased cortisol function Decreased estrogen function Decreased cross-linking Increased solubility Increased tissue growth Increased cellular protection Increased proteasome enzymes Decreased strength
Ripening	Rapid progression	Decreased progesterone function Increased estrogen function Increased prostaglandin function Increased cortisol function Increased hyaluronic acid function Increased hydration Increased vascularization
Dilating	Opening	Maximum decrease in strength to allow baby to pass with pressure
Repair	Healing	Increased synthesis of collage Decreased hyaluronic acid function Increased matricellular proteins Increased neutrophils and macrophages

Table 9: Collagen remodeling in the cervix.

As cortisol levels rise, we begin to see changes in the cervix. Cortisol raises the production of proteasome enzymes, enzymes that break down proteins. These protease enzymes begin to degrade Type III collagen fibers.[258] The rise in cortisol also degrades collagen Type I through lysosome-mediated pathways.[259] To top it all off, elevations in cortisol degrade progesterone receptors.

All these pathways of cortisol stimulation cause an overall remodeling of the collagen fibers and a softening of the collagen tissue by decreasing the Type I collagen and increasing softened collagen fibers and a more fluid structure.

Nutritional Deficiencies and Cervix Remodeling

This inflammatory structure-changing process is a normal part of childbirth that begins around 28 weeks gestation. It's crazy to think that by 30 weeks the body is preparing for childbirth.

As maternity functional medicine practitioners, our goal is to help women make this switch toward a functional childbirth through support and balance. The rising cortisol changes the function of progesterone and supports the changing structure of the cervix. This is normal, natural, and necessary.

This increasing inflammation needs to be countered by anti-inflammatories and antioxidants to prevent the early ripening of the cervix and preterm labor. Of course, nutrition plays a role.

Maternal malnutrition is associated with premature cervical remodeling. This is new and exciting. In a 2017 article published in the *Journal of Obstetric, Gynecologic and Neonatal Nursing*, doctors set out to link nutritional deficiencies with an increased risk of premature cervical remodeling. What they found was that women who had lower dietary intakes of zinc, calcium, and vitamins A, B9, D, and E were at a higher risk of premature cervical softening and ripening.[260]

Of these, zinc, calcium, and vitamin E consumption had the highest correlation to preterm cervical remodeling risk.

Zinc is a component of metalloproteinase enzymes that work to degrade and remodel collagen in wound healing. Zinc is also important for protecting collagen from excessive degradation.[261] A Cochran Database review found evidence to support zinc supplementation in the prevention of preterm labor.[262] The balance of these actions is not isolated to zinc but is also highly dependent on other nutrients for regulation.

In cases of malnutrition, the actions of metalloproteinase enzymes are upregulated, causing an excess of collagen degradation, which can result in premature cervical remodeling and early onset of labor. Calcium helps to regulate the activity of these enzymes. When calcium is low, activity is high; when calcium is high, activity is low.[263]

Hypocalcemia is underreported in pregnancy, mostly because women who are deficient in calcium are typically asymptomatic. In a study from India, more than 66 percent of women were diagnosed with hypocalcemia, yet they were all asymptomatic.[264] This deficiency increased the probability of preterm labor and preeclampsia.

Vitamin E is amazing at reducing oxidative stress, and we know that the process of softening and ripening the cervix is highly inflammatory and full of ROS production. The activity of metalloproteinase enzymes increases the production of these compounds. The ability of vitamin E to neutralize ROS is the primary driver of how it functions in preventing preterm cervical remodeling. Vitamin E also helps to regulate the expression of metalloproteinase.[265]

When working with mothers, understanding the unique needs that begin to change in the third trimester is important for allowing her body to begin to facilitate labor. This is where standard prenatal vitamins and prenatal nutrition truly fail mothers. The goal of these standards and supplements continues to be to support the growing baby and less for the function of the mother's body as she gears up for a functional childbirth.

It's a balancing act but one that must occur because every step from then on is built upon the action before it. This linear increase in inflammation from 28 weeks to delivery must occur in the mother for her body to respond functionally to the other cues given for the initiation of birth.

Prostaglandins and Cervical Ripening

The next step in cervical remodeling is ripening, and the main stars of cervical ripening are the prostaglandins. The study of prostaglandins in labor is not new with early studies nearly 60 years old. Knowledge of the effects of prostaglandins on the cervix has been used to help prevent preterm labor and initiate labor when necessary (and when not).

Prostaglandin receptors in the myometrium and the cervix helps to make natural changes that are required for the ripening of the cervix to allow for a functional childbirth. This mechanism is normal and, in a healthy mother, well-regulated with antioxidants and anti-inflammatory fatty acids.

Prostaglandins are small, hormone-like peptides that help to maintain body homeostasis and regulate inflammation. In the progression of labor, the primary prostaglandins we focus on are the 2-series prostaglandins.

There are four major forms of 2-series prostaglandins: prostaglandin E2 (PGE2), prostacyclin (PGI2), prostaglandin D2 (PGD2), and prostaglandin F2α (PGF2α).

The production of prostaglandins and the expression of receptors is tightly controlled by the steroid hormones throughout pregnancy. Increases in estrogen and progesterone help to signal the increase of PGE2 and PGF2α from their precursor prostaglandin, prostaglandin H2 (PGH2).

Progesterone seems to signal the increase in the expression of receptors for prostaglandins, while estrogen signals the increase in the production of prostaglandins. At the onset of pregnancy, when progesterone spikes, there is a sharp increase in the production of receptors and, as the fetus and placenta mature to produce more estrogen, there is an increase in the production of prostaglandins.[266]

Toward the end of pregnancy, a combination of changes in estrogen and progesterone ratios plus increasing glucocorticoid production from the placenta increases the synthesis of prostaglandins in the amniotic environment, specifically PGH2.[267] As the prostaglandin production increases, so does the production of estrogen and oxytocin.

Estrogen and prostaglandins have a cyclical relationship during the progression to labor. The rising levels of estrogen have been associated with the regulation of the prostaglandin synthetase complex, which alters ratios between PGE2 and PGF2α[268], and as the prostaglandin levels rise, they stimulate aromatase expression that increases estrogen production.[269]

This cyclical production continues and triggers other reactions and processes in maternal physiology, culminating in childbirth.

The Other Prostaglandins

Thromboxane is in a family of fats known as eicosanoids that are formed through the same pathways as prostaglandins from the same PGH2 precursor as PGE2 and PGF2α. Thromboxane stimulates platelet aggregation and blood clotting.[270]

Thromboxanes are higher in maternal blood than in nonpregnant women and increase even more at the onset of labor. Outside of pregnancy, thromboxane is produced by platelets, but during pregnancy, the uterine-placental unit is also a source.

Studies show that thromboxane is the primary vasoconstrictor at delivery, helping to seal off the blood vessels as they detach with the placenta.[271]

The active form of thromboxane is the A2 form (TXA2). Studies show that TXA2 is nearly 1,000 times more effective as a vasoconstrictor during labor than PGE2 or PGF2α. PGE2 and PGF2α are vasoconstrictors during labor—research confirms this—they just may not be the primary drivers. TXA2 is second to prostacyclin (PGI2) in its vasoconstriction and blood-clotting abilities during labor.[272]

The production and balance of these lipid compounds are reliant on the dietary consumption of essential fatty acids, both omega-3s and omega-6s.

Dietary Fats and Prostaglandin Formation and Function

All prostaglandins are derived from arachidonic acid (AA), which is, in turn, derived from dietary linoleic acid. (LA) is an essential omega-6 fatty acid, meaning we must consume it in the diet.

In the body, LA forms portions of the cell membranes and is used in many processes in the body. The body cannot store prostaglandins; they are made, used, and metabolized on demand. What the body does store is the precursor LA.

LA has been a hot fat topic in the nutrition world, mostly regarding the ratio to omega 3s in the diet. When the ratio is off, we get more inflammatory responses in the body and less balancing anti-inflammatory responses. During labor, we need both. If there is a balance, then the natural processes will do what they need to do. If we consume *too* much omega-3, just as when we consume too much omega-6, we can have a negative impact.

The use of isolated DHA supplementation during pregnancy has increased in recent decades after studies showed cognitive improvements in infants of mothers who consumed more dietary and supplemental DHA. For those of you who don't know what DHA is, it is one of two main types of long-chain polyunsaturated omega-3 fatty acids: eicosapentaenoic acid (EPA) and docosahexaenoic acid (DHA).

EPA and DHA are found together in animal products; the best known is fish. These acids can also be converted in the body as needed from alpha-linoleic acid (ALA) found in plants. Hundreds of studies have shown the increased health benefits of consuming foods rich in these compounds and taking supplements rich in these compounds in pregnancy and fetal development.

Something we tend to do in natural medicine and dietary supplementation is when we find a positive correlation on a specific nutrient, we tend to isolate it from its natural combinations. This is what happened with the supplementation of omega-3 fatty acids in pregnancy: isolated DHA supplementation.

EPA and DHA work differently in the body and work better when balanced. EPA is not found in high levels in the brain, while DHA is, which is why DHA helps to increase brain health in babies. EPA and AA compete in the conversion of prostaglandins. Notice the "eicosa-" part of the name of EPA, and do you remember that prostaglandins and thromboxanes are members of the eicosanoid family?

Linoleic acid (becoming arachidonic acid) and EPA can be used in the production of prostaglandins and thromboxanes.[273] EPA is used in the production of 3-series prostaglandins and is important in the balance of the 2-series prostaglandins.

It doesn't suppress them completely but balances their function with 3-series prostaglandins, and the balance is crucial to the proper function of the body and the health of the baby.

EPA also upregulates the proteins needed to increase cell affinity for DHA. Studies show that DHA-only supplementation neglects the EPA functions required for correct fatty acid balance, including a reduction of DHA transport to the fetus—the whole reason mothers are taking DHA.[274]

The Inuit populations of the Arctic are known for their high intake of EPA and DHA in the form of fish and marine sea animals. Based on these heavy omega-3 diets, a study was done to assess cord blood levels of DHA in correlation with maternal DHA/AA ratios. The maternal DHA was related to the amount of DHA in cord blood. Higher DHA levels were associated with longer gestations and healthier babies.[275] What they didn't note in the study was that the intake of EPA was also greater and that DHA was not consumed on its own.

DHA, on the other hand, cannot enter the prostaglandin cycle but it still affects it. It affects the receptor sites, specifically, the TXA2 receptors. Remember that this is the primary vasoconstrictor and blood-clotting factor during delivery. Studies have shown that DHA is exceptionally good at binding to the TXA2 receptor and blocking platelet aggregation, thus thinning the blood and decreasing clotting.[276]

Did you read that?

Now, there is no study that links isolated DHA supplementation to increased risks of bleeding during labor because the studies done on fish oils in pregnancy used both EPA and DHA together but only measure for DHA.

In the diet, EPA and DHA are found together, or the precursor ALA is consumed and converted in the body to required EPA and DHA. Nowhere in the diet, and even in cultures that consume high amounts of fish and marine life, do you see isolated DHA consumption except in supplementation and especially in pregnancy.

No, I have no proof—no study to back my theory—but it is a concept that I've thought about. In my own practice, I recommend fish oil supplements that contain *both* EPA and DHA. The EPA component is crucial to the function of the DHA, and its actions have a balancing effect on the body. Without EPA, DHA is less likely to cross the placenta and enter the cord and baby, and more likely to affect the blood platelets and TXA2 receptors.

The mechanisms and actions of EPA and DHA in their ability to reduce blood clotting are not well-understood, with research studies showing both an increased risk and no increased risk. Together, EPA and DHA do not have the scientific backing to associate intake with increased risk of bleeding, but separate? Maybe.

This is just a hunch I've developed throughout the years. It is not possible that this one factor is the cause of the rise in postpartum hemorrhaging in the United States. I suspect, like every other condition I've discussed in this book, there are multiple patterns, multiple causes, and probably a multitude of combinations of patterns that are associated with the increased risk of bleeding in childbirth. I just propose that this could be a contributing factor. It seems coincidental that the studies on DHA in fetal brain development and increased use of isolated DHA supplements in pregnancy also coincide with the increase in childbirth bleeding, but so do other things, such as increasing rates of induction, both with Pitocin and cervical ripening prostaglandins.

Hyaluronic Acid – The Forgotten Component of Cervical Ripening

Hyaluronic acid (HA) is more popular as an anti-wrinkle serum than a cervical ripening agent, but without it, the cervix does not soften or ripen. HA is found in cartilage and soft tissues and makes up a large part of synovial fluid in the body. It has a high affinity for water molecules and is a hydrator and softener of the skin, cartilage, and joints.

It is synthesized in several different ways: estrogen synthesis, bacterial fermentation of starches in the gut, and direct consumption through hyaluronic-rich animal products.

So, I mentioned this study that compared induction methods . . . well, one of the methods reviewed was direct injection of HA into the cervix. Those in the HA group were significantly less likely to need additional induction medication (Pitocin), had increased cervical dilation as compared to cervical ripening medications, and no adverse effects were reported. Yet it was deemed a weak option for induction because of the process of injecting HA into the cervix.[277] Let's all cringe like a man who just watched a video of a kid hitting a ball into another man's testicles.

What this study confirmed is what other studies had discovered years before: The influx of HA into the cervix was a primary trigger of ripening.

During pregnancy, the concentration of HA in the cervix is low. The cervix needs to be firm and tight to hold the pregnancy. From 28 weeks, when we see a rise in cortisol, estrogen, and prostaglandins (specifically PGF2α), we start to see small changes in HA production, with a sharp rise in the last weeks of pregnancy.

HA has a high affinity for water molecules, as I mentioned, but it doesn't absorb them into cells. Instead, it suspends them in animation, so to speak, holding them in place and adding intracellular moisture to softening the tissue. The space created by the reconstruction of the collagen fibers, from a knotted nest of fibers to a more parallel fiber structures, gives space for the HA to bring fluid into the tissues.

At the onset of labor, maternal serum levels of HA jump. A study looked at serum HA levels in women at term but not in labor and at term in labor: Women at term but not in labor had serum HA levels of 46.9 +/- 7.9 ng/mL, while women at term and in labor had serum HA levels of 100.4 +/- 11.3 ng/mL. These values doubled at the onset of labor.[278]

HA stimulates the enzyme collagenase.

Collagenase is an enzyme that breaks down the bonds in collagen. As the bonds break, there are bigger gaps for the HA-bound water molecules to penetrate and accumulate, adding to the softening and ripening that occurs in active labor. HA also stimulates the enzymes gelatinase and elastase that help to break down the connective tissue of the cervix and soften the tendons and ligaments of the pelvis.

HA production is also a positive feedback mechanism. Estrogen and PGF2α are necessary for HA synthesis. HA stimulates the production of PGF2-alpha, so each is responsible for increasing levels of the other. The enzymes that synthesize HA are dependent on both magnesium and manganese[279] and precursor sugar molecules. There's that nutritional component.

So, as you can see, without adequate amounts of HA, the cervix cannot effectively soften, leading to slow or no progression in labor. Low HA production could also be a cause for "failed inductions." If you are adding in the oxytocin and prostaglandins and yet there is no cervical ripening occurring, there is a good chance that at some level of HA synthesis there is a deficiency, possibly magnesium or manganese. This deficiency could have occurred months prior as the body slowly increased production and softened the cervix before the initiation of labor.

Studies show that magnesium deficiency has a significant effect on the concentrations of HA.[280] With an estimated 60 percent of American women of reproductive age not consuming the minimum dietary requirements for magnesium, this could be more of a contributing factor than is commonly discussed.

Oxytocin and Protein

Oxytocin is one of the key players in the birthing game. Without oxytocin, the uterus cannot contract, the cervix cannot efface or dilate, and natural birth does not occur. Oxytocin is Elvis— labor doesn't start until Elvis enters the room; he's the star of the show. Oxytocin has many other important functions in the body other than the stimulation of contractions during childbirth, but for now, let's focus on birth.

Oxytocin is a peptide hormone (protein-based), much like prolactin and relaxin. It is produced in the hypothalamus and stored in the pituitary. As a peptide hormone, it is created by combining nine different amino acids. Most of these amino acids are produced in the body, but two of the components are essential amino acids, meaning we cannot make them, and they must be consumed in the diet. They are leucine and isoleucine.

Right away, we can make the conclusion that if a mother does not have enough protein in her diet, especially leucine and isoleucine, then she will not be able to make efficient oxytocin. Proteins are particularly important in pregnancy because they fuel many different chemical processes and enzymes as well as fuel the growth of the baby, and they are also important to produce this essential hormone. (See Figure 10.)

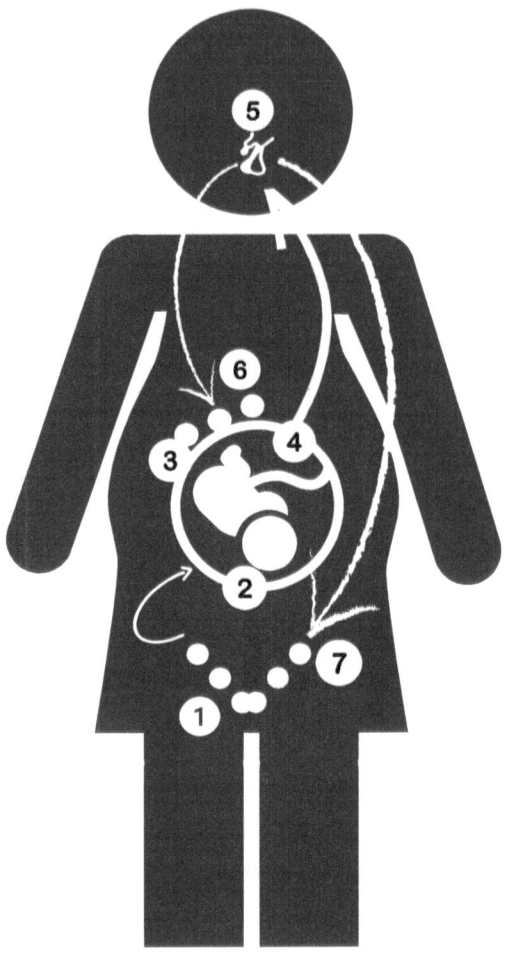

Figure 10: 1) Starting around 28 weeks gestation, the cervix begins to remodel in response to the rise in hormones. 2) The increase in prostaglandins and changes in the cervix trigger an increase in internal oxytocin production. 3) The increase in internal oxytocin stimulates an increase in the production of oxytocin and prostaglandin receptors. 4) At term, the mature baby secretes surfactants that trigger the placenta to stimulate the pituitary. 5) In response to placental signals, the pituitary releases oxytocin. 6) Oxytocin stimulates uterine contractions. 7) Oxytocin stimulates an increase in prostaglandin and HA production.

Childbirth is not as simple as oxytocin causing contractions. When the placenta begins to produce CRH, the pituitary is stimulated to release oxytocin. Oxytocin works on a positive feedback mechanism. When the oxytocin binds to receptors, it sends signals to produce more oxytocin, as does the natural increase in estrogen. As the receptors dissolve, the amount of oxytocin produced decreases.

It's also not as simple as oxytocin binding to receptors.

Oxytocin Physiology in Labor

The production of oxytocin doesn't happen just at the onset of labor. Like the other factors that play into the progression of childbirth, we see that oxytocin production and receptor formation occurs at a gradual increase throughout gestation and culminates in a peak at childbirth.[281]

When you read about oxytocin production in childbirth, most articles and texts discuss the production of oxytocin from the pituitary, but oxytocin can also be produced by the uterine lining and the placenta.[282]

In the early stages of the third trimester, oxytocin is primarily produced by the placenta in response to rising estrogen levels[283] and CRH. CRH is produced by the hypothalamus as well as the placenta. Elevated cortisol levels decrease the production of CRH from the mother and increase the production from the placenta and uterine tissues, which increases oxytocin production from the uterine tissues and not the pituitary.

This rise in oxytocin produces minute contractions within the uterus and triggers the production of PGF2α prostaglandins.[284] This is amplified during active labor.

PGF2α then stimulates the formation of oxytocin receptors on the uterus as well as more prostaglandin receptors on the cervix.[285] The formation of oxytocin receptors begins around 28 weeks as the cascade of events that signals the linear path to childbirth begins.

NUTRIENT HIGHLIGHT: VITAMIN A

Vitamin A comes in two dietary forms: provitamin A carotenoids (beta-carotene, alpha-carotene, beta-cryptoxanthin) and preformed vitamin A retinoids (retinol, retinal, retinoic acid).

There are also synthetic versions of vitamin A. These forms are often used in supplementation and in research. They tend to be more water-soluble and easier to regulate in trials but also more toxic.

There are over 750 carotenoids found in plants with only beta-carotene, alpha-carotene, and beta-cryptoxanthin being able to convert to retinol. Beta-carotene is the one most referenced.

On their own, carotenoids are potent antioxidants that help neutralize toxins in the body and reduce oxidative stress, specifically in the reproductive organs. To function, though, they must be converted to retinol. Their main dietary function is to serve as a source of retinol because retinol is the true vitamin A.

Carotenoids in the diet are converted to retinol in the liver. The liver stores vitamin A in an alcohol-based form called retinyl esters, which is why it is such a nutritional powerhouse for vitamin A. These dietary esters are converted to retinol in the small intestines.

There is a negative feedback mechanism in place that "measures" the levels of retinol in the liver. When there are adequate levels of stored vitamin A in the body, there is an inhibition of absorption from the diet and a decrease in the conversion to retinol in the liver. Conversion is also limited in the presence of other nutritional deficiencies, such as zinc.

When you hear "vitamin A" what you should really be hearing is "retinol." This is the usable form of vitamin A in the body. It is essential for human health and development. Retinol conversion to retinal or retinoic acid depends on the body's need. Retinol functions on a cellular level, controlling cellular development and growth, and plays an important part in the development of embryos. Retinal is used in eye health and development. Retinoic acid is necessary for hormone function and genetic expression as well as tooth and bone growth—all important functions for pregnancy, childbirth, and fetal development.

Oxytocin and the War on Prenatal Vitamin A

Multiple studies have highlighted that oxytocin increases with the administration of vitamin A and estrogen. These two together upregulated the genetic expression of oxytocin and oxytocin receptors.[286][287]

Toward the end of pregnancy, we see a nearly six-fold increase in the number of vitamin A receptors on the uterus, and vitamin A has been linked with the increase in oxytocin gene expression seen in the last weeks of pregnancy.[288]

Yet we have a war against the dietary consumption and use of vitamin A in pregnancy. One of the richest foods in vitamin A, liver, is one of the pregnancy diet's no-nos, with the fear of consumption causing birth defects.

I wrote an article many years ago that discussed my top 10 foods for preparing for labor. In that article, I mentioned both chicken and beef livers. I had a comment on the page that berated me a bit. The lady accused me of giving out harmful advice that could cause serious birth defects. This was perfect! I needed a jumping-off spot for another article on the consumption of liver in pregnancy and its safety, and she gave it to me.

The dietary intake of organ meat has been vilified for the past 60 years, with no real merit behind it. Cultures all around the world have prized the organs of animals. They provide a nutrient-dense animal food source, more than the meat itself. Not long ago, western cultures still consumed the organs of animals in meals, and many other countries still do. In fact, in the Masai tribes of Africa, women are only allowed to eat organ meat

I remember my grandfather cooking liver and onions as a kid. He loved it because he had grown up eating it. He said he would crave it and would often make it just for himself. No one else *really* loved it as he did. My kids and he would have gotten along great. I've never met two children that love organ meat as much as they do, probably because liver was one of the first foods we fed them.

What happened to make us hate liver and organ meat so much?

Bad science.

Liver began to fall out of favor decades ago as science discovered many of its functions, such as body detoxification. It was assumed that because the liver detoxified chemicals, hormones, and medications, that it was a harborer of toxins itself and that eating the liver would, in turn, be eating an accumulation of toxic chemicals.

We now know this is false. The liver produces enzymes, and these enzymes break down these chemicals and expel them through the bowels and the kidneys. It does not store them. What it does store is a large amount of nutrients needed to make these enzymes and for these enzymes to function.

In 1995, an article written in *The New York Times* stirred the prenatal nutrition pot. This article by Jane E. Brody and titled *Study Links Excess Vitamin A to Birth Defects* created a swirl of thought and discussion over the dietary intake of vitamin A, like liver. The article stated:

> *"Women who consume excessive amounts of vitamin A during the early months of pregnancy can cause serious birth defects in their unborn children, a large new study has shown.... The study showed that 1 baby in 57 born to women taking doses of* vitamin A *above 10,000 international units daily was damaged as a result.... The higher the doses consumed, the greater the risk, the researchers found. Babies born to women who consumed more than 10,000 international units of the vitamin daily were 2.4 times as likely to be born with such defects as babies exposed to 5,000 international units or less. But babies exposed to 20,000 international units during the first three months of gestation were about four times as likely to be born with defects that included cleft lip, cleft palate, hydrocephalus and major heart malformations."*

The specific study that was mentioned in *The New York Times* was a survey study done at Boston University School of Medicine. The researchers interviewed 22,748 women during their pregnancies, analyzing the supplements they were taking and the foods they were eating. It found that 98.6 percent of the women interviewed were well under the toxic amount of vitamin A. Those who were consuming higher amounts received most of their vitamin A in a synthetic form from prenatal vitamins and fortified foods. When you read the actual article published in *The New England Journal of Medicine*, little of the vitamin A supplied was through food sources. The majority was via supplementation.

This isn't the only study that has been done. In fact, there have been several, dating back to 1967. The findings in these studies vary based on the methods used, but there are some key features.

The first thing to note about the research studies published between 1967 and 1986—those most referenced in support of no liver and vitamin A consumption during pregnancy—is that they were done using a synthetic and isolated form of vitamin A. This form was water-soluble, and if you remember, natural vitamin A is fat-soluble. This meant that it did not accumulate in the tissues the same as dietary vitamin A and was easier to regulate for testing. But because it did not accumulate, it did not activate the natural negative feedback mechanism that helps to regulate vitamin A metabolism in the liver. Interesting. This synthetic form has a long history of being linked to birth defects in lab animals and in humans.

In one study,[289] dosages of 35,000 IU were given daily during the first 10 days of a rat's gestation cycle. Gestation is 16 weeks long. The study noticed defects in the offspring, including cleft palate and various eye defects. That is a ridiculously large amount of vitamin A per weight. I can't even do the math on how much vitamin A you would need to consume to get to the equivalent of what they did to these rats.

Because dietary liver is a rich source of retinol, it has been the black sheep of the prenatal diet since the first study linked high levels of vitamin A to birth defects. The amount of vitamin A stored in the liver is not static and can range from 3,000 IU per 3 oz to 12,000 IU per 3 oz., with some sources, depending on region and diet, being upward of 25,000 IU per ounce serving. This includes cod liver oil supplements.

Some concern with the dietary consumption of liver has popped up again as there is an increased craze in dietary supplements of liver and cod liver oil, especially in the first few weeks of pregnancy. These defects are only seen when high doses of vitamin A are consumed in the first trimester. To elicit birth defects, the dosage needed to be maintained at high levels daily over the course of weeks to months.

The link between dietary vitamin A and birth defects is literally nonexistent. In fact, you would need to consume more than 20,000 IU per day of retinol, not beta-carotene, over the course of weeks or months to induce an overdose dietarily. If you are eating that much liver, you like liver way more than I am giving the population credit for. Not a single study links beta-carotene consumption to birth defects. There is still debate over whether dietary retinol could even cause toxicity due to the negative feedback mechanism that controls vitamin A absorption and metabolism.

To answer the question and concern about the fear of liver consumption, excess vitamin A, and the possibility that I was giving out dangerous information when I recommended liver consumption in preparation for labor: The answer is that consuming liver in the last couple of weeks of pregnancy *will not* cause birth defects in the baby. Liver is fair game in the preparation for childbirth.

In fact, research is showing that *deficiencies* in vitamin A, specifically at the end of gestation, have a direct effect on oxytocin production and function.[290] With an estimated 50 percent of women not consuming the minimum requirements for vitamin A, this may be a factor in the increased rates of labor complications associated with poor oxytocin production and function.

Are You the Key Master?

Cell receptors are proteins in the cell walls that work like doors. Some have locks, others just need the right-sized molecule. Oxytocin cell receptors need a key to unlock the door and allow oxytocin to enter the cells. The key to unlocking the oxytocin receptor is two-fold: You need *both* magnesium and cholesterol. If you are lacking in either, the door will not open.

Magnesium is the key master and the receptor is the gatekeeper (name that movie). Deficiencies in magnesium decrease the affinity of oxytocin receptors for oxytocin by 1,500-fold.[291] That's big.

Magnesium has many functions in the body, but regarding oxytocin and labor, it is the molecule that transports oxytocin through the receptors. Magnesium not only transports oxytocin into cells but also the electrolytes needed to contract and relax the muscle cells. Without enough magnesium, the muscles are nutritionally weak. This can cause abnormal contracting and spasming and increase pain perception. It's painful enough; let's not make it worse. Magnesium helps to create smooth, fluid, strong, and functional contractions.

With an estimated 60-plus percent of American women of reproductive age not consuming enough magnesium, this is a possible factor for weak contractions and other issues with oxytocin function.

Cholesterol levels rise in pregnancy to be the precursor to steroid hormones and help stabilize the oxytocin receptors, increasing their longevity.[292] [293]

What About Baby?

From 28 weeks on, the mother's body has been preparing for childbirth. Her body has remodeled and softened her cervix, raised estrogen to raise prostaglandins that stimulated oxytocin in the uterus that increased prostaglandins again that made oxytocin receptors, and round and round her body went until something triggered this preparation and prodromal phase to become active labor.

In 2004, it was first suggested that fetal lung maturity was the signal for the activation of childbirth.[294]

Surfactants are inflammatory proteins that are produced by the lungs of the maturing baby. Cortisol helps to stimulate the maturation of the fetal lungs. Just as we see cortisol beginning to rise in the third trimester, and the resulting maternal cascades, we also see a rise in surfactant production by the baby. Surfactants can be detected in the amniotic fluid between 28 and 32 weeks gestation, and the concentration increases five-fold by 37 weeks.[295] These inflammatory proteins work like a hormonal signal. A specific surfactant, named surfactant protein A (SP-A), has become the most researched of the known types. SP-A increases the production of macrophages. As the baby breathes in the amniotic fluid, it breathes out these proteins. SP-A and other surfactants bind to the macrophages, travel through the amniotic fluid to the amniotic sac and the placenta and embed themselves in the tissue. This increases inflammatory responses. Once the inflammatory responses are, well, too inflammatory, the maternal body signals the expulsion of the body, a.k.a. birth.

Studies have shown that the injection of SP-A into mice causes preterm labor and that injecting an antibody against SP-A causes a delay in delivery.[296] [297]

There is an intricate ballet of sorts that is occurring in the mother's body throughout pregnancy and in preparation for childbirth. Actions that start in the early third trimester culminate in a cascade of reactions between multiple organ systems and two independent humans.

To help women achieve their birth goals, we need to focus on both the prenatal and maternity sides of care. We need to have a healthy baby, but we also need to have a healthy and functional mother who has been able to support her body throughout the third trimester to allow these processes to occur the way they are intended.

Preparing for labor doesn't happen at 36 weeks as most women and practitioners believe. It starts at the beginning. It starts the moment a mother believes she is pregnant. The way her placenta develops, the genetic expression of her baby, the nutrient intake she accumulates at the correct stages of pregnancy to prepare for the next. In the maternity functional medicine clinic, the support of a healthy baby is always important, but our true endgame goal is a healthy mother who has been given the support and guidance she needs to succeed in childbirth.

An Illusion of Control

No two births are the same, even within the same mother. We are never the same person, physically, mentally, and structurally throughout our lives. With maternity functional medicine, we can set up a mother nutritionally to be able to function her absolute best, but each mother has a different best.

Each mother comes with genetics, developmental structure, trauma, and other aspects that can affect her birth outcomes. We also have that other person in this journey: the baby. The genetics, health, and position of the baby influences the childbirth process just as much as the work a mother puts into the story.

As maternity functional medicine providers, our goal is to set the mother up for the most functional experience her body and baby can have. She can do everything right and still need a cesarean because the baby decided to engage in a malposition, or the genetics expressed during her own fetal development can predispose her to structural or hormonal defects. These are the possibilities we cannot affect. The relationship we have with our patients should emphasize our limitations as well as our strengths.

There are only some things we can control. When we are unable to control them, we manage them, knowing that we cannot change fetal position and that the genetic structure of the mother is established and out of our control. We can still help these mothers though. We can help them understand their unique body and set them up for nutritional success that spans far past the months of gestation and birth—setting the foundation for their new child to help prevent the same complications in future generations.

Chapter 13

Why the Method of Birth Matters

The way in which a birth occurs does matter. It matters to the mother, and it matters for the health of the child. Little attention has been given to the effects that the method of birth has on both, yet research shows that this single act makes a significant and long-lasting impact.

There are scenarios where surgical delivery is the safest and best option for a mother to deliver, and that is still an amazing and wonderful birth. In these birth scenarios, it is important, though, to acknowledge the difference in the birth method and the effects it has on postpartum recovery as well as the health of the baby. By understanding, respecting, and not ignoring these occurrences we can help these mothers and babies achieve health success in postpartum recovery.

The Catecholamine Surge

Studies show that the hormonal changes that occur during labor not only facilitate the delivery of the mature baby but also are crucial to stimulating physiologic changes in the baby at birth. The chemical processes of birth have evolved over millions of years, and if you haven't noticed, nothing in the body happens without a clear reason or connection. These maternal physiological changes during childbirth are connected and crucial for the maternal physiology of postpartum and physiological changes that babies need to enter the world beyond the womb.

After months and weeks of maternal physiologic extremes, the trigger for functional labor is the maturity of the baby's lungs. Labor is physically stressful and rises in cortisol are a normal part of the process of labor. With these rises in cortisol, we see a rise in neurotransmitters, each with a job to do in the maternal and fetal physiology to help the mother and child survive birth and life outside the womb.

During active labor, there is a catecholamine surge. These neurotransmitters spike in the second stage of labor, after the mother's cervix has fully effaced and changed but before she has the natural urge to push. There is a period of rest that occurs, where a mother naturally sleeps between (and sometimes during) contractions. As a doula, I've seen so many women, when allowed to enter this mental and physical space, literally sleep through the transitional phase of labor. Then it is as if a switch has been turned on and she becomes awake, energized, and the urge to push occurs. This is the surge in catecholamines that gives her the energy she needs to push but also prepares the baby for its entrance into the world.

This rise in norepinephrine and epinephrine has been shown to control fetal circulation during transition and pushing when blood oxygen levels are lowest, maintain glucose supply to the fetal heart and brain, prepare the lungs to breathe air, and increase the alertness and wakefulness of the baby at birth.[298]

There is an interesting balance between oxytocin and catecholamines. When the catecholamines surge, there is a drop in oxytocin, often causing more spacing between contraction at the pushing phase, and once delivery occurs and the surge is over, oxytocin rises again to clamp down on the uterus as the placenta detaches.

Cool fact: It is the drop in these catecholamines that makes moms shaky postpartum. Elevated catecholamines, which can occur due to stress in the delivery room, can inhibit oxytocin and increase the risk of hemorrhage.

Possible Impact of Scheduled Birth on Baby's Brain

A scheduled delivery is a planned cesarean with no trial of labor. This means that mom did not have an onset of natural labor before the surgical procedure. For many women, the decision to have a cesarean is not really a decision; it is a medical choice based on the health risks of their pregnancy going further or their risk of complications during childbirth. This is the way she needs to deliver and that is okay. We would be remiss, however, if we did not discuss the facts and implications of this type of deviation from the natural processes of birth and the effects it has on the baby.

Babies born via cesarean before the onset of natural labor tend to struggle with transitioning to the outside world. Their rates of admission to neonatal care units for respiratory problems are higher. Each week earlier than term (40 weeks) doubles the risk of admission to neonatal units.[299] These babies also require higher rates of oxygen supplementation and resuscitation.[300]

These babies never received the catecholamine surge that would have occurred during labor to increase their lung function and alertness.

Another interesting take is the effect that the squishing of the baby's head and brain has on brain development. In both animal studies and human studies, we see that the pressure on the head as it passes through the birth canal has positive impacts on the development of the brain.

Animal models show that the natural pressure pauses normal cellular death.

Every day we have cells that die, but when a baby is born vaginally, this cell death is paused.[301] Babies born via cesarean have no delay in cell death and have a greater loss of brain cells over time. Cesarean babies also have changes in vocalizations that hint at a change in neurological function.[302]

A possible connection to this change in cell death rates is that cesarean-delivered babies have significantly lower white matter, myelination, development in the brain after birth compared to vaginally delivered babies.[303] This difference in myelination corrects itself over time and is not seen in older cesarean-delivered children. The consequences of this are still unknown.

The Microbiome

The microbiome is a city of bacteria, viruses, yeasts, and who knows what else that colonizes the digestive system and vaginal cavity. Each microbe has a job to do in the system and each of our microbiomes is unique. Just like a big city, the gut has good and bad microbes—some that just go about their day doing their jobs, others that rob, steal, and kill, and others that regulate the microbe world.

In a healthy body, there is balance in this system. If the system is disturbed by stress, pathogenic invasion, infections, medications, or poor diets, we see a dysbiosis, and the city implodes into chaos that creates damage and breaks down the city.

There has been great attention given to the role of microbes in digestive health because, well, they are found in the digestive system. The microbiome, when in balance, keeps the naturally occurring "bad" bacteria from over-colonizing and creating problems such as inflammation, gas, bloating, diarrhea, constipation, etc.

It is also an important part of the breakdown and assimilation of numerous vitamins in the diet. For example, the key enzymes required for the breakdown and absorption of B12 are produced by microbial fermentation, which is why fermented foods like kombucha are so high in B12.

Many of the vitamins we have talked about being essential for the hormones and processes of labor and delivery are not usable in their natural form. They must be broken down or changed into a form that our body can utilize. Vitamin K is a great example of how plant-based nutrients need to be broken down by gut bacteria to get their full health potential.

The microbiome is also our first line of defense against the outside world. It is considered a part of the immune system in that it helps to stimulate immune responses to invading pathogens and toxins. In fact, 70–80 percent of our immune system is found in the gut.

Not only do the bacteria directly attack and consume invading microorganisms, but they also digest the fiber in our food to form short-chain fatty acids, which are then used as an energy source for the cells that line our digestive system and prevent invaders from passing into the blood.

Large colonies of healthy bacteria and yeasts are found in the gut. The colon is devoid of oxygen, and it is here that the anaerobic bacteria thrive. These bacteria are the police of the gut and help to prevent the colonization of negative microbe species. These species are our primary immune regulation team and include *Bifidobacterium, Lactobacillus,* and many others. With the gut housing 10–100 trillion different organisms, identifying and understanding their actions is a science unto itself.

Mom's Diet and Microbiome Health

The microbiome is our first line of defense against pathogens and is an important modulator of different processes in the body. The research around the microbiome is fascinating and early, but what we already know is that the diet plays a critical role in the health of the microbiome and the body.

The diet affects the microbiome at an acute and chronic level. Changes in the microbiome can be seen within 24 hours of dietary shifts.[304]

Several studies have investigated the effects of different macronutrients, micronutrients, minerals, and combinations of each, and how they affect the microbiome. Proteins are a big piece of the microbiome puzzle.

Diets that rely heavily on meat-based proteins and less on plant-based proteins show higher levels of *Bacteroides, Alistipes, Bilophila,* and *Clostridium* and less *Lactobacillus* and *Bifidobacterium*.[305] Pea proteins, specifically, are shown to increase positive microbes, *Lactobacillus* and *Bifidobacterium,* and a decrease in *Clostridium*.[306]

Certain fats have been shown to improve microbiome health as well. Salmon and foods containing polyunsaturated and monounsaturated fats help to increase *Lactobacillus* and decrease the *Clostridium* species. While high amounts of rancid and trans-fats, like those found in fried and processed foods, decrease the positive bacteria and increase the production of negative species.[307]

Dairy is a complex of different sugars, fats, proteins, vitamins, minerals, and more. Studies show contradictory interactions in the gut. In some studies, we see that dairy consumption increases the growth of the *Clostridium* species, and in others we see an increase in short-chain fatty acids that are anti-inflammatory. Dairy contains fats called conjugated linoleic acids (CLAs). These dietary fats are anti-inflammatory and provide numerous health benefits. CLA is consumed in the diet but also produced by the *Bifidobacterium* species of bacteria. Much of the anti-inflammatory effects of dairy are associated with this CLA component. The source of the dairy and the type of dairy used make a significant difference in the reactions seen in the gut. The foods highest in CLA are sheep milk, yogurt, and certain types of cheese. We also see a difference in CLA concentrations in dairy from cows fed exclusively grass versus cows kept indoors on grains.[308] CLA is only found in the fat of dairy, so low-fat and nonfat milk provides only lactose that feeds negative bacteria.

Carbohydrates are digested based on their structure, with more complex forms taking longer to break down, and some forms, such as fibers, not being digested at all. These different types of carbohydrates and sugars affect the microbiome very differently.

Overall, the standard American diet, with its higher protein, negative fat, low-fat dairy, and high sugar amounts is poised to create dysbiosis in the gut microbiome.[309]

When comparing different dietary patterns with their correlation to gut dysbiosis and the prevalence of certain microbes in the gut, the key take-home message is that no matter the ratio of macronutrients, the driver is the abundance of plant-based food sources. The more plants in the diet, the better the gut health.

Polyphenols are phytonutrients found in fruits and vegetables. They are not vitamins or minerals and are often left out in the analysis of nutrition and nutrient density. These phytonutrients are a crucial part of the diet that must be present for proper health. Many of the benefits we see, across all aspects of nutrition, are related to the presence of phytochemicals and not the nutrients themselves. Many nutrients are absorbed and function differently in their food-based sources than in supplements and in isolation due to the interactions between the phytonutrients and these vitamins and minerals. In the treatment of dysbiosis, the introduction of polyphenols through the diet is important for changing the gut microbiome.

Yet these changes are only temporary, meaning once a mother returns to a poor diet, her microbiome returns to its established dysbiosis. The primary microbiome developmental phase is the acute "window of opportunity" between birth and the first few years of life. This time fame seems to establish the foundation of the microbiome health that can be influenced by supplements and diet but not fully changed. Not yet.[310]

Group B Strep and Antibiotics in Labor

Group B strep (GBS) is a common and normal bacterium of the digestive and vaginal microbiome. It is passed from mother to daughter and if the mother is positive, the daughter will most likely be positive as a carrier as well. Twenty-five percent of women are carriers. Being a carrier does not mean that a woman has an infection or disease; all it means is that her body carries this bacterium in her normal flora. She received it from her own mother at vaginal birth.

In women who are carriers and have healthy microbiomes, the GBS is balanced by other microbes. In most women, it is harmless and just a normal part of the gut and vaginal environment. In women who are carriers and who have an unhealthy microbiome, the GBS becomes overabundant. This overabundance of GBS can cause complications in labor, such as premature rupture of membranes or preterm labor, but the biggest worry is that of the health of the newborn.

Sidenote: I was a GBS baby and spent a few weeks in the neonatal intensive care unit (NICU) with a lung infection, so it can be a serious complication if not identified, managed, and treated correctly. This does not mean routine antibiotics for all. This means a clear understanding of pathogenesis and the risk of infections based on time of membrane rupture and length of labor.

It takes about 12 hours for the bacteria to migrate up into the sac and colonize. If the rupture of membranes occurs during labor, the risk of infection is significantly reduced. The risk to the newborn is significantly higher in those who were not aware that their membranes had ruptures (leaking fluids) or had a rupture of membranes without the onset of labor.[311]

GBS in newborns can cause sepsis, pneumonia, and meningitis—all serious conditions. My mother had been leaking fluid for a full week before it was detected by her physician—plenty of time for bacteria to migrate into the womb and infect the amniotic fluid.

The standard of care is to administer antibiotics during labor to decrease the amount of GBS present at the birth. This opens another round of issues.

The antibiotics used not only decrease GBS but also destroy the vaginal microbiome, limiting the exposure of positive vaginal microbes to the baby.

Until recently, the connection between the routine use of antibiotics during childbirth and the effects on infant microbiomes was not well documented if at all. A study published in 2019 finally linked the use of these routine medications with changes in the infant microbiome, showing that the use of these medications did, in fact, change the initial inoculation of vaginal microbes to the baby.[312] These changes mimicked those seen in cesarean deliveries.

The use of antibiotics in the prevention of GBS infections is based on three studies that included 500 women. These studies showed a cumulative 83 percent reduction in infant GBS infections. Cochrane reviews of these studies found severe bias and a lack of evidence to recommend routine antibiotic administration.[313]

The GBS load that is detectable can be changed. We see this clinically and in research. A mother can be negative at one time of testing and positive at another time of testing. Currently, one in four women are carriers, and

20–30 percent of women receive antibiotics during labor. In these mothers, maternal functional medicine may play a role in maintaining a healthy microbiome that decreases the risk of GBS overgrowth and, thus, decreases the need for antibiotic use during childbirth.

Birth Method and the Microbiome

The initial colonization of the gut happens at birth: vaginal birth.

In early life is a window of opportunity in which we can change the foundation of the microbiome. In fact, 20 minutes after birth, the baby's microbiome is identical to the vaginal microbiome of the mother, while cesarean-delivered babies have gut microbiomes that mimic skin microbiomes.[314]

The vaginal microbiome mimics the gut microbiome and is heavily dominated by different *Lactobacillus* species,[315] while the skin microbiome is variant.

In the hospital setting, the *Clostridium* family is prevalent. Studies show that cesarean babies tend to have higher amounts of this family after birth and through the first several years of life, during the window of immune development.[316] Members of the Clostridium family produce neurotoxins that affect the function of brain chemistry.[317] Cesarean delivery carries with it an increased risk of infant and child neurological conditions, such as autism and attention deficit disorder.[318] Is it the only factor to these conditions? No, but it is a contributing factor that should be taken seriously.

In the initial year of life, the two different methods of birth have a drastic effect on the gut microbiome as do other factors, such as whether a mother breastfeeds or not, the introduction of rice cereal as a primary food source, the child's diet, and the exposure to pathogens. Each of these lifestyle markers changes the genetic expression of the microbiome and sets the foundation for the overall health of the individual for the rest of their life.

By the age of three, there is no measurable difference in the guts of virginally birthed and cesarean-birthed children. The question becomes, during this window of opportunity, what are the long-term effects of dysbiosis as the immune system develops?

Health Risks in Cesarean-delivered Babies

The long-term risks that cesarean delivery has on the lifetime health of children and adults is poorly understood. With the limited research available, there seems to be a correlation with method of birth and the increased propensity for certain health conditions later in life.

The risk of asthma and allergies has been the most connected to birth method and primarily to the changes in the gut microbiome that occurs in the prime window of immune development.[319]

The immune systems of cesarean-delivered children appear to also be weaker, predisposing them to increased hospitalization rates from viral and bacterial infections, specifically affecting the lungs and gut.[320] The researchers said the link between cesarean birth and the increased risk of infection reflected the differences in the microbiomes of these children during critical immunological times.

A 2019 study found a direct correlation between the method of delivery and the risk of obesity at the age of two.[321] Specifically, planned cesareans were associated with a greater risk of childhood obesity. These correlations could directly affect the risk of early cardiovascular disease and unknown health consequences.

Similar studies found a correlation among women, specifically, their method of birth, and their risk of obesity and type 2 diabetes. Women born via cesarean were nearly 50 percent more likely to develop type 2 diabetes compared to women born vaginally.[322] This new study, published in 2020, shows a link among method of delivery, the increased risk of pregnancy complications, and health complications, such as diabetes, and the increased risk of delivering via cesarean—perpetuating a vicious cycle of increasing risk, maternal complications, and the need for medical and surgical intervention.

Cesarean Risks for Mom

Cesareans are serious surgical procedures that come with risks. Many practitioners, and countries at this point, have high rates of cesarean delivery with the whole cascade of consequences. This is not a procedure to be taken lightly for the health of both the baby and the mother.

In hospitals and countries with high resources, the risk of death during cesarean is low. But if mothers are delivering in lower-income communities and countries[323], their risk is greater. Studies show that this risk increases no matter where a woman lives or her socioeconomic standing with repeat cesareans.[324]

Several studies have also linked cesarean delivery with an increased risk of complications, such as hemorrhage, hysterectomy, uterine rupture, complications associated with anesthetics, obstetric shock, cardiac arrest, acute renal failure, assisted ventilation or intubation, puerperal venous thromboembolism, major puerperal infection, in-hospital wound disruption, and hematoma. Some of those risks are not truly birth-related, but surgically related, and would be risks for any surgical procedure.[325]

These are the short-term risks to mom; there are also long-lasting risks to surgical delivery. Pelvic adhesions, small bowel obstruction, sexual dysfunction, subfertility, urinary incontinence, pelvic organ prolapse, hernia,[326] and secondary infertility are all long-term complications associated with surgical delivery.[327]

The current trend of surgical delivery in the United States is rising, with nearly 30 percent of all births being surgical deliveries. Some of these deliveries are unavoidable but many are not and, this number will never be zero. Many cesarean deliveries are scheduled and elective with no medical backing. Others are decided during labor due to complications that could have been mitigated through proper functional medicine support throughout pregnancy to increase the mother's ability to birth naturally.

The effects of surgical delivery are vast and much of the effects are still unknown.

Conclusion

Take the Next Steps

I did not expect to answer all your questions in this book. While I was in the early stages of writing this book, I did a meditation workshop that had me seek my book through a meadow and ask it one question. My question was, "How do I fit it all in?" My book answered, "You don't."

Now, anyone who knows me knows I don't meditate. I should, but I don't. I'm a go-go-go type of person, meaning I cannot sit down and my brain is always working. Rest is hard for me. This was an exercise specifically for writers like me that was designed to be a visual meditation that got you thinking.

There were so many more small and big topics I wanted and thought about putting in here, which gives you the ability to do what I've been doing: ask the right questions and seek the answers through valid research, exploration, and good ol' connect-the-dots.

You are in a prime position to make change, no matter who you are. You do not need a degree in biochemistry or medicine to pick up a book or a medical journal and read. It sure helps, but I've taught these concepts to patients and practitioners whose medical base is limited.

Using this Information in the Clinic

Let's be honest, this is what you are kind of hoping you would get at some point in the book—an approach to using this in practice. A bit of a protocol, so to speak. I don't like protocols because it really misses that unique biochemical individual approach, but there is something nice about having a loose protocol that helps you find those biochemical differences.

In any functional medicine intake and treatment, there are steps you need to take to truly assess and care for someone's unique presentation. In pregnancy, we must dig even deeper sometimes.

Here are my steps to maternity functional medicine assessment and care:

- Comprehensive Pre-pregnancy Medical History
- Previous Pregnancy History
- Current Pregnancy History
- Patient's Own Pregnancy and Birth
  (Mother of the Mother's Pregnancy and Birth)
- Patient's Childhood
- Lab Testing
- Treatment Design
- Guidance

These steps are designed to help you assess and accurately diagnose your patients, create a unique treatment approach that encompasses the individual and the condition, not just the condition, and guide your patient through the vast changes that are occurring week to week in her body.

These treatment steps are different than working with a nonpregnant functional medicine patient because the body of the patient is changing drastically week to week, and so then does your plan and treatment design. You must recognize the phase at which the mother is when she is seen in addition to the conditions. For this reason, if you are a mother reading this book, you should always seek out a professional who is trained to support these complicated changes. Supplements are great, but the wrong one can be an issue.

When taking the patient's history, it is imperative to understand her birth experience. Understanding what her own mother did during the pregnancy that was the developmental phase of the mother you are seeing can help you determine possible epigenetic issues or predispositions to conditions. There are familial and genetic connections to disease in pregnancy. If a mother struggled with childbirth, her daughter has a higher risk of labor complications as well. A woman who grew up on a poorer diet during the developmental years may have more of a risk of pelvic shape issues. These are all considerations that we must contemplate when assessing each patient.

If the mother is a multigravida, we want to know her previous pregnancy history. What complications and complaints did she experience? How were her birth experiences? How far apart were her pregnancies? This is all good information to help us formulate some areas that may be deficient. A mother who is pregnant with number five and has four under the age of eight may be coming into this pregnancy nutritionally depleted due to lack of recovery between multiple pregnancies.

Interestingly, many traditional cultures understood that a mother could not have the nutritional reserves to reproduce frequently. Many cultures timed their pregnancies to ensure ample nutrient reserves for both mother and baby. Nomadic and hunter-gatherer cultures, specifically, had longer intervals between births. There were several reasons behind this, but much centered around the fact that a mother could not nutritionally support the nursing infant and another pregnancy. The resulting infant would be weaker and the mother would be weaker.[328]

Lab testing is a tool, and there is a multitude of extravagant testing options out there. Many commonly used functional medicine tests are overkill in pregnancy and often not accurate due to the unique changes in maternal biochemistry and physiology. Some common testing that has been well established in prenatal care can be used to assess for maternal function. Often these are reduced to the most basic of lab tests, but when used correctly, these can give a wealth of information on overall function.

The plan you produce is not fluid and is ever-changing. This requires constant supervision. In my clinic, a mother is never left alone; she has complete access to my guidance. I am available during the ever-changing weeks to help her assess shifts in symptoms and reassess her nutritional and supplemental regimens. Guidance is crucial. Unlike some conditions where you give your patient a supplemental protocol and check in six months later, maternity care requires constant adjustment and reassessments through different phases of gestation.

If you are planning on working with mothers, you need to be prepared to work with mothers. You need to be available at the drop of a hat to answer questions and give them guidance. You need to be available in the last couple of months when her body is being stressed more than it will ever be at any other time in her life. This is a collaborative feat, and we are only a part of this guidance.

The Death of Philosophical Debate in Medicine

Science is about exploration and discovering what we cannot see. Instead of telling graduating medical professionals, "We've given you everything you need to go out and do your job, so do it." We should be telling them, "We've given you a base to start doing your job, go out and learn more."

The conversation shouldn't be a "my science is better than yours" argument, but a philosophical debate based on the information presented. This is how we truly decode the body and discover its mysteries.

Medicine is riddled with the disease of arrogance, and I'm not just talking about western medicine. The line in the sand that has been drawn by both the conventional and the alternative sides of medicine is thick, with little sign of coming together in peaceful conversation.

One of the things I absolutely love about science, and especially anatomy and physiology, is that we don't know everything about it. We think we do, but we don't. Every year, there is something new to add to the story of us, and every year, there are new advances in medicine—both conventional and alternative.

Like our country, medicine is divided into who is right and who is wrong, each side believing they have the right approach and that their mindset is the only right way. Both sides use science as their defense, and less about true exploration and discovery. In this process of justifying our beliefs, we've become bitter, angry, and defensive, leaving little room for conversation.

Throughout history, great minds have sat around and discussed, pondered, and explored an array of possibilities. New ideas were brought to the table, analyzed, and debated. This philosophical approach to medicine helped to create medical advances in procedures, medications, and theories of how the body works. Without the idea of philosophical debate and questioning in medicine, we would still be drilling holes in our heads when we sneezed. (If you're like me, that's a lot of holes—dang allergies!) Things like germ theory would never have existed without the questioning, exploring, and conversations between intelligent minds.

Philosophy literally means "love of wisdom." The reason most of us decided to pursue paths in the fields we did was because of this: love of wisdom. We wanted to learn.

The path we each took to get where we are was full of unique and wonderful experiences, studies, and mentors. These different journeys offer us different views of the same concept.

It is like the elephant meme.

You know the meme cartoon where an elephant is standing and there are a bunch of blind men feeling it and trying to describe it? They all describe it differently, but in the end, they are all describing the same thing from different perspectives. This to me signifies the medical world.

Considering the different branches of medicine: conventional, functional, traditional Chinese, chiropractic, naturopathic, etc., we are all describing the same beautiful physiology from different perspectives, journeys, and views, yet we are all describing the same thing.

Instead of coming together and discussing our findings and putting the entire picture together, we have all put a hard line in the sand. Conventional medicine looks down on alternative practices as pseudoscience, while the alternative medicine practitioners condemn the methods of conventional medicine. Each modality is wrought with the same disease: arrogance. Only their medicine is the right path. They have the answers patients have been looking for.

No medical modality has all the answers. We are each flawed in some way in the treatment of our patients. Together, though, we could be unstoppable. If we could all erase the lines and come to the middle to begin debating—not yelling and not accusing but actually debating our medical philosophies—think of the advances in patient care we could make. How amazing would it be if we dropped our guard and listened to our fellow practitioners and discovered what they knew, and each added to the story?

Collaboration in medical care instead of solidarity.

Don't Stop Here

What I've given you is just the beginning, the foundation to fuel your passion to learn more. My goal was to educate and inspire you to take the next steps in your journey. You are here because you wanted to have more advanced tools to help your patients or yourself. Maybe this is the spur that gets you excited to go do some more research. That's great, I love it, and do it.

We need more people trying to piece the puzzles together. We need more philosophical debate with more viewpoints on the same subject to unravel the many mysteries the body still has hidden for us.

I invite you to continue your education by seeking out mentorships and continuing education courses and subscribing to an array of medical journals.

I offer courses, classes, and mentorship workshops to practitioners and patients alike. I don't believe that this knowledge should be limited to professionals. I believe that the women should understand how their bodies work and how they can care for themselves. As the resources for them are limited and the practitioners offering guidance are few and far between, women are required to take their health into their own hands.

The more maternity functional medicine practitioners there are to offer guidance to these women, the more women we have the potential to save. Together we can create a safe and supportive community for women around the world to have access to nutritional guidance that is backed by science and offers real nutrient therapy for overall function. Every woman deserves to be fully supported in her maternity journey, regardless of socioeconomic status, previous health, or other measures.

I believe we live in an amazing time for both conventional medicine and alternative medicine as advances in research and science bridge the two worlds together. I feel blessed to be where I am and when I am in history as science advances and begins to connect what we know in biochemistry and physiology to what we have always known through culture and traditions. Scientific progress and research into epigenetics, diet, and lifestyle on the effects of overall health and function is capable of not just helping the women we see in our offices but also the women we will one day see in our offices. We are healing the mothers of today to heal the mothers of tomorrow. I believe this medicine can save future women from childbirth trauma, complications, and death. Maternity health must become a priority in healthcare.

Together, we can make a difference. Join me.

Appendix A

Prenatal Dietary Reference Intakes

Knowing the symptoms of deficiency and excess can help you assess the nutritional status of patients without the use of excessive lab testing. The recommended nutrient intakes are a bit confusing. These are, really, educated guesses on what the average required amount is for the general population.

In pregnancy, I consider these minimums but know that people's unique biochemistry means they have unique nutrient needs. Symptoms associated with nutritional deficiencies are more common than we typically think, and many of the commonly dismissed pregnancy complaints are signs of nutritional insufficiencies.

Dietary Reference Intakes (DRI) are a set of reference values used to assess the nutrient intakes of individuals. These values vary based on age, sex, lifestyle, and reproductive status (a.k.a. pregnancy). These values include the Recommended Daily Allowance (RDA), Adequate Intake (AI), and Tolerable Upper Intake Limit (UL).

The RDA is the *average* amount of nutrients that a healthy person should consume each day. This value is for those who are not deficient. This is the daily amount needed to maintain health. RDAs are developed by the Food and Nutrition Board at the Institute of Medicine of the National Academy of Sciences. These values are primarily based on studies from the 1950s and have not been updated.

The AI is used when there is not sufficient evidence to support the establishment of an RDA for the nutrient. The value is an assumption of need to maintain health.

Prenatal Dietary Reference Intakes

The UL is the largest daily intake that is considered safe for *most* people. These values also do not acknowledge physical size, structure, and preexisting conditions that can change the individuals' required intake.

This information is for resource purposes. All RDA recommended values were taken from the *Food and Nutrition Board, Institute of Medicine – National Academy of Sciences Dietary Reference Intakes: Recommendations for Individuals.* (Institute of Medicine 2000) These values are outdated.[329]

For a comprehensive list of food sources for these nutrients, please visit my website and download this reference material for free.

Vitamin A	
RDA/AI Pregnancy	
14 – 18 years 19 – 50 years	2,500 IU 2,567 IU
UL	10,000 IU[330]
General Def. Symptoms (SXS)	Night blindness, vision changes, frequent colds, gut inflammation, dry skin and eyes, slow wound healing, vaginal dryness, recurrent miscarriage
Def. in Pregnancy	Deficiencies are more common during the third trimester and are associated with birth defects, preterm labor, anemia, and childbirth complications.[331] [332]
General Excess SXS	Headache, rash, coarse hair, hair loss, especially of the eyebrows, cracked lips, irritability, nausea and vomiting, liver damage, birth defects *Birth defects in association with dietary vitamin A are controversial. >15,000 IU per day for extended time in preconception and first trimester only of synthetic or a combination of synthetic and dietary have been associated with fetal birth defects.* See chapter 12.
Excess in Pregnancy	This is a controversial subject, see chapter 12 for more information, but excess vitamin A in the first trimester is associated with birth defects.

This information is for resource purposes. All RDA recommended values were taken from the Food and Nutrition Board, Institute of Medicine – National Academy of Sciences Dietary Reference Intakes: Recommendations for Individuals. (Institute of Medicine 2000) These values are outdated.

Prenatal Dietary Reference Intakes

	Vitamin D
RDA/AI Pregnancy	
14 – 50 years	600 IU *It has been well established in the literature that this amount is nowhere near the amount needed for pregnancy function. 4,000 IU is the minimum required amount needed to sustain a healthy pregnancy. Serum vitamin D testing should be used to assess the individual's status and need.*
UL	4,000 IU *Newer research indicates that doses greater than this are safe and often required to positively affect health. There is no data on ULs in pregnancy and studies show a new higher RDA for pregnancy should be established.*
General Def. SXS	Fatigue, joint pain, frequent colds, depression, anxiety, blood sugar dysregulation, changes in bone health, irregular menstrual cycles, recurrent miscarriage
Def. in Pregnancy	Deficiency is associated with preeclampsia, neonatal hypocalcemia, low birth weight, intrauterine growth restriction (IUGR), small for gestational age (SGA), gestational diabetes, placental insufficiency, placental calcification, prolonged labor and increased risk of cesarean delivery, postpartum hemorrhage, placental atony, and prenatal and postpartum depression.[333] *Up to 50 percent of women are vitamin D deficient during pregnancy.*[334]
General Excess SXS	Hypercalcemia, nausea and vomiting, weakness, frequent urination, kidney stones, gallbladder stones
Excess in Pregnancy	There are no known cases of vitamin D excess in pregnancy causing maternal or fetal complications. Fetal hypercalcemia is no longer associated with direct vitamin D supplementation but a genetic condition that changes vitamin D metabolism. Studies show that a maternal 25-OH vitamin D of a minimum of 40 ng/mL is required for a healthy and functional pregnancy.[335]

This information is for resource purposes. All RDA recommended values were taken from the Food and Nutrition Board, Institute of Medicine – National Academy of Sciences Dietary Reference Intakes: Recommendations for Individuals. (Institute of Medicine 2000) These values are outdated.

Vitamin E	
RDA/AI Pregnancy	
14 – 50 years	22.5 IU or 15 mg
UL	1,500 IU or 1,000 mg
General Def. SXS	Numbness in the arms and legs, muscle weakness, vision changes, increased inflammation, frequent colds, blood clotting, PMS, lower progesterone levels
Def. in Pregnancy	Deficiency is associated with an increased risk of gestational hypertension, placental insufficiency, early placental calcification, vascular damage, placental abruption, IUGR, SGA, premature delivery and retained placenta.[336]
General Excess SXS	Poor blood clotting, easy bruising, fatigue, nausea and vomiting, headache, diarrhea, abdominal cramping, increased creatinine in urine
Excess in Pregnancy	Early rupture of membranes at term[337]

This information is for resource purposes. All RDA recommended values were taken from the Food and Nutrition Board, Institute of Medicine – National Academy of Sciences Dietary Reference Intakes: Recommendations for Individuals. (Institute of Medicine 2000) These values are outdated.

Prenatal Dietary Reference Intakes

Vitamin K	
RDA/AI Pregnancy	
14 – 18 years 19 – 50 years	(AI) 75 mcg (AI) 90 mcg
UL	No Limit *No adverse effects have been associated with vitamin K consumption from food or supplements in humans or animals. No UL has been developed. (Institute of Medicine 2001)*
General Def. SXS	Easy bruising, poor blood clotting, heavy menstrual bleeding, blood in urine or stools, easy nose bleeds, heavier menstrual bleeding
Def. in Pregnancy	Lower prothrombin levels causing issues with blood clotting and increased risk of bleeding in both mother and baby. Cholestasis in pregnancy can be a cause of vitamin K deficiency and is associated with an increased risk of postpartum hemorrhaging.[338]
General Excess SXS	No established symptoms of toxicity *Vitamin K excess is not seen with dietary intake. It has been documented with the use of a K3 derivative that was used in baby formula. These symptoms included blood clotting, excess bilirubin, hemolytic anemia.*[339]
Excess in Pregnancy	No known issues

This information is for resource purposes. All RDA recommended values were taken from the Food and Nutrition Board, Institute of Medicine – National Academy of Sciences Dietary Reference Intakes: Recommendations for Individuals. (Institute of Medicine 2000) These values are outdated.

Vitamin B1	
RDA/AI Pregnancy	
14 – 50 years	1.4 mg
UL	No limit
General Def. SXS	Fatigue, irritability, poor memory, loss of appetite, sleep issues, abdominal pain, numbness and tingling, slower than normal heart rate, blurry vision, blood sugar regulation issues and in severe cases, beriberi, premenstrual syndrome
Def. in Pregnancy	Preconception thiamine deficiency and severe pregnancy nausea are the primary causes of deficiency. Deficiency is associated with IUGR, SGA, weight loss, and gestational diabetes. Wernicke's encephalopathy is an extreme outcome of thiamine deficiency associated with HG. *Thiamine deficiency preconception is more common with concurrent pregnancies.*
General Excess SXS	No established symptoms of toxicity *The body can reduce absorption and secrete excess thiamine through the urine, reducing the risk of toxicity.*
Excess in Pregnancy	No known issues

This information is for resource purposes. All RDA recommended values were taken from the Food and Nutrition Board, Institute of Medicine – National Academy of Sciences Dietary Reference Intakes: Recommendations for Individuals. (Institute of Medicine 2000) These values are outdated.

Prenatal Dietary Reference Intakes

Vitamin B2	
RDA/AI Pregnancy	
14 – 50 years	1.4 mg
UL	No limit
General Def. SXS	Lesion in the corners of the mouth, swelling of the tongue, mouth, or throat, swollen and cracked lips, hair loss, chronic sore through, loss of or hoarse voice, ringing in the ears, headaches, itchy and dry eyes, skin rash, anemia
Def. in Pregnancy	Preeclampsia
General Excess SXS	Yellowing of the urine can occur as excess riboflavin is excreted. High doses (greater than 400 mg/day) can also cause diarrhea or increased urination.
Excess in Pregnancy	No known issues

This information is for resource purposes. All RDA recommended values were taken from the Food and Nutrition Board, Institute of Medicine – National Academy of Sciences Dietary Reference Intakes: Recommendations for Individuals. (Institute of Medicine 2000) These values are outdated.

Vitamin B3	
RDA/AI Pregnancy **14 – 50 mg**	18 mg
UL	35 mg
General Def. SXS	Rash that occurs after exposure to sunlight or at areas of pressure points, such as the bottoms of the feet and around the hands like gloves, swelling in the mouth with pain, bright red tongue, headache, nausea and vomiting, diarrhea, fatigue, depression, confusion, poor memory, history of painful periods, miscarriages, and in severe cases, pellagra
Def. in Pregnancy	Birth defects and pregnancy gingivitis
General Excess SXS	Skin flushing, increased heart rate, itching, nausea and vomiting, abdominal pain, diarrhea, gout, liver damage, stroke
Excess in Pregnancy	No known issues *Serious adverse effects have not been documented until doses reach much higher amounts of 3,000 mg or more per day over a long time.*[340]

This information is for resource purposes. All RDA recommended values were taken from the Food and Nutrition Board, Institute of Medicine – National Academy of Sciences Dietary Reference Intakes: Recommendations for Individuals. (Institute of Medicine 2000) These values are outdated.

Prenatal Dietary Reference Intakes

	Vitamin B5
RDA/AI Pregnancy	
14 – 50 years	(AI) 6 mg
UL	No limit *B5 has been well tolerated in studies using up to 1,200 mg/day with only mild gastric side effects.
General Def. SXS	Numbness and tingling in the hands and feet, headaches, extreme fatigue, irritability, restlessness, sleep issues, stomach pain, heartburn, diarrhea, nausea and vomiting, loss of appetite, muscle cramps
Def. in Pregnancy	Deficiency in early pregnancy is associated with pregnancy loss.
General Excess SXS	Symptoms of upset stomach and diarrhea have been seen at doses of 1,000–1,200 mg/day, but overdosing on dietary intake or normal supplementation doses have not been observed.
Excess in Pregnancy	No known issues

This information is for resource purposes. All RDA recommended values were taken from the Food and Nutrition Board, Institute of Medicine – National Academy of Sciences Dietary Reference Intakes: Recommendations for Individuals. (Institute of Medicine 2000) These values are outdated.

	Vitamin B6
RDA/AI Pregnancy	
14 – 50 years	1.9 mg
UL	80–100 mg *Dependent on age*
General Def. SXS	Depression and anxiety, mental confusion, poor memory, dandruff, irritations, and rashes in the folds of the skin, dry and cracked lips and corners of the mouth, painful and shiny tongue, anemia, history of irregular menstrual cycles
Def. in Pregnancy	Deficiency is associated with pregnancy nausea, prenatal and postpartum depression, preeclampsia, and preterm labor. *Some studies show that B6 deficiency is one of the most common causes of anemia in pregnancy.*[341]
General Excess SXS	Sensitivity to light, tingling in the extremities, buzzing sensation in the feet *No toxicity symptoms have been seen in studies where dosages were below 200 mg/day. Toxicity symptoms are typically seen in greater than 500 mg/day doses.*[342]
Excess in Pregnancy	No known issues

This information is for resource purposes. All RDA recommended values were taken from the Food and Nutrition Board, Institute of Medicine – National Academy of Sciences Dietary Reference Intakes: Recommendations for Individuals. (Institute of Medicine 2000) These values are outdated.

Prenatal Dietary Reference Intakes

	Vitamin B7
RDA/AI Pregnancy	
14 – 50 years	(AI) 30 mcg
UL	No limit *Studies have shown that doses up to 200 mg are safe, with no adverse effects.*
General Def. SXS	Hair thinning and loss throughout the whole body, scaly rash around body openings (mouth, eyes, nose, perineum, ears), conjunctivitis, increased lactic acid production, increased acid in the urine, brittle nails, depression, fatigue, insomnia
Def. in Pregnancy	Birth defects and pregnancy loss can be seen in marginal biotin deficiency when general symptoms are not present.[343] It is also associated with gestational diabetes. *There is 50 percent reduction in biotin in the first trimester.*[344]
General Excess SXS	High doses of biotin have been known to interfere with thyroid lab results, mimicking Graves' disease and can persist for days after doses.[345]
Excess in Pregnancy	No known issues

This information is for resource purposes. All RDA recommended values were taken from the Food and Nutrition Board, Institute of Medicine – National Academy of Sciences Dietary Reference Intakes: Recommendations for Individuals. (Institute of Medicine 2000) These values are outdated.

Vitamin B9	
RDA/AI Pregnancy	
14 – 50 years	600 mcg
UL	1,000 mcg *Studies show that the upper limit for folate is based on flawed studies.*[346]
General Def. SXS	Fatigue, premature gray hair, mouth sores, tongue swelling, depression, anemia, fatigue, pale skin, central nail ridge, irritability, shortness of breath, recurrent miscarriages, increased homocysteine, heavy menstrual bleeding
Def. in Pregnancy	Birth defects, premature birth, low birth weight, placental abruption, and preeclampsia
General Excess SXS	Excess folate is excreted through the urine. High doses can mask B12 deficiency, and some patients with genetic methylation issues do worse on folate supplements. *Unmetabolized folate has unknown side effects.*
Excess in Pregnancy	Excess amounts of unmetabolized folic acid are associated with an increased risk of asthma and autism in newborns. These same risks have not been verified with dietary folate or natural folate use.

This information is for resource purposes. All RDA recommended values were taken from the Food and Nutrition Board, Institute of Medicine – National Academy of Sciences Dietary Reference Intakes: Recommendations for Individuals. (Institute of Medicine 2000) These values are outdated.

Prenatal Dietary Reference Intakes

Vitamin B12	
RDA/AI Pregnancy	
14 – 50 years	2.6 mcg
UL	No limit
General Def. SXS	Pale and yellow tinged skin, painful and sore tongue, mouth ulcers, tingling in the extremities, vision changes, irritability, depression, anemia, headaches, tinnitus, lightheadedness and dizziness, extreme fatigue, geographic tongue, deep tongue fissures, gray-brown nails, history of amenorrhea as well as heavy menstrual bleeding
Def. in Pregnancy	Birth defects, pregnancy loss, preterm labor, IUGR, SGA, placental insufficiency, HELLP syndrome, and preeclampsia
General Excess SXS	Increased acne and rosacea *There are certain, rare conditions where B12 supplementation is not recommended, such as Leber hereditary optic neuropathy aka Leber's Disease.
Excess in Pregnancy	No known issues

This information is for resource purposes. All RDA recommended values were taken from the Food and Nutrition Board, Institute of Medicine – National Academy of Sciences Dietary Reference Intakes: Recommendations for Individuals. (Institute of Medicine 2000) These values are outdated.

Vitamin C	
RDA/AI Pregnancy	
14 – 18 years 19 – 50 years	80 mg 85 mg
UL	2,000 mg
General Def. SXS	Rough and bumpy skin patches, changes in hair structure, weak hair, bright red hair follicles, spoon-shaped fingernails, red spots in fingernails, dry and weak skin, easy bruising, slow wound healing, joint pain, bleeding gums and gum inflammation, frequent colds, anemia, history of heavy menstrual bleeding
Def. in Pregnancy	Birth defects, preterm labor, placental insufficiency, IUGR, SGA, stillbirth, premature rupture of membranes and preeclampsia, placental abruption *Up to 13 percent of pregnant women are deficient in vitamin C, even when taking a prenatal vitamin supplement.*[347]
General Excess SXS	Diarrhea, nausea and vomiting, heartburn, abdominal cramps, headache, insomnia, increased estrogen
Excess in Pregnancy	Some studies link excess vitamin C intake, primarily through supplementation, with preterm labor.

This information is for resource purposes. All RDA recommended values were taken from the Food and Nutrition Board, Institute of Medicine – National Academy of Sciences Dietary Reference Intakes: Recommendations for Individuals. (Institute of Medicine 2000) These values are outdated.

Choline	
RDA/AI Pregnancy	
14 – 50 years	(AI) 450 mg
UL	3,500 mg
General Def. SXS	Anxiety, fatigue, reduced ability to problem solve, difficulty in retaining new information, muscle aches, tingling in the extremities, restlessness, liver inflammation, increasing homocysteine
Def. in Pregnancy	Fetal growth issues and gestational diabetes *Ninety-five percent of pregnant women are not meeting the RDA requirements for choline, with >50 percent being confirmed deficient with blood analysis.*
General Excess SXS	Low blood pressure, sweating, excessive salivation, diarrhea, fishy body odor
Excess in Pregnancy	No known issues

This information is for resource purposes. All RDA recommended values were taken from the Food and Nutrition Board, Institute of Medicine – National Academy of Sciences Dietary Reference Intakes: Recommendations for Individuals. (Institute of Medicine 2000) These values are outdated.

Chromium	
RDA/AI Pregnancy	
14 – 18 years **19 – 50 years**	(AI) 29 mcg (AI) 30 mcg
UL	No limit *Some researchers suggest an UL of 1,000 mcg, yet some other studies show that doses of 1,000 mcg are required to elicit the desired effects. Currently, there is no known UL and few side effects are linked to higher chromium doses.*
General Def. SXS	Craving for sweets, depression, weight gain, poor metabolic function, elevated cholesterol, numbness and tingling in the extremities, anxiety, fatigue, muscle weakness, history of PCOS
Def. in Pregnancy	Gestational diabetes
General Excess SXS	No established symptoms of toxicity *Known toxicity symptoms are caused by the hexavalent chromium compounds found in workplace environments and most toxicity is related to inhalation. Dietary and supplemental chromium is not associated with these same toxicity symptoms.*
Excess in Pregnancy	Studies show that excess chromium can increase oxidative stress and affect fetal growth.[348]

This information is for resource purposes. All RDA recommended values were taken from the Food and Nutrition Board, Institute of Medicine – National Academy of Sciences Dietary Reference Intakes: Recommendations for Individuals. (Institute of Medicine 2000) These values are outdated.

Prenatal Dietary Reference Intakes

Copper	
RDA/AI Pregnancy	
14 – 18 years	1 mg
UL	10 mg *Excess copper is excreted through the urine and stools; excess is more common in patients with chronic liver diseases such as hepatitis.
General Def. SXS	Fatigue, frequent colds, brittle teeth and bones, arthritis and joint pain, sensitivity to cold, pale skin, premature gray hair, vision changes, easy bruising, anemia, symptoms mimic B vitamin deficiency symptoms
Def. in Pregnancy	Pregnancy loss and birth defects in the first trimester, poor fetal lung development
General Excess SXS	Yellowing of the skin and eyes (jaundice), Kayser-Fleischer rings around the eyes, abdominal cramps with black stools and diarrhea, headaches, depression, sudden and unexplained changes in mood
Excess in Pregnancy	Excess copper has been associated with an increased risk of preeclampsia secondary to a buildup in the liver, IUGR and small for gestational age due to oxidative stress in the placenta.[349]

This information is for resource purposes. All RDA recommended values were taken from the Food and Nutrition Board, Institute of Medicine – National Academy of Sciences Dietary Reference Intakes: Recommendations for Individuals. (Institute of Medicine 2000) These values are outdated.

Iodine	
RDA/AI Pregnancy	
14 – 50 years	220 mcg
UL	900–1,000 mcg *Depending on age*
General Def. SXS	Swelling of the neck, unexpected weight gain, fatigue, hair loss, dry skin, feeling cold, slow heart rate, lightheadedness and dizziness, poor memory, hypothyroidism, recurrent miscarriage, heavy or irregular menses
Def. in Pregnancy	Fetal hypothyroidism, pregnancy loss, birth defects, stillbirth, IUGR, SGA, placental insufficiency, and poor cognition in children
General Excess SXS	Nausea and vomiting, metallic taste in the mouth, burning pain in the mouth, coughing, gum, and tooth pain
Excess in Pregnancy	Severe vomiting, fetal goiter *This was seen in a single case study where a patient was taking 62.5x the RDA for iodine in pregnancy.*[350]

This information is for resource purposes. All RDA recommended values were taken from the Food and Nutrition Board, Institute of Medicine – National Academy of Sciences Dietary Reference Intakes: Recommendations for Individuals. (Institute of Medicine 2000) These values are outdated.

Prenatal Dietary Reference Intakes

	Iron
RDA/AI Pregnancy	
14 – 50 mg	27 mg
UL	45 mg
General Def. SXS	Extreme fatigue, weakness, pale complexion, rapid heart rate, shortness of breath, headaches, lightheadedness and dizziness, cold hands and feet, inflammation and soreness of the tongue, brittle nails and hair, central nail ridge or groove, spoon-shaped nails, restless leg, anemia
Def. in Pregnancy	Anemia, low birth weight, larger placenta to fetus size ratio, preeclampsia, placenta previa, placental abruption, premature labor, prenatal and postpartum depression, and reduced milk supply postpartum
General Excess SXS	Stomach cramping, nausea and vomiting, fever and chills, diarrhea with blood, back and groin pain, flushing, numbness and tingling in the extremities, metallic taste in the mouth
Excess in Pregnancy	Gestational diabetes and oxidative stress that is associated with hypertension and preeclampsia

This information is for resource purposes. All RDA recommended values were taken from the Food and Nutrition Board, Institute of Medicine – National Academy of Sciences Dietary Reference Intakes: Recommendations for Individuals. (Institute of Medicine 2000) These values are outdated.

Phosphorus	
RDA/AI Pregnancy	
14 – 18 years 19 – 50 years	1,250 mg 700 mg
UL	4,000 mg
General Def. SXS	Weak bones and teeth, joint pain and stiffness, bone pain, fatigue, lack of appetite, frequent colds, anemia *Deficiency is rare and is seen in severe cases of malnutrition.*
Def. in Pregnancy	Increased phosphorus excretion is seen in preeclampsia, placental calcification, and poor fetal development.[351] [352] *There is little to no research on the effects of low phosphorus on the increased risk of pregnancy complications.*
General Excess SXS	Muscle cramps and spasms, numbness and tingling around the mouth, bone pain, itchy skin *Excess phosphorus in the diet and through supplementation is rare; excess blood phosphorus is more likely to occur in cases of kidney disease, excess vitamin D, and ketogenic diets.*
Excess in Pregnancy	Calcium and phosphate are the primary components of placental calcification, yet excess dietary intake have not been connected as a cause of calcification. Other factors seem to be at play and this condition is not directly associated with excess intake.

This information is for resource purposes. All RDA recommended values were taken from the Food and Nutrition Board, Institute of Medicine – National Academy of Sciences Dietary Reference Intakes: Recommendations for Individuals. (Institute of Medicine 2000) These values are outdated.

Prenatal Dietary Reference Intakes

	Potassium
RDA/AI Pregnancy	
14 – 18 years 19 – 50 years	(AI) 2,600 mg (AI) 2,900 mg *Outside of pregnancy, the RDA for potassium is 4,700 mg. There is no good information on why the AI is less in pregnancy. This is another value that needs revision.
UL	No limit
General Def. SXS	Fatigue, weakness, muscle cramps and spasms, muscle twitching, edema, constipation and bloating with normal to loose stools, heart palpitations, hypertension, poor circulation, numbness and tingling, shortness of breath, increased urination of profuse clear urine
Def. in Pregnancy	Gestational diabetes, preeclampsia, and HELLP syndrome
General Excess SXS	Shortness of breath, pain in the chest, unusual heart rate *Extra potassium is removed via the kidneys and excess is uncommon. The most common causes of excess potassium in the blood are dehydration, diabetes, kidney disease, medications, Addison's disease, and anemia.
Excess in Pregnancy	Higher blood values of potassium in the first trimester are associated with a greater risk of preeclampsia and gestational diabetes. *These higher values are not due to excess potassium intake but other mechanisms that change potassium metabolism and balance in the body.[353]

This information is for resource purposes. All RDA recommended values were taken from the Food and Nutrition Board, Institute of Medicine – National Academy of Sciences Dietary Reference Intakes: Recommendations for Individuals. (Institute of Medicine 2000) These values are outdated.

Magnesium	
RDA/AI Pregnancy	
14 – 18 years 19 – 30 years 31 – 50 years	400 mg 350 mg 360 mg
UL	350 mg *There is some conflict with the RDA for pregnancy, and doses needed during pregnancy are often significantly greater. There is also conflict over this UL as it is based on the dose that may cause diarrhea and is not based on supplement form, which varies on its effects on the gut.
General Def. SXS	Calf cramps and charley horses, muscle twitching, restless leg, muscle fatigue, reduced emotion (not depression, but a lack of emotional response), hypertension, irregular heart rate, history of painful periods
Def. in Pregnancy	Pregnancy nausea, gestational hypertension, preeclampsia, IUGR/small for gestational age (SGA), and impaired placental development and function
General Excess SXS	Nausea, vomiting, diarrhea, hypotension *Overdose is rare and seen in patients with kidney disease or when IV magnesium is used.
Excess in Pregnancy	Hypotension

This information is for resource purposes. All RDA recommended values were taken from the Food and Nutrition Board, Institute of Medicine – National Academy of Sciences Dietary Reference Intakes: Recommendations for Individuals. (Institute of Medicine 2000) These values are outdated.

Prenatal Dietary Reference Intakes

Manganese	
RDA/AI Pregnancy	
14 – 50 years	(AI) 2 mg
UL	11 mg
General Def. SXS	Glucose dysregulation, metabolic changes, brittle teeth and bones, history of fertility issues
Def. in Pregnancy	IUGR, SGA *Little is known about how deficiencies and excesses of manganese in pregnancy affects both mother and baby. Studies do find deficiency connections to IUGR and SGA. Studies not specific to pregnancy showed lower HA concentrations in manganese deficiency.[354]
General Excess SXS	No established symptoms of toxicity *Toxicity is commonly seen in workplaces that use manganese. Symptoms are associated with inhalation where the mineral is transported directly to the brain and liver, causing liver damage and neurological changes. Neurological symptoms, like Parkinson's disease, have been seen with manganese-contaminated water.
Excess in Pregnancy	No known issues *No known issues with dietary consumption. Environmental manganese is associated with neurological issues in babies, including lower dopamine levels.[355]

This information is for resource purposes. All RDA recommended values were taken from the Food and Nutrition Board, Institute of Medicine – National Academy of Sciences Dietary Reference Intakes: Recommendations for Individuals. (Institute of Medicine 2000) These values are outdated.

Molybdenum	
RDA/AI Pregnancy	
14 – 50 years	50 mcg
UL	2,000 mcg
General Def. SXS	No known *Deficiency is rare, and the only documented cases are in patients with Crohn's disease receiving parenteral nutrition.
Def. in Pregnancy	No known *Secondary molybdenum deficiency can be seen genetically and is commonly diagnosed during pregnancy. This condition affects the fetus and not the mother. There has only been one case of deficiency known, and it was in a patient requiring parenteral nutrition.
General Excess SXS	No established symptoms of toxicity *There has only been one documented case of toxicity from dietary and supplemental intake that resulted in hallucination, seizures, and neurological symptoms. The UL was determined by assessing reproductive function in rats given high doses.
Excess in Pregnancy	No issues *Excess molybdenum interferes with copper levels and can cause copper deficiency. (Institute of Medicine 1990)

This information is for resource purposes. All RDA recommended values were taken from the Food and Nutrition Board, Institute of Medicine – National Academy of Sciences Dietary Reference Intakes: Recommendations for Individuals. (Institute of Medicine 2000) These values are outdated.

Selenium	
RDA/AI Pregnancy	
14 – 50 years	60 mcg
UL	400 mcg *The UL is set based on the prevention of weakening hair and nails in early selenium toxicity.*
General Def. SXS	Fatigue, hypothyroidism, hair loss, mental fog, muscle weakness, frequent colds, history of infertility
Def. in Pregnancy	Hypothyroidism, low birth weight, pregnancy loss, IUGR, SGA, birth defects, and retained placenta.[356]
General Excess SXS	Weakening of the hair and nails, skin rashes, fatigue, irritability, garlic breath odor
Excess in Pregnancy	There are no cases of toxicity in pregnancy; all cases and studies have been done in nonpregnancy individuals.[357]

This information is for resource purposes. All RDA recommended values were taken from the Food and Nutrition Board, Institute of Medicine – National Academy of Sciences Dietary Reference Intakes: Recommendations for Individuals. (Institute of Medicine 2000) These values are outdated.

Sodium	
RDA/AI Pregnancy	
14 – 50 years	(AI) 1,500 mg
UL	2,300 mg
General Def. SXS	Restlessness, headaches, muscle weakness and cramps, confusion, poor balance, lightheadedness, sluggishness, nausea, hypotension *Sodium deficiency is more often caused by overhydration and lack of sodium in the diet.*
Def. in Pregnancy	Deficiency is associated with nausea and vomiting, excessive heat, hypotension, early-stage preeclampsia, and an increased risk of hemorrhage.[358][359]
General Excess SXS	Edema, nausea, vomiting and stomach cramping, hypertension and hypotension dependent on cause, kidney stones
Excess in Pregnancy	Excess sodium, whether due to excess in the diet, or deficiencies in other electrolytes is associated with edema and gestational hypertension (not preeclampsia) and gestational diabetes although the gestational diabetes mellitus (GDM) causes elevations in sodium.

This information is for resource purposes. All RDA recommended values were taken from the Food and Nutrition Board, Institute of Medicine – National Academy of Sciences Dietary Reference Intakes: Recommendations for Individuals. (Institute of Medicine 2000) These values are outdated.

Prenatal Dietary Reference Intakes

	Zinc
RDA/AI Pregnancy	
14 – 18 years **19 – 50 years**	12 mg 11 mg
UL	34–40 mg *Dependent on age*
General Def. SXS	Weight loss, poor wound healing, decreased sense of smell and taste, diarrhea, loss of appetite, depression, anemia, blood sugar dysregulation, transverse depression across the nail from lack of nail growth period, white spots in nails, recurrent miscarriages, infertility
Def. in Pregnancy	Birth defects, pregnancy loss, IUGR, SGA, placental insufficiency, gestational diabetes, preeclampsia, preterm labor, prolonged labor, and retained placenta[360]
General Excess SXS	Metallic taste in the mouth, increased sweating, stomach pain, diarrhea, headaches, low copper, anemia, low white blood cells *There is no storage of zinc and symptoms disappear after removal of high-dose supplements if diagnosed early. Ignoring early signs and continuing dosing can lead to more systemic issues such as lower HDL cholesterol, impaired immune function, and anemia. These symptoms are typically seen in doses greater than 100 mg/day.* [361]
Excess in Pregnancy	Excess zinc in supplemental form can cause deficiencies in copper.

This information is for resource purposes. All RDA recommended values were taken from the Food and Nutrition Board, Institute of Medicine – National Academy of Sciences Dietary Reference Intakes: Recommendations for Individuals. (Institute of Medicine 2000) These values are outdated.

Appendix B

Glossary of Terms

Acetylation – The addition of an acetic acid somewhere in chemistry.

Alternative Medicine – A range of medicinal approaches that are not part of the conventional/western medical model.

Anabolic Metabolism – The energetic action that creates larger molecules from smaller molecules, as in the storage of glucose and fatty acids as triglycerides.

Antiemetic – Preventing vomiting.

Antioxidants – Innate and dietary substances that inhibit oxidation.

Apoptosis – Programmed and controlled cell death.

Assimilation – The biological absorption and processing of dietary nutrients.

Bisphenol-A – A synthetic, organic compound used in the manufacturing of plastics.

Catabolic Metabolism – The breakdown of stored larger molecules into smaller units.

Cellular Metabolism – The chemical changes in which basic chemicals are broken down into energy while other chemicals are removed.

Conventional/Western Medicine – Modern medical approach consisting of scientific diagnosis of disease and treatment with medications and surgical procedures.

Elucidate – To explain or make clear by explanation of analysis.

Glossary of Terms

Epigenetics – The study of modifications to genetic code versus alterations to the genetic code.

Erythropoiesis – The chemical formation of red blood cells.

Etiology – The origin of disease.

Fetal Programming – The effects of maternal influences and environment on the genetic transcription of genes during embryonic and fetal development.

Fluoridation – The addition of fluoride to water, food, or other substrates.

Gestation – The time between conception and birth that an infant is carried in the womb.

Gluconeogenesis – The process by which glucose is generated from noncarbohydrate sources, such as the breakdown of protein.

Glycogenolysis – The process by which glycogen is broken down into simple glucose.

Hemolysis – The disintegration and destruction of red blood cells due to various causes.

Hyperinsulinemia – An elevation of insulin in the blood, with or without the diagnosis of diabetes.

Hypoglycemia – Clinical and measurable decrease of sugar in the bloodstream.

In Vitro Fertilization – A medical procedure in which an egg is fertilized outside of the womb and implanted once embryonic development has begun.

Insulin Resistance – A dysfunctional cellular response to insulin that results in elevated levels of blood glucose levels.

Methylation – The addition of a methyl group somewhere in chemistry.

Nucleic Acid – A complex of nucleotides.

Nucleotides – The basic structural unit of nucleic acids.

Oxidation – A chemical reaction that gains an oxygen and changes the chemical structure of a substance.

Parturition – The processes and actions of giving birth.

Peroxidation – A chain reaction of oxidization reactions that degrades lipids.

Phosphorylation – The addition of a phosphate group somewhere in chemistry.

Phytonutrients – A nonvitamin substance found in plants that has been shown to have beneficial effects in human health.

Reactive Oxygen Species – Highly reactive chemicals that create oxidation.

Steroidogenesis – The biological process in which reproductive and steroid hormones are created.

Surfactants – A complex mixture of fats, carbohydrates, and proteins that affects and reduces the surface tension of liquids lining the alveoli, allowing for lung expansion.

Traditional Chinese Medicine – A form of medicine, originating from China, that is based on Confucianism and the observations of nature to describe and treat medical conditions.

Vasodilation – To open, expand, or dilate blood vessels.

Notes

1 Fallon S, Enig M. *Nourishing Traditions.* Revised 2nd Edition. Brandywine, MD: New Trends Publishing; 2001.

2 GBD 2015 Maternal Mortality Collaborators. Global, regional, and national levels of maternal mortality, 1990–2015: a systematic analysis for the global burden of disease study 2015. *Lancet.* 2016;388(10053):1775–1812. doi:10.1016/S0140-6736(16)31470-2

3 Main EK, Menard MK. Maternal mortality: time for national action. *Obstet Gynecol.* 2013 Oct;122(4):735–736. doi:10.1097/AOG.0b013e3182a7dc8c

4 Adams KM, Lindell KC, Kohlmeier M, Zeisel SH. Status of nutrition education in medical schools. *Am J Clin Nutr.* 2006;83(4):941S-944S. doi:10.1093/ajcn/83.4.941S

5 Adams KM, Butsch WS, Kohmeier M. The state of nutrition education at US medical schools. J. Biomed. Edu. 2015;357627. doi: 10.1155/2015/357627

6 Vetter ML, Herring SJ, Sood M, Shah NR, Kalet AL. What do resident physicians know about nutrition: An evaluation of attitudes, self-perceived proficiency, and knowledge. *J Am Coll Nutr.* 2008;27(2):287–298. doi:10.1080/07315724.2008.10719702

7 Centers for Disease Control and Prevention. School health guidelines to promote healthy eating and physical activity. *MMWR.* 2011;60(RR05):1–76. Available at https://www.cdc.gov/healthyschools/npao/strategies.htm

8 Food and Nutrition Board; Board on Children, Youth, and Families; Institute of Medicine. *Nutrition Education in the K-12 Curriculum: The Role of National Standards: Workshop Summary.* Washington (DC): National Academies Press (US); 2013. Available from: https://www.ncbi.nlm.nih.gov/books/NBK202128/?term=Nutrition%20Education%20in%20the%20K-12%20Curriculum

9 US Department of Health and Human Services and US Department of Agriculture. *2015–2020 Dietary Guidelines for Americans. 8th Edition.* December 2015. Available at http://health.gov/dietaryguidelines/2015/guidelines/external icon

10 Eagle TF, Gurm R, Goldberg CS, DuRussel-Weston J, Kline-Rogers E, Palma-Davis L, Aaronson S, Fitzgerald CM, Mitchell LR, Rogers B, Bruenger P, Jackson EA, Eagle KA. Health status and behavior among middle-school children in a Midwest community: What are the underpinnings of childhood obesity? *Am Heart J.* 2019;160(6):1185–1189. doi:10.1016/j.ahj.2010.09.019

11 Mayer-Davis EJ, Lawrence JM, Dabelea D, et al. Incidence trends of type 1 and type 2 diabetes among youths, 2002–2012. *N Engl J Med.* 2017;376(15):1419–1429. doi:10.1056/NEJMoa1610187

12 McKenna MJ, Murray BF. Vitamin D dose response is underestimated by Endocrine Society's Clinical Practice Guideline. *Endocr Connect.* 2013;2(2):87–95. Published 2013 Apr 12. doi:10.1530/EC-13-0008

13 Holick MF, Binkley NC, Bischoff-Ferrari HA, Gordon CM, Hanley DA, Heaney RP, Murad MH, Weaver CM. Evaluation, treatment, and prevention of vitamin D deficiency: An Endocrine Society clinical practice guideline. *J Clin Endocrinol Metab.* 2011;96:1191–1930. doi:10.1210/jc.2011-0385

14 Hollis BW, Wagner CL. *Vitamin D in pregnancy and lactation: A new paradigm.* 2nd ed. Springer Intl Publishing; 2018:32. https://link.springer.com/chapter/10.1007%2F978-3-319-90988-2_4.

15 Raghupathi W, Raghupathi V. An Empirical study of chronic diseases in the United States: A visual analytics approach. *Int J Environ Res Public Health.* 2018;15(3):431. Published 2018 Mar 1. doi:10.3390/ijerph15030431

16 Roberts JM, Balk JL, Bodnar LM, Belizán JM, Bergel E, Martinez A. Nutrient involvement in preeclampsia. *J Nutr.* 2003;133(5):1684S–1692S. doi:10.1093/jn/133.5.1684S

17 Ikem, E, Halldorsson, TI, Birgisdóttir, BE, Rasmussen, MA, Olsen, SF, Maslova, E. Dietary patterns and the risk of pregnancy-associated hypertension in the Danish national birth cohort: a prospective longitudinal study. *BJOG.* 2019; 126:663–673. doi:10.1111/1471-0528.15593

18 Zhu Z, Cao F, Li X. Epigenetic programming and fetal metabolic programming. *Front Endocrinol.* 2019;10:764. doi:10.3389/fendo.2019.00764

19 Ravelli GP, Stein ZA, Susser MW. Obesity in young men after famine exposure in utero and early infancy. *N Engl J Med.* 1976;295:349–353. doi:10.1056/NEJM197608122950701

20 Hemond J, Robbins RB, Young PC. The effects of maternal obesity on neonates, infants, children, adolescents, and adults. *Clin Obstet Gynecol.* 2016;59:216–227. doi:10.1097/GRF.0000000000000179

21 Aiken CE, Tarry-Adkins JL, Penfold NC, Dearden L, Ozanne SE. Decreased ovarian reserve, dysregulation of mitochondrial biogenesis, and increased lipid peroxidation in female mouse offspring exposed to an obesogenic maternal diet. *FASEB J.* 2016;30:1548–1556. doi:10.1096/fj.15-280800

22 Nguyen LT, Saad S, Tan Y, Pollock C, Chen H. Maternal high-fat diet induces metabolic stress response disorders in offspring hypothalamus. *J Mol Endocrinol.* 2017;59:81–92. doi:10.1530/JME-17-0056

23 Wang Q, Huang R, Yu B, Cao F, Wang H, Zhang M, et al. Higher fetal insulin resistance in Chinese pregnant women with gestational diabetes mellitus and correlation with maternal insulin resistance. *PLoS ONE.* 2013;8:e59845. doi:10.1371/journal.pone.0059845

24 Pinney SE, Simmons RA. Metabolic programming, epigenetics, and gestational diabetes mellitus. *Curr Diab Rep.* 2012;12:67–74. doi:10.1007/s11892-011-0248-1

25 Menezo Y, Clément P, Dale B. DNA Methylation Patterns in the early human embryo and the epigenetic/imprinting problems: A plea for a more careful approach to human assisted reproductive technology (ART). *Int J Mol Sci.* 2019;20(6):1342. doi:10.3390/ijms20061342

26 Warita K, Mitsuhashi T, Ohta K, et al. Gene expression of epigenetic regulatory factors related to primary silencing mechanism is less susceptible to lower doses of bisphenol A in embryonic hypothalamic cells. *J Toxicol Sci.* 2013;38(2):285–289. doi:10.2131/jts.38.285

27 McKillop DJ, McNulty H, Scott JM, McPartlin JM, Strain JJ, Bradbury I, Girvan J, Hoey L, McCreedy R, Alexander J, Patterson BK, Hannon-Fletcher M, Pentieva K. The rate of intestinal absorption of natural food folates is not related to the extent of folate conjugation. *Am J Clin Nutr.* 2006;84(1):167–173. doi:10.1093/ajcn/84.1.167

28 Wallace TC, Fulgoni VL. Usual Choline Intakes Are Associated with Egg and Protein Food Consumption in the United States. *Nutrients.* 2017;9(8):839. doi:10.3390/nu908083

29 Christensen KE, Mikael LG, Leung KY, Lévesque N, Deng L, Wu Q, Malysheva OV, Best A, Caudill MA, Greene NDE, Rozen R. High folic acid consumption leads to pseudo-MTHFR deficiency, altered lipid metabolism, and liver injury in mice. *Am J Clin Nut.* 2015;101(3): 646–658. doi:10.3945/ajcn.114.086603

30 DeSoto MC, HItlan R. Synthetic folic acid supplementation during pregnancy may increase the risk of developing autism. *J Pediatr Biochem.* 2012;2:251–261. doi:10.3233/JPB-120066

31 Wiens D, DeSoto MC. Is High Folic Acid Intake a Risk Factor for Autism?—A Review. *Brain Sciences.* 2017;7(11):149. doi:0.3390/brainsci7110149

32 Zhu Z, Cao F, Li X. Epigenetic programming and fetal metabolic programming. *Front Endocrinol.* 2019;10:764. doi:10.3389/fendo.2019.00764

33 Seto E, Yoshida M. Erasers of histone acetylation: the histone deacetylase enzymes. *Cold Spring Harb Perspect Biol.* 2014;6(4):a018713. doi:10.1101/cshperspect.a018713

34 Puppala S, Li C, Glenn JP, Saxena R, Gawrieh S, Quinn A, et al. Primate fetal hepatic responses to maternal obesity: epigenetic signaling pathways and lipid accumulation. *J Physiol.* 2018;596:5823–5837. doi:10.1113/JP275422

35 Aagaard-Tillery KM, Grove K, Bishop J, Ke X, Fu Q, McKnight R, et al. Developmental origins of disease and determinants of chromatin structure: maternal diet modifies the primate fetal epigenome. *J Mol Endocrinol.* 2008; 41:91–102. doi:10.1677/JME-08-0025

36 Begum G, Stevens A, Smith EB, Connor K, Challis JR, Bloomfield F, et al. Epigenetic changes in fetal hypothalamic energy regulating pathways are associated with maternal undernutrition and twinning. *FASEB J.* 2012;26:1694–1703. doi:10.1096/fj.11-198762

37 Stevens A, Begum G, Cook A, Connor K, Rumball C, Oliver M, et al. Epigenetic changes in the hypothalamic proopiomelanocortin and glucocorticoid receptor genes in the ovine fetus after periconceptional undernutrition. *Endocrinology.* 2010;151:3652–3664. doi:10.1210/en.2010-0094

38 Ramon-Krauel M, Pentinat T, Bloks VW, Cebria J, Ribo S, Perez-Wienese R, et al. Epigenetic programming at the Mogat1 locus may link neonatal overnutrition with long-term hepatic steatosis and insulin resistance. *FASEB J.* 2018;32:6025–6037. doi:10.1096/fj.201700717RR

39 Shin JS, Choi MY, Longtine MS, Nelson DM. Vitamin D effects on pregnancy and the placenta. *Placenta.* 2010;31(12):1027–1034. doi:10.1016/j.placenta.2010.08.015

40 Schmidt M, Dogan C, Birdir C, et al. Placental growth factor: a predictive marker for preeclampsia? *Gynakol Geburtshilfliche Rundsch.* 2009;49(2):94–99. doi:10.1159/000197908

41 Wilson RL, Leemaqz SY, Goh Z, et al. Zinc is a critical regulator of placental morphogenesis and maternal hemodynamics during pregnancy in mice. *Sci Rep.* 2017;7(1):15137. doi:10.1038/s41598-017-15085-2

42 Thorsell A, Nätt D. Maternal stress and diet may influence affective behavior and stress-response in offspring via epigenetic regulation of central peptidergic function. *Environ Epigenet.* 2016;2(3):dvw012. doi:10.1093/eep/dvw012

43 Price, W. A. *Nutrition and physical degeneration; a comparison of primitive and modern diets and their effects.* New York, London: P.B. Hoeber. 1939

44 Duncan FE, Que EL, Zhang N, Feinberg EC, O'Halloran TV, Woodruff TK. The zinc spark is an inorganic signature of human egg activation. *Sci Rep.* 2016;6:24737. doi:10.1038/srep24737

45 Sandström B., Cederblad A. Zinc absorption from composite meals. Ii. Influence of the main protein source. *Am J Clin Nutr.* 1980;33:1778–1783. doi:10.1093/ajcn/33.8.1778

46 Lopez HW, Duclos V, Coudray C, et al. Making bread with sourdough improves mineral bioavailability from reconstituted whole wheat flour in rats. *Nutrition.* 2003;19(6):524–530. doi:10.1016/s0899-9007(02)01079-1

47 Mailloux RJ, Hamel R, Appanna VD. Aluminum toxicity elicits a dysfunctional TCA cycle and succinate accumulation in hepatocytes. J Biochem Mol Toxicol. 2006;20(4):198–208. doi:10.1002/jbt.20137

48 Lammi-Keefe C, Couch S, Kirwan J. *Handbook of Nutrition and Pregnancy. 2nd Edition.* Humana Press; 2018.

49 Voorhees JL, Rao GV, Gordon TJ, Brooks CL. Zinc binding to human lactogenic hormones and the human prolactin receptor. *FEBS Lett.* 2011;585(12):1783–1788. doi:10.1016/j.febslet.2011.04.019

50 Sussman D, van Eede M, Wong MD, Adamson SL, Henkelman M. Effects of a ketogenic diet during pregnancy on embryonic growth in the mouse. *BMC Pregnancy Childbirth.* 2013;13:109. doi:10.1186/1471-2393-13-109

51 Bartels Ä, Egan N, Broadhurst DI, et al. Maternal serum cholesterol levels are elevated from the 1st trimester of pregnancy: a cross-sectional study. *J Obstet Gynaecol.* 2012;32(8):747–752. doi:10.3109/01443615.2012.714017

52 Edison RJ, Berg K, Remaley A, et al. Adverse birth outcome among mothers with low serum cholesterol. *Pediatrics.* 2007;120(4):723–733. doi:10.1542/peds.2006-1939

53 Grimes SB, Wild R. *Effect of Pregnancy on Lipid Metabolism and Lipoprotein Levels. [Updated 2018 Feb 20].* In: Feingold KR, Anawalt B, Boyce A, et al., editors. Endotext [Internet]. South Dartmouth (MA): MDText.com, Inc.; 2000. Available from: https://www.ncbi.nlm.nih.gov/books/NBK498654/

54 Haruna M, Matsuzaki M, Ota E, et al. Positive correlation between maternal serum coenzyme Q10 levels and infant birth weight. *Biofactors.* 2010;36(4):312–318. doi:10.1002/biof.104

55 Kawamukai M. Biosynthesis and bioproduction of coenzyme Q(10) by yeasts and other organisms. *Biotechnol Appl Biochem.* 2010;53:217–226. doi:10.1042/BA20090035

56 Saini R. Coenzyme Q10: The essential nutrient. *J Pharm Bioallied Sci.* 2011;3(3):466–467. doi:10.4103/0975-7406.84471

57 Bentov Y, Hannam T, Jurisicova A, Esfandiari N, Casper RF. Coenzyme Q10 supplementation and oocyte aneuploidy in women undergoing IVF-ICSI treatment. *Clin Med Insights Reprod Health.* 2014;8:31–36. doi:10.4137/CMRH.S14681

58 Teran E, Hernández I, Tana L, et al. Mitochondria and Coenzyme Q10 in the Pathogenesis of Preeclampsia. *Front Physiol.* 2018;9:1561. doi:10.3389/fphys.2018.01561

59 Martinefski MR, Cocucci SE, Di Carlo MB, et al. Fetal coenzyme Q10 deficiency in intrahepatic cholestasis of pregnancy. *Clin Res Hepatol Gastroenterol.* 2020;44(3):368–374. doi:10.1016/j.clinre.2019.07.006

60 Giannubilo SR, Tiano L, Cecchi S, Principi F, Tranquilli AL, Littarru GP. Plasma coenzyme Q10 is increased during gestational diabetes. *Diabetes Res Clin Pract.* 2011;94(2):230–235. doi:10.1016/j.diabres.2011.07.007

61 Lopez MJ, Mohiuddin SS. *Biochemistry, Essential Amino Acids. [Updated 2020 Apr 26].* In: StatPearls [Internet]. Treasure Island (FL): StatPearls Publishing; 2020 Jan. Available from: https://www.ncbi.nlm.nih.gov/books/NBK557845/

62 Seong WJ. Chong GO, Hong DG, Lee TH, Lee YS, Cho YL, Chun SS, Park IS. Clinical significance of serum albumin level in pregnancy-related hypertension. *Gynecol Obstet Res.* 2010;36(6)1165–1173. doi:10.1111/j.1447-0756.2010.01296.x

63 Zeng Z, Liu F, Li S: Metabolic Adaptations in Pregnancy: A Review. *Ann Nutr Metab.* 2017;70:59–65. doi:10.1159/000459633

64 Napso T, Yong HEJ, Lopez-Tello J, Sferruzzi-Perri AN. The role of placental hormones in mediating maternal adaptations to support pregnancy and lactation. *Front Physiol.* 2018;9:1091. doi:10.3389/fphys.2018.01091

65 Hanukoglu I. Antioxidant protective mechanisms against reactive oxygen species (ROS) generated by mitochondrial P450 systems in steroidogenic cells. *Drug Metab Rev.* 2006;38(1–2):171–196. doi:10.1080/03602530600570040

66 Young FM, Luderer WB, Rodgers RJ. The antioxidant beta-carotene prevents covalent cross-linking between cholesterol side-chain cleavage cytochrome P450 and its electron donor, adrenodoxin, in bovine luteal cells. *Mol Cell Endocrinol.* 1995;109(1):113–118. doi:10.1016/0303-7207(95)03491-o

67 Starks MA, Starks SL, Kingsley M, Purpura M, Jäger R. The effects of phosphatidylserine on endocrine response to moderate intensity exercise. *J Int Soc Sports Nutr.* 2008;5:11. doi:10.1186/1550-2783-5-11

68 Lundqvist J. Vitamin D as a regulator of steroidogenic enzymes [version 1; peer review: 1 approved, 1 approved with reservations]. *F1000Research.* 2014;3:155. doi:10.12688/f1000research.4714.1

69 Su EJ, Cheng YH, Chatterton RT, Lin ZH, Yin P, Reierstad S, Innes J, Bulun SE. Regulation of 17-beta hydroxysteroid dehydrogenase type 2 in human placental endothelial cells, *Biol Reprod.* Sept 2007;77(3):517–525. doi:10.1095/biolreprod.106.059451

70 Valk EE, Hornstra G. Relationship between vitamin E requirement and polyunsaturated fatty acid intake in man: a review. *Int J Vitam Nutr Res.* 2000;70(2):31–42. doi:10.1024/0300-9831.70.2.31

71 Barnes MM, Smith AJ. The effects of vitamin E deficiency on some enzymes of steroid hormone biosynthesis. *Int J Vitam Nutr Res.* 1975;45(4):396–403. PMID: 1213866

72 Shirakawa H, Ohsaki Y, Minegishi Y, et al. Vitamin K deficiency reduces testosterone production in the testis through down-regulation of the Cyp11a a cholesterol side chain cleavage enzyme in rats. *Biochim Biophys Acta.* 2006;1760(10):1482–1488. doi:10.1016/j.bbagen.2006.05.008

73 Lundqvist J. Vitamin D as a regulator of steroidogenic enzymes [version 1; peer review: 1 approved, 1 approved with reservations]. *F1000Research.* 2014;3:155. doi:10.12688/f1000research.4714.1

74 Lundqvist J. Vitamin D as a regulator of steroidogenic enzymes [version 1; peer review: 1 approved, 1 approved with reservations]. *F1000Research*. 2014;3:155. doi:10.12688/f1000research.4714.1

75 Hollis BW, Wagner CL. *Vitamin D in pregnancy and lactation: A new paradigm*. 2nd ed. Springer Intl Publishing; 2018:32

76 Hollis BW, Hulsey TC, Ebeling M, Wagner CL. Vitamin D supplementation during pregnancy: double-blind, randomized clinical trial of safety and effectiveness. *J Bone Miner Res*. 2011;26(10):2341-2357

77 Hollis BW, Hulsey TC, Ebeling M, Wagner CL. Vitamin D supplementation during pregnancy: double-blind, randomized clinical trial of safety and effectiveness. *J Bone Miner Res*. 2011;26(10):2341-57

78 Wagner CL, McNeil R, Hamilton SA, et al. A randomized trial of vitamin D supplementation in 2 community health center networks in South Carolina. *Am J Obstet Gynecol*. 2013;208(2):137.e1-137.13. doi:10.1016/j.ajog.2012.10.888

79 Sablok A, Batra A, Thariani K, et al. Supplementation of vitamin D in pregnancy and its correlation with feto-maternal outcome. *Clin Endocrinol (Oxf)*. 2015;83(4):536–541. doi:10.1111/cen.12751

80 Mojibian M, Soheilykhah S, Fallah Zadeh MA, Jannati Moghadam M. The effects of vitamin D supplementation on maternal and neonatal outcome: A randomized clinical trial. *Iran J Reprod Med*. 2015;13(11):687–696. PMID: 26730243

81 Hollis BW, Wagner CL. *Vitamin D in pregnancy and lactation: A new paradigm*. 2nd ed. Springer Intl Publishing; 2018:32. doi:10.1002/jbmr.463

82 Halvorsen K. Vitamin E and progesterone. *Acta Pathologica Microbiologica Scandinavica*. 1944;(3):510–516. doi:10.1111/j.1699-0463.1944.tb04964.x

83 Tal R, Taylor HS, Burney RO, et al. *Endocrinology of Pregnancy*. [Updated 2021 Mar 18]. In: Feingold KR, Anawalt B, Boyce A, et al., editors. Endotext [Internet]. South Dartmouth (MA): MDText.com, Inc.; 2000. Available from: https://www.ncbi.nlm.nih.gov/books/NBK278962/

84 Berkane N, Liere P, Oudinet JP, Hertig A, Lefèvre G, Pluchino N, Schumacher M, Chabbert-Buffet N. From pregnancy to preeclampsia: A key role for estrogens. *Endocr Rev.* April 2017;38(2):123–144. doi:10.1210/er.2016-1065

85 Bai J, Qi QR, Li Y, et al. Estrogen receptors and estrogen-induced uterine vasodilation in pregnancy. *Int J Mol Sci.* 2020;21(12):4349. doi:10.3390/ijms21124349

86 Bai J, Qi QR, Li Y, et al. Estrogen receptors and estrogen-induced uterine vasodilation in pregnancy. *Int J Mol Sci.* 2020;21(12):4349. doi:10.3390/ijms21124349

87 University of Maryland at Baltimore. Science Daily. https://www.sciencedaily.com/releases/1997/03/970321141042.htm. Published March 21, 1997. Accessed February 14, 2021.

88 Kallak TK, Hellgren C, Skalkidou A, et al. Maternal and female fetal testosterone levels are associated with maternal age and gestational weight gain. *Eur J Endocrinol.* 2017;177(4):379–388. doi:10.1530/EJE-17-0207

89 Troisi R, Potischman N, Roberts JM, Harger G, Markovic N, Cole B, Lykins D, Siiteri P, Hoover RN. Correlation of serum hormone concentrations in maternal and umbilical cord samples. *Cancer Epidemiol Biomarkers Prev.* 2003; 12:452–456. PMID: 12750241

90 Quinn T, Greaves R, Badoer E, Walker D. DHEA in prenatal and postnatal Life: Implications for brain and behavior. *Vitam Horm.* 2018;108:145–174. doi:10.1016/bs.vh.2018.03.001

91 Leff-Gelman P, Flores-Ramos M, Carrasco A.E.Á. Cortisol and DHEA-S levels in pregnant women with severe anxiety. *BMC Psychiatry.* 2020;393. doi:10.1186/s12888-020-02788-6

92 Tagawa N, Hidaka Y, Takano T, Shimaoka Y, Kobayashi Y, Amino N. Serum concentrations of dehydroepiandrosterone and dehydroepiandrosterone sulfate and their relation to cytokine production during and after normal pregnancy. *Clin Chim Acta.* 2004;340(1–2):187–193. doi:10.1016/j.cccn.2003.10.018

93 Kota SK, Gayatri K, Jammula S, et al. Endocrinology of parturition. *Indian J Endocrinol Metab.* 2013;17(1):50–59. doi:10.4103/2230-8210.107841

94 Jung C, Ho JT, Torpy DJ, Rogers A, Doogue M, Lewis JG, Czajko RJ, Inder WJ. A longitudinal study of plasma and urinary cortisol in pregnancy and postpartum. *J Clin Endocrinol Metab.* 2011;96(5):1533–1540. doi:10.1210/jc.2010-2395

95 Golf SW, Happel O, Graef V, Seim KE. Plasma aldosterone, cortisol and electrolyte concentrations in physical exercise after magnesium supplementation. *J Clin Chem Clin Biochem.* 1984;22(11):717–721. doi:10.1515/cclm.1984.22.11.717

96 Sartori SB, Whittle N, Hetzenauer A, Singewald N. Magnesium deficiency induces anxiety and HPA axis dysregulation: modulation by therapeutic drug treatment. *Neuropharmacology.* 2012;62(1):304–312. doi:10.1016/j.neuropharm.2011.07.027

97 Cuciureanu MD, Vink R. Magnesium and stress. In: Vink R, Nechifor M, editors. *Magnesium in the Central Nervous System* [Internet]. Adelaide (AU): University of Adelaide Press; 2011. Available from: https://www.ncbi.nlm.nih.gov/books/NBK507250/

98 Keller-Wood M, Feng X, Wood CE, et al. Elevated maternal cortisol leads to relative maternal hyperglycemia and increased stillbirth in ovine pregnancy. *Am J Physiol Regul Integr Comp Physiol.* 2014;307(4):R405-R413. doi:10.1152/ajpregu.00530.2013

99 Verbeeten DK, Ahmet AH. The role of corticosteroid-binding globulin in the evaluation of adrenal insufficiency. *J Pediatr Endocrinol Metab.* 2017;31(2):107–115. doi:10.1515/jpem-2017-0270

100 Liggins GC. The role of cortisol in preparing the fetus for birth. *Reprod Fertil Dev.* 1994;6(2):141–150. doi:10.1071/rd9940141

101 Li J, Liu A, Liu H, et al. Maternal TSH levels at first trimester and subsequent spontaneous miscarriage: a nested case-control study. Endocr Connect. 2019;8(9):1288–1293. doi:10.1530/EC-19-0316

102 Kolanu BR, Vadakedath S, Boddula V, Kandi V. Activities of serum magnesium and thyroid hormones in pre-, peri-, and post-menopausal women. *Cureus.* 2020;12(1):e6554. doi:10.7759/cureus.6554

103 Kralik A, Eder K, Kirchgessner M. Influence of zinc and selenium deficiency on parameters relating to thyroid hormone metabolism. *Horm Metab Res.* 1996;28(5):223–226. doi:10.1055/s-2007-979169

104 Freake HC, Govoni KE, Guda K, Huang C, Zinn SA. Actions and interactions of thyroid hormone and zinc status in growing rats. *J Nutr.* 2001;131(4):1135–1141. doi:10.1093/jn/131.4.1135

105 Betsy A, Binitha M, Sarita S. Zinc deficiency associated with hypothyroidism: an overlooked cause of severe alopecia. *Int J Trichology.* 2013;5(1):40–42. doi:10.4103/0974-7753.114714

106 Fairweather-Tait SJ, Collings R, Hurst R. Selenium bioavailability: current knowledge and future research requirements. *Am J Clin Nutr.* 2010;91(5):1484S–1491S. doi:10.3945/ajcn.2010.28674J

107 Ventura M, Melo M, Carrilho F. Selenium and thyroid disease: from pathophysiology to treatment. *Int Journal of Endocrinology.* 2017. doi:10.1155/2017/1297658

108 Dunn JT. What's happening to our iodine? *J Clin Endocrin Metab.* 1998;83:3398–3400. doi:10.1210/jcem.83.10.5209

109 *How Molecular Iodine Attacks Breast Cancer.* Oncology Times: December 25, 2016;38(24):34. doi:10.1097/01.COT.0000511599.52147.f1

110 Wolff J, Chaikoff. Plasma inorganic iodide as a homeostatic regulator of thyroid function. *J Biol Chem.* 1948;174(2):555–564. doi:10.1016/S0021-9258(18)57335-X

111 Zava TT, Zava DT. Assessment of Japanese iodine intake based on seaweed consumption in Japan: A literature-based analysis. Thyroid Res. 2011;4:14. Published 2011 Oct 5. doi:10.1186/1756-6614-4-14

112 Patrick L. Iodine: Deficiency and therapeutic considerations. *Altern MedRev.* 2008;13:116–127. PMID: 18590348

113 Ahad F, Ganie SA. Iodine, Iodine metabolism and Iodine deficiency disorders revisited. *Indian J Endocrinol Metab.* 2010;14(1):13–17. PMID: 21448409

114 Foley TP Jr. The relationship between autoimmune thyroid disease and iodine intake: a review. *Endokrynol Pol.* 1992;43 Suppl 1:53–69. PMID: 1345585

115 Norman K. The persistence of methyl bromide residues in rice, dried fruit, seeds and nuts following laboratory fumigation. *Pest Manag Sci.* 2000;56:154–158. doi:10.1002/(SICI)1526-4998(200002)56

116 Buchberger W, Holler W, Winsauer K. Effects of sodium bromide on the biosynthesis of thyroid hormones and brominated/iodinated thyronines. *J Trace Elem Electrolytes Health Dis*. 1990;4(1):25–30. PMID: 2135954

117 Allain P, Berre S, Krari N, et al. Bromine and thyroid hormone activity. *J Clin Pathol*. 1993;46(5):456–458. doi:10.1136/jcp.46.5.456

118 Pavelka S. Metabolism of bromide and its interference with the metabolism of iodine. *Physiol Res*. 2004;53 Suppl 1:S81-S90. PMID: 15119938

119 Kheradpisheh Z, Mirzaei M, Mahvi AH, et al. Impact of drinking water fluoride on human thyroid hormones: A case-control study. *Sci Rep*. 2018;8(1):2674. doi:10.1038/s41598-018-20696-4

120 Clinical Thyroidology. Is fluoridated drinking water associated with a higher prevalence of hypothyroidism? American Thyroid Association. June 2015;8(6):3. https://www.thyroid.org/patient-thyroid-information/ct-for-patients/volume-8-issue-6/vol-8-issue-6-p-3/. Assessed 2/24/2021

121 Iddah MA, Macharia BN. Autoimmune thyroid disorders. *Int Sch Res Notices*. 2013. doi:10.1155/2013/509764

122 Kim D. The Role of Vitamin D in Thyroid Diseases. *Int J Mol Sci*. 2017;18(9):1949. doi:10.3390/ijms18091949

123 Prietl B., Treiber G., Pieber T.R., Amrein K. Vitamin D and immune function. *Nutrients*. 2013;5:2502–2521. doi:10.3390/nu5072502

124 Baeke F., Takiishi T., Korf H., Gysemans C., Mathieu C. Vitamin D: Modulator of the immune system. *Curr Opin Pharmacol*. 2010;10:482–496. doi:10.1016/j.coph.2010.04.001

125 Stagnaro-Green A, Roman SH, Cobin RH, el-Harazy E, Alvarez-Marfany M, Davies TF. Detection of at-risk pregnancy by means of highly sensitive assays for thyroid autoantibodies. *JAMA*. 1990;264(11):1422–1425. PMID: 2118190

126 Galofre JC, Davies TF. Autoimmune thyroid disease in pregnancy: a review. *J Womens Health (Larchmt)*. 2009;18(11):1847–1856. doi:10.1089/jwh.2008.1234

127 Negro R. Mangieri T. Coppola L, et al. Levothyroxine treatment in thyroid peroxidase antibody-positive women undergoing assisted reproduction technologies: A prospective study. *Hum Reprod.* 2005;20:1529–1533. doi:10.1093/humrep/deh843

128 Glinoer D. The regulation of thyroid function in pregnancy: Pathways of endocrine adaptation from physiology to pathology. *Endocr Rev.* 1997;18 (3):404–433. doi:10.1210/edrv.18.3.0300

129 Roti E, Fang SL, Emerson CH, Braverman LE. Human placenta is an active site of thyroxine and 33',5-triiodothyronine tyrosyl ring deiodination. *J Clin Endocrinol Metab.* 1981;53:498–501. doi:10.1210/jcem-53-3-498

130 Ayyavoo A, Derraik JG, Hofman PL, et al. Severe hyperemesis gravidarum is associated with reduced insulin sensitivity in the offspring in childhood. *J Clin Endocrinol Metab.* 2013;98(8):3263–3268. doi:10.1210/jc.2013-2043

131 Depue RH, Bernstein L, Ross RK, Judd HL and Henderson BE. Hyperemesis gravidarum in relation to estradiol levels, pregnancy outcome, and other maternal factors: a seroepidemiologic study. *Am J Obstet Gynecol.* 1986;156:1137–1141. doi:10.1016/0002-9378(87)90126-8

132 Järnfelt-Samsioe A, Samsioe G, Velinder GM. Nausea and vomiting in pregnancy—a contribution to its epidemiology. *Gynecol Obstet Invest.* 1983;16(4):221–229. doi:10.1159/000299262

133 Goodwin TM, Montoro M and Mestman JH. Transient hyperthyroidism and hyperemesis gravidarum: clinical aspects. *Am J Obstet Gynecol.* 1992;167:648–652. doi:10.1016/s0002-9378(11)91565-8

134 Forbes S. Pregnancy sickness and parent-offspring conflict over thyroid function. *J Theor Biol.* 2014;355:61–67. doi:10.1016/j.jtbi.2014.03.041

135 Lee NM, Saha S. Nausea and vomiting of pregnancy. *Gastroenterol Clin North Am.* 2011;40(2):209-vii. doi:10.1016/j.gtc.2011.03.009

136 Reymunde A, Santiago N, Perez L. Helicobacter pylori and severe morning sickness. *Am J Gastroenterol.* 2001;96(7):2279–2280. doi:10.1111/j.1572-0241.2001.03991.x

137 Wilson EA, Jawad MJ. Stimulation of human chorionic gonadotropin secretion by glucocorticoids. *Am J Obstet Gynecol.* 1982;142(3):344–349. doi:10.1016/0002-9378(82)90741-4

138 Matok I, Clark S, Caritis S, et al. Studying the antiemetic effect of vitamin B6 for morning sickness: pyridoxine and pyridoxal are prodrugs. *J Clin Pharmacol.* 2014;54(12):1429–1433. doi:10.1002/jcph.369

139 Harker N, Montgomery A, Fahey T. Treating nausea and vomiting during pregnancy: case progression. *BMJ.* 2004;328:337.

140 Fejzo MS, Sazonova OV, Sathirapongsasuti JF, et al. Placenta and appetite genes GDF15 and IGFBP7 are associated with hyperemesis gravidarum. *Nat Commun.* 2018;9(1):1178. Published 2018 Mar 21. doi:10.1038/s41467-018-03258-0

141 Petry CJ, Ong KK, Burling KA, et al. Associations of vomiting and antiemetic use in pregnancy with levels of circulating GDF15 early in the second trimester: A nested case-control study. *Wellcome Open Res.* 2018;3:123. doi:10.12688/wellcomeopenres.14818.1

142 Liu Y, Wu M, Ling J, et al. Serum IGFBP7 levels associate with insulin resistance and the risk of metabolic syndrome in a Chinese population. *Sci Rep.* 2015;5:10227. doi:10.1038/srep10227

143 Imagawa A, Hata H, Nakatsu M, et al. Peppermint oil solution is useful as an antispasmodic drug for esophagogastroduodenoscopy, especially for elderly patients. *Dig Dis Sci.* 2012;57(9):2379–2384. doi:10.1007/s10620-012-2194-4

144 Mei Z, Cogswell ME, Looker AC, Pfeiffer CM, Cusick SE, Lacher DA, et al. Assessment of iron status in US pregnant women from the National Health and Nutrition Examination Survey (NHANES), 1999–2006. *Am J Clin Nutr.* 2011;93:1312–1320. doi 10.3945/ajcn.110.007195

145 Moras M, Lefevre SD, Ostuni MA. From Erythroblasts to Mature Red Blood Cells: Organelle Clearance in Mammals. *Front Physiol.* 2017;8:1076. doi:10.3389/fphys.2017.01076

146 Koury MJ, Ponka P. New insights into erythropoiesis: the roles of folate, vitamin B12, and iron. *Annu Rev Nutr.* 2004;24:105–131. doi:10.1146/annurev.nutr.24.012003.132306

147 Aguree S. Gernand AD. Plasma volume expansion across healthy pregnancy: a systematic review and meta-analysis of longitudinal studies. *BMC Pregnancy Childbirth*. 2019;19:508. doi:10.1186/s12884-019-2619-6agui

148 Soma-Pillay P, Nelson-Piercy C, Tolppanen H, Mebazaa A. Physiological changes in pregnancy. *Cardiovasc J Afr*. 2016;27(2):89–94. doi:10.5830/CVJA-2016-021.

149 Best CM, Pressman EK, Cao C, et al. Maternal iron status during pregnancy compared with neonatal iron status better predicts placental iron transporter expression in humans. *FASEB J*. 2016;30(10):3541–3550. doi:10.1096/fj.201600069R. 2016.

150 Monsen ER. Iron nutrition and absorption: dietary factors which impact iron bioavailability. *J Am Diet Assoc*. 1988;88(7):786–790. PMID: 3290310. 1988.

151 Rehu M, Punnonen K, Ostland V, Heinonen S, Westerman M, Pulkki K, Sankilampi U. Maternal serum hepcidin is low at term and independent of cord blood iron status. *Eur J Haematol*. 2010;85:345–52. doi:10.1111/j.1600-0609.2010.01479.x

152 Ikeda Y, Tajima S, Izawa-Ishizawa Y, et al. Estrogen regulates hepcidin expression via GPR30-BMP6-dependent signaling in hepatocytes. *PLoS One*. 2012;7(7):e40465. doi:10.1371/journal.pone.0040465. 2012.

153 Guo W, Bachman E, Li M, Roy CN, Blusztajn J, Wong S, Chan SY, Serra C, Jasuja R, Travison TG, et al. Testosterone administration inhibits hepcidin transcription and is associated with increased iron incorporation into red blood cells. *Aging Cell*. 2013;12:280–291. doi:10.1111/acel.12052

154 O'Brien KO, Thomas CE. *Iron Requirements and Adverse pregnancy outcomes. Handbook of Nutrition in Pregnancy*. 2nd ed. Springer Intl Publishing; 2018:32.

155 Fernández-Ballart JD. Iron Metabolism during Pregnancy. *Clin. Drug Investig*. 2000;19:9–19 (2000). doi:10.2165/00044011-200019001-00002

156 Nemeth E, Ganz T. Anemia of inflammation. *Hematol Oncol Clin North Am*. 2014;28(4):671-vi. doi:10.1016/j.hoc.2014.04.005

157 Yoshihito Iuchi (2012). *Anemia Caused by Oxidative Stress*, Anemia, Dr. Donald Silverberg (Ed.), ISBN: 978-953-51-0138-3, InTech, Available from: http://www.intechopen.com/books/anemia/anemia-caused-by-oxidative-stress

158 Mannaerts D, Faes E, Cos P, Briedé JJ, Gyselaers W, Cornette J, et al. Oxidative stress in healthy pregnancy and preeclampsia is linked to chronic inflammation, iron status and vascular function. *PLoS ONE*. 2018;13(9):e0202919. doi:10.1371/journal.pone.0202919

159 Chai W, Liebman M. Effect of different cooking methods on vegetable oxalate content. *J Agric Food Chem*. 2005;53(8):3027–3030. doi:10.1021/jf048128d

160 Lee S, Guillet R, Cooper EM, et al. Maternal inflammation at delivery affects assessment of maternal iron status. *J Nutr*. 2014;144(10):1524–1532. doi:10.3945/jn.114.191445

161 Fukushima T, Horike H, Fujiki S, Kitada S, Sasaki T, Kashihara N. Zinc deficiency anemia and effects of zinc therapy in maintenance hemodialysis patients. *Ther Apher Dial*. 2009;13(3):213–219. doi:10.1111/j.1744-9987.2009.00656.x

162 Soma-Pillay P, Nelson-Piercy C, Tolppanen H, Mebazaa A. Physiological changes in pregnancy. *Cardiovasc J Afr*. 2016;27(2):89–94. doi:10.5830/CVJA-2016-021.

163 O'Malley EG, Cawley S, Kennedy RAK, Reynolds CME, Molloy A, Turner MJ. Maternal anaemia and folate intake in early pregnancy. *J Public Health (Oxf)*. 2018;40(3):e296-e302. doi:10.1093/pubmed/fdy013

164 Govindappagari S, Nguyen M, Gupta M, Hanna RM, Burwick RM. Severe Vitamin B12 Deficiency in Pregnancy Mimicking HELLP Syndrome. *Case Rep Obstet Gynecol*. 2019;2019:4325647. doi:10.1155/2019/4325647

165 Smith EM, Tangpricha V. Vitamin D and anemia: insights into an emerging association. *Curr Opin Endocrinol Diabetes Obes*. 2015;22(6):432–438. doi:10.1097/MED.0000000000000199

166 Michelazzo FB, Oliveira JM, Stefanello J, Luzia LA, Rondó PH. The influence of vitamin A supplementation on iron status. *Nutrients*. 2013;5(11):4399–4413. doi:10.3390/nu5114399

167 Sebastiani G, Herranz Barbero A, Borrás-Novell C, et al. The Effects of Vegetarian and Vegan Diet during Pregnancy on the Health of Mothers and Offspring. *Nutrients*. 2019;11(3):557. doi:10.3390/nu11030557

168 American College of Obstetrics and Gynecologists. ACOG practice bulletin No. 95: anemia in pregnancy. *Obstet Gynecol*. 2008;112:201–207. doi:10.1097/AOG.0b013e3181809c0d

169 Siu AL, U.S Preventive Services Task Force. Screening for iron deficiency anemia and iron supplementation in pregnant women to improve maternal health and birth outcomes: U.S. Preventive Services Task Force Recommendation Statement. *Ann Intern Med*. 2015;163:529–536. doi:10.7326/M15-1707

170 Gavin NI, Gaynes BN, Lohr KN, Meltzer-Brody S, Gartlehner G, Swinson T. Perinatal depression: a systemic review of prevalence and incidence. *Obstet Gynecol*. 2005;106(5 Pt 1:1071–1083. doi:10.1097/01.AOG.0000183597.31630.db

171 Ramachandran Pillai R, Wilson AB, Premkumar NR, Kattimani S, Sagili H, Rajendiran S. Low serum levels of High-Density Lipoprotein cholesterol (HDL-c) as an indicator for the development of severe postpartum depressive symptoms. *PLoS ONE*. 2018;13(2):e0192811. doi:10.1371/journal.pone.0192811

172 Ernst E, Saradeth T, Seidl S, Resch KL, Frischenschlager O. Cholesterol and Depression. *Arch Intern Med*. 1994;154(10):1166. doi:10.1001/archinte.1994.00420100153025

173 Schultz BG, Patten DK, Berlau DJ. The role of statins in both cognitive impairment and protection against dementia: a tale of two mechanisms. *Transl Neurodegener*. 2018;7:5. Published 2018 Feb 27. doi:10.1186/s40035-018-0110-3

174 Bjorkhem I, Meaney S. Brain cholesterol: long secret life behind a barrier. *Arterioscler Thromb Vasc Biol*. 2004;24:806–815. doi:10.1161/01.ATV.0000120374.59826.1b

175 Williams MR, Sharma P, Macdonald C, Pearce RKB, Hirsch SR, Maier M. Axonal myelin decrease in the splenium in major depressive disorder. *Eur Arch Psychiatry Clin Neurosci*. 2019;269(4):387–395. doi:10.1007/s00406-018-0904-4

176 Kim J, Wessling-Resnick M. Iron and mechanisms of emotional behavior. J Nutr Biochem. 2014;25(11):1101–1107. doi:10.1016/j.jnutbio.2014.07.003

177 Bae YJ, Kim SK. Low dietary calcium is associated with self-rated depression in middle-aged Korean women. *Nutr Res Pract*. 2012;6(6):527–533. doi:10.4162/nrp.2012.6.6.527

178 Young SN. Folate and depression—a neglected problem. *J Psychiatry Neurosci*. 2007;32(2):80–82. PMID: 17353937

179 Eby GA, Eby KL, Murk H. Magnesium and major depression. In: Vink R, Nechifor M, editors. *Magnesium in the Central Nervous System* [Internet]. Adelaide (AU): University of Adelaide Press; 2011. Available from: https://www.ncbi.nlm.nih.gov/books/NBK507265/

180 Hvas AM, Juul S, Bech P, Nexø E. Vitamin B6 level is associated with symptoms of depression. *Psychother Psychosom*. 2004;73(6):340–343. doi:10.1159/000080386

181 Gasperi V, Sibilano M, Savini I, Catani MV. in the Central Nervous System: An Update of Biological Aspects and Clinical Applications. *Int J Mol Sci*. 2019;20(4):974. Published 2019 Feb 23. doi:10.3390/ijms20040974

182 Amin OA, Abouzeid SM, Ali SA, Amin BA, Alswat KA. Clinical association of vitamin D and serotonin levels among patients with fibromyalgia syndrome. *Neuropsychiatr Dis Treat*. 2019;15:1421–1426. doi:10.2147/NDT.S198434

183 Ranjbar E, Kasaei MS, Mohammad-Shirazi M, et al. Effects of zinc supplementation in patients with major depression: a randomized clinical trial. *Iran J Psychiatry*. 2013;8(2):73–79. PMID: 24130605

184 Plevin D, Galletly C. The neuropsychiatric effects of vitamin C deficiency: a systematic review. *BMC Psychiatry*. 2020;20(1):315. doi:10.1186/s12888-020-02730-w

185 Brown RR, Yess N, Price JM, Linkswiler H, Swan P, Hankes LV. Vitamin B6 depletion in man: urinary excretion of quinolinic acid and niacin metabolites. J Nutr. 1965;87(4):419–423. doi:10.1093/jn/87.4.419

186 Sharkey JT, Puttaramu R, Word RA, Olcese J. Melatonin synergizes with oxytocin to enhance contractility of human myometrial smooth muscle cells. *J Clin Endocrinol Metab.* 2009;94(2):421–427. doi:10.1210/jc.2008-1723

187 Barker SA. N, N-Dimethyltryptamine (DMT), an Endogenous Hallucinogen: Past, Present, and Future Research to Determine Its Role and Function. *Front Neurosci.* 2018;12:536. Published 2018 Aug 6. doi:10.3389/fnins.2018.00536

188 Bajpai A, Verma AK, Srivastava M, Srivastava R. Oxidative stress and major depression. *J Clin Diagn Res.* 2014;8(12):CC04-CC07. doi:10.7860/JCDR/2014/10258.5292

189 O'Shaughnessy RW, Scott GD, Iams JD, Zuspan FP. Plasma catecholamines in normal pregnancy and in pregnancies complicated by mild chronic hypertension. *Clin Exp Hypertens B.* 1983;2(1):113–121. doi:10.3109/10641958309023464

190 Holzman C, Senagore P, Tian Y, et al. Maternal catecholamine levels in midpregnancy and risk of preterm delivery. *Am J Epidemiol.* 2009;170(8):1014–1024. doi:10.1093/aje/kwp218

191 Alehagen S, Wijma K, Lundberg U, et al. Catecholamines and cortisol reactions to childbirth. *Int. J. Behav. Med.* 2001;8:50–65. doi: 10.1207/S15327558IJBM0801_04

192 Apter-Levy Y, Zagoory-Sharon O, Feldman R. Chronic Depression Alters Mothers' DHEA and DEHA-to-Cortisol Ratio: Implications for Maternal Behavior and Child Outcomes. *Front Psychiatry.* 2020;11:728. doi:10.3389/fpsyt.2020.00728

193 Leff-Gelman, P., Flores-Ramos, M., Carrasco, A.E.Á. et al. Cortisol and DHEA-S levels in pregnant women with severe anxiety. *BMC Psychiatry* 20, 393 (2020). https://doi.org/10.1186/s12888-020-02788-6

194 Sripada R. Marx C. King A. et al. DHEA Enhances Emotion Regulation Neurocircuits and Modulates Memory for Emotional Stimuli. *Neuropsychopharmacol.* 2013;38:1798–1807. doi:10.1038/npp.2013.79

195 Hypertension Prevalence Among Adults Aged 18 and Over: United States, 2017–2018. Center for Disease Control and Prevention. Updated 4/24/2020. Accessed 3/21/2021

196 High Blood Pressure during Pregnancy. Center for Disease Control and Prevention. Updated May 6 2021. Accessed 8/27/2021

197 Facts About Hypertension. Center for Disease Control and Prevention. Updated July 19, 2021. Accessed 8/27/2021

198 Ndanuko RN, Tapsell LC, Charlton KE, Neale EP, Batterham MJ. Dietary Patterns and Blood Pressure in Adults: A Systematic Review and Meta-Analysis of Randomized Controlled Trials. *Adv Nutr*. 2016;7(1):76–89. doi:10.3945/an.115.009753

199 Ikem E, Halldorsson TI, Birgisdóttir BE, Rasmussen MA, Olsen SF, Maslova E. Dietary patterns and the risk of pregnancy-associated hypertension in the Danish National Birth Cohort: a prospective longitudinal study. *BJOG*. 2019;126(5):663–673. doi:10.1111/1471-0528.15593

200 Pistollato F, Sumalla Cano S, Elio I, Masias Vergara M, Giampieri F, Battino M. Plant-Based and Plant-Rich Diet Patterns during Gestation: Beneficial Effects and Possible Shortcomings. *Adv Nutr*. 2015;6(5):581–591. doi:10.3945/an.115.009126

201 Ali AA, Rayis DA, Abdallah TM, Elbashir MI, Adam I. Severe anaemia is associated with a higher risk for preeclampsia and poor perinatal outcomes in Kassala hospital, eastern Sudan. *BMC Res Notes*. 2011;4:311. doi:10.1186/1756-0500-4-311

202 Mentese A, Güven S, Demir S, et al. Circulating parameters of oxidative stress and hypoxia in normal pregnancy and HELLP syndrome. *Adv Clin Exp Med*. 2018;27(11):1567–1572. doi:10.17219/acem/74653

203 Adam I, Elhassan EM, Haggaz AE, Ali AA, Adam GK. A perspective of the epidemiology of malaria and anaemia and their impact on maternal and perinatal outcomes in Sudan. *J Infect Dev Ctries*. 2011;5(2):83–87. doi:10.3855/jidc.1282

204 Zamudio S, Plamer SK, Regensteiner JG, Moore LG. High altitude and hypertension during pregnancy. *Am J Hum Biol*. 1995;7(2):183–193. doi:10.1002/ajhb.1310070206

205 Bolin M, Åkerud H, Cnattingius S, Stephansson O, Wikström AK. Hyperemesis gravidarum and risks of placental dysfunction disorders: a population-based cohort study. *BJOG*. 2013;120(5):541–547. doi:10.1111/1471-0528.12132

206 Iqbal S, Klammer N, Ekmekcioglu C. The Effect of Electrolytes on Blood Pressure: A Brief Summary of Meta-Analyses. *Nutrients.* 2019;11(6):1362. doi:10.3390/nu11061362

207 Iqbal S, Klammer N, Ekmekcioglu C. The Effect of Electrolytes on Blood Pressure: A Brief Summary of Meta-Analyses. *Nutrients.* 2019;11(6):1362. doi:10.3390/nu11061362

208 Yılmaz ZV, Akkaş E, Türkmen GG, Kara Ö, Yücel A, Uygur D. Dietary sodium and potassium intake were associated with hypertension, kidney damage and adverse perinatal outcome in pregnant women with preeclampsia. *Hypertens Pregnancy.* 2017;36(1):77–83. doi:10.1080/10641955.2016.1239734

209 Bera S, Siuli RA, Gupta S, et al. Study of serum electrolytes in pregnancy induced hypertension. *J Indian Med Assoc.* 2011;109(8):546–548. PMID: 22315860

210 Bara M, Guiet-Bara A, Durlach J. Regulation of sodium and potassium pathways by magnesium in cell membranes. *Magnes Res.* 1993;6(2):167–177. PMID: 8274363

211 Zarean E, Tarjan A. Effect of Magnesium Supplement on Pregnancy Outcomes: A Randomized Control Trial. *Adv Biomed Res.* 2017;6:109. doi:10.4103/2277-9175.213879

212 Dalton LM, Ní Fhloinn DM, Gaydadzhieva GT, Mazurkiewicz OM, Leeson H, Wright CP. Magnesium in pregnancy. *Nutr Rev.* 2016;7(9):549–557. doi:10.1093/nutrit/nuw018

213 Fu ZM, Ma ZZ, Liu GJ, Wang LL, Guo Y. Vitamins supplementation affects the onset of preeclampsia. *J Formos Med Assoc.* 2018;117(1):6–13. doi:10.1016/j.jfma.2017.08.005

214 Behjat Sasan S, Zandvakili F, Soufizadeh N, Baybordi E. The Effects of Vitamin D Supplement on Prevention of Recurrence of Preeclampsia in Pregnant Women with a History of Preeclampsia. *Obstet Gynecol Int.* 2017;2017:8249264. doi:10.1155/2017/82492647

215 Cardús A, Parisi E, Gallego C, Aldea M, Fernández E, Valdivielso JM. 1,25-Dihydroxyvitamin D3 stimulates vascular smooth muscle cell proliferation through a VEGF-mediated pathway. *Kidney Int.* 2006;69(8):1377–1384. doi:10.1038/sj.ki.5000304

216 Hirschler V, Molinari C, Maccallini G, Intersimone P, Gonzalez CD. Vitamin D Levels and Cardiometabolic Markers in Indigenous Argentinean Children Living at Different Altitudes. *Glob Pediatr Health*. 2019;6. doi:10.1177/2333794X18821942

217 Schwalfenberg G. Not enough vitamin D: health consequences for Canadians. *Can Fam Physician*. 2007;53(5):841–854. PMID: 17872747

218 Wacker J, Frühauf J, Schulz M, Chiwora FM, Volz J, Becker K. Riboflavin deficiency and preeclampsia. *Obstet Gynecol*. 2000;96(1):38–44. doi:10.1016/s0029-7844(00)00847-4

219 Hofmeyr GJ, Lawrie TA, Atallah AN, Duley L, Torloni MR. Calcium supplementation during pregnancy for preventing hypertensive disorders and related problems. Cochran *Database Syst Rev*. 2014;6. doi:10.1002/14651858.CD001059

220 Villar J, Abdel-aleem H, Merialdi M, Mathai M, Ali MM, Zaveleta N, et al. World Health Organization randomized trial of calcium supplementation among low calcium intake pregnant women. *Am J Obst Gynecol*. 2006;194(3):639-649. doi:10.1016/j.ajog.2006.01.068

221 Mujawar SA, Patil VW, Daver RG. Study of serum homocysteine, folic Acid and vitamin b(12) in patients with preeclampsia. *Indian J Clin Biochem*. 2011;26(3):257–260. doi:10.1007/s12291-011-0109-3

222 Wu X, Yang K, Tang X, et al. Folate metabolism gene polymorphisms MTHFR C677T and A1298C and risk for preeclampsia: a meta-analysis. *J Assist Reprod Genet*. 2015;32(5):797–805. doi:10.1007/s10815-014-0408-8

223 Apicella C, Ruano CSM, Méhats C, Miralles F, Vaiman D. The Role of Epigenetics in Placental Development and the Etiology of Preeclampsia. *Int J Mol Sci*. 2019;20(11):2837. doi:10.3390/ijms20112837

224 Possomato-Vieira JS, Khalil RA. Mechanisms of endothelial dysfunction in hypertensive pregnancy and preeclampsia. *Adv Pharmacol*. 2016; 77:361–431. doi: 10.1016/bs.apha.2016.04.008

225 Stillman IE, Karumanchi SA. The glomerular injury of preeclampsia. J Am Soc Nephrol. 2007;18(8):2281–2284. doi:10.1681/ASN.2007020255

226 Owusu Darkwa E, Djagbletey R, Sottie D, et al. Serum nitric oxide levels in healthy pregnant women: a case- control study in a tertiary facility in Ghana. *Matern Health Neonatol Perinatol.* 2018;4:3. doi:10.1186/s40748-017-0072-y

227 Krupp J, Boeldt DS, Yi FX, Grummer MA, Bankowski Anaya HA, Shah DM, Bird IM. The loss of sustained Ca(2+) signaling underlies suppressed endothelial nitric oxide production in preeclamptic pregnancies: implications for new therapy. *Am J Physiol Heart Circ Physiol.* 2013;305:H969–H979. doi: 10.1152/ajpheart.00250.2013

228 Motta C, Grosso C, Zanuzzi C, Molinero D, Picco N, Bellingeri R, Alustiza F, Barbeito C, Vivas A, Romanini MC. Effect of sildenafil on pre-eclampsia-like mouse model induced by L-name. *Reprod Domest Anim.* 2015; 50:611–616. doi: 10.1111/rda.12536

229 Goodman RP, Killam AP, Brash AR, Branch RA. Prostacyclin production during pregnancy: comparison of production during normal pregnancy and pregnancy complicated by hypertension. *Am J Obstet Gynecol.* 1982; 142:817–822. doi:10.1016/s0002-9378(16)32525-x

230 Downing I, Shepherd GL, Lewis PJ. Reduced prostacyclin production in pre-eclampsia. *Lancet.* 1980; 2:1374. doi: 10.1016/s0140-6736(80)92443-5

231 Chavarría ME, Lara-González L, González-Gleason A, García-Paleta Y, Vital-Reyes VS, Reyes A. Prostacyclin/thromboxane early changes in pregnancies that are complicated by preeclampsia. *Am J Obstet Gynecol.* 2003; 188:986–992.a. doi:10.1067/mob.2003.203

232 Hansson SR, Naav A, Erlandsson L. Oxidative stress in preeclampsia and the role of free fetal hemoglobin. *Front Physiol.* 2014;5:516. doi:10.3389/fphys.2014.00516

233 Roberts LJ 2nd, Oates JA, Linton MF, et al. The relationship between dose of vitamin E and suppression of oxidative stress in humans. *Free Radic Biol Med.* 2007;43(10):1388–1393. doi:10.1016/j.freeradbiomed.2007.06.019frumb

234 Roberts JM, Myatt L, Spong CY, et al. Vitamins C and E to prevent complications of pregnancy-associated hypertension. *N Engl J Med.* 2010;362(14):1282–1291. doi:10.1056/NEJMoa0908056

235 Rumbold A, Duley L, Crowther CA, Haslam RR. Antioxidants for preventing pre-eclampsia. *Cochrane Database Syst Rev.* 2008;2008(1):CD004227. doi:10.1002/14651858.CD004227.pub3

236 Aguirre JD, Culotta VC. Battles with iron: manganese in oxidative stress protection. *J Biol Chem.* 2012;287(17):13541–13548. doi:10.1074/jbc.R111.312181

237 Yamakura F, Kobayashi K, Furukawa S, Suzuki Y. In vitro preparation of iron-substituted human manganese superoxide dismutase: possible toxic properties for mitochondria. *Free Radic Biol Med.* 2007;43(3):423–430. doi:10.1016/j.freeradbiomed.2007.04.024

238 Lee YK, Lyu ES, Oh SY, et al. Daily Copper and Manganese Intakes and Their Relation to Blood Pressure in Normotensive Adults. *Clin Nutr Res.* 2015;4(4):259–266. doi:10.7762/cnr.2015.4.4.259

239 Liu T, Hivert MF, Rifas-Shiman SL, et al. Prospective Association Between Manganese in Early Pregnancy and the Risk of Preeclampsia. *Epidemiology.* 2020;31(5):677–680. doi:10.1097/EDE.0000000000001227

240 Liu T, Zhang M, Guallar E, et al. Trace Minerals, Heavy Metals, and Preeclampsia: Findings from the Boston Birth Cohort. *J Am Heart Assoc.* 2019;8(16):e012436. doi:10.1161/JAHA.119.012436

241 Mahadik KV, Sina SA. Study of serum levels of superoxide dismutase in preeclampsia and eclampsia: role of the test as a predictive tool. *J Obstet Gynaecol Res.* 2003;29(4):262–267. doi:10.1046/j.1341-8076.2003.00105.x

242 Tsay HJ, Wang P, Wang SL, Ku HH. Age-associated changes of superoxide dismutase and catalase activities in the rat brain. *J Biomed Sci.* 2000;7(6):466–474. doi:10.1007/BF02253362

243 Tatone C, Carbone MC, Falone S, et al. Age-dependent changes in the expression of superoxide dismutases and catalase are associated with ultrastructural modifications in human granulosa cells. *Mol Hum Reprod.* 2006;12(11):655–660. doi:10.1093/molehr/gal080

244 Grum T, Hintsa S, Hagos G. Dietary factors associated with preeclampsia or eclampsia among women in delivery care services in Addis Ababa, Ethiopia: a case-control study. *BMC Res Notes.* 2018;11(1):683. doi:10.1186/s13104-018-3793-8

245 Teran E, Hernández I, Tana L, et al. Mitochondria and Coenzyme Q10 in the Pathogenesis of Preeclampsia. *Front Physiol.* 2018;9:1561. doi:10.3389/fphys.2018.01561

246 Teran E, Hernandez I, Nieto B, Tavara R, Ocampo JE, Calle A. Coenzyme Q10 supplementation during pregnancy reduces the risk of pre-eclampsia. *Int J Gynaecol Obstet.* 2009;105(1):43–45. doi:10.1016/j.ijgo.2008.11.033

247 Teran E, Chedraui P, Racines-Orbe M, et al. Coenzyme Q10 levels in women with preeclampsia living at different altitudes. *Biofactors.* 2008;32(1–4):185–190. doi:10.1002/biof.5520320122

248 Kahveci B, Melekoglu R, Evruke IC, Cetin C. The effect of advanced maternal age on perinatal outcomes in nulliparous singleton pregnancies. *BMC Pregnancy Childbirth.* 2018;18(1):343. doi:10.1186/s12884-018-1984-x

249 Teran E, Racines-Orbe M, Vivero S, Escudero C, Molina G, Calle A. Preeclampsia is associated with a decrease in plasma coenzyme Q10 levels. *Free Radic Biol Med.* 2003;35(11):1453–1456. doi:10.1016/j.freeradbiomed.2003.08.004

250 Price, W. A. *Nutrition and physical degeneration; a comparison of primitive and modern diets and their effects.* New York, London: P.B. Hoeber. 1939

251 Richter ON, Kübler K, Schmolling J, et al. Oxytocin receptor gene expression of estrogen-stimulated human myometrium in extracorporeally perfused non-pregnant uteri. *Mol Hum Reprod.* 2004;10(5):339–346. doi:10.1093/molehr/gah039

252 Mozurkewich, E.L., Chilimigras, J.L., Berman, D.R. *et al.* Methods of induction of labour: a systematic review. *BMC Pregnancy Childbirth* 11, 84 (2011). https://doi.org/10.1186/1471-2393-11-84

253 Danforth DN. The fibrous nature of the human cervix, and its relation to the isthmic segment in gravid and nongravid uteri. *Am J Obstet Gynecol.* 1947;53(4):541–560. doi:10.1016/0002-9378(47)90273-1

254 Iwahashi M, Muragaki Y, Ooshima A, Umesaki N. Decreased Type I Collagen Expression in Human Uterine Cervix during Pregnancy. *J Clin Endocrinol Metab.* 2013;88(5):2231–2235. doi:10.1210/jc.2002-021213

255 Word RA, Li XH, Hnat M, Carrick K. Dynamics of cervical remodeling during pregnancy and parturition: mechanisms and current concepts. *Semin Reprod Med.* 2007;25(1):69–79. doi:10.1055/s-2006-956777

256 Shi JW, Lai ZZ, Yang HL, et al. Collagen at the maternal-fetal interface in human pregnancy. *Int J Biol Sci.* 2020;16(12):2220–2234. Published 2020 May 25. doi:10.7150/ijbs.45586

257 House M, Tadesse-Telila S, Norwitz ER, Socrate S, Kaplan DL. Inhibitory effect of progesterone on cervical tissue formation in a three-dimensional culture system with human cervical fibroblasts. *Biol Reprod.* 2014;90(1):18. Published 2014 Jan 30. doi:10.1095/biolreprod.113.112540

258 Akins ML, Luby-Phelps K, Bank RA, Mahendroo M. Cervical softening during pregnancy: regulated changes in collagen cross-linking and composition of matricellular proteins in the mouse. *Biol Reprod.* 2011;84(5):1053–1062. doi:10.1095/biolreprod.110.089599

259 Shi JW, Lai ZZ, Yang HL, et al. Collagen at the maternal-fetal interface in human pregnancy. *Int J Biol Sci.* 2020;16(12):2220–2234. Published 2020 May 25. doi:10.7150/ijbs.45586

260 Koenig MD, McFarlin BL, Steffen AD, et al. Decreased Nutrient Intake Is Associated with Premature Cervical Remodeling. *J Obstet Gynecol Neonatal Nurs.* 2017;46(1):123–134. doi:10.1016/j.jogn.2016.08.006

261 Osorio R, Yamauti M, Osorio E, et al. Zinc reduces collagen degradation in demineralized human dentin explants. *J Dent.* 2011;39(2):148–153. doi:10.1016/j.jdent.2010.11.005

262 Ota E, Mori R, Middleton P, et al. Zinc supplementation for improving pregnancy and infant outcome. *Cochrane Database Syst Rev.* 2015;2015(2):CD000230. Published 2015 Feb 2. doi:10.1002/14651858.CD000230.pub5

263 Meraz-Cruz N, Ortega A, Estrada-Gutierrez G, et al. Identification of a calcium-dependent matrix metalloproteinase complex in rat chorioallantoid membranes during labour. *Mol Hum Reprod.* 2006;12(10):633–641. doi:10.1093/molehr/gal072

264 Kumar A, Agarwal K, Devi SG, Gupta RK, Batra S. Hypocalcemia in pregnant women. *Biol Trace Elem Res.* 2010;136(1):26–32. doi:10.1007/s12011-009-8523-6

265 Hantke B, Lahmann C, Venzke K, et al. Influence of flavonoids and vitamins on the MMP- and TIMP-expression of human dermal fibroblasts after UVA irradiation. *Photochem Photobiol Sci.* 2002;1(10):826–833. doi:10.1039/b207731k

266 Blesson CS, Büttner E, Masironi B, Sahlin L. Prostaglandin receptors EP and FP are regulated by estradiol and progesterone in the uterus of ovariectomized rats. *Reprod Biol Endocrinol.* 2012;10:3. doi:10.1186/1477-7827-10-3

267 Methods of induction of labour: a systematic review. BMC Pregnancy Childbirth Olson DM. The role of prostaglandins in the initiation of parturition. *Best Pract Res Clin Obstet Gynaecol.* 2003;17(5):717–730. doi:10.1016/s1521-6934(03)00069-5

268 Ham EA, Cirillo VJ, Zanetti ME, Kuehl Fr. Estrogen-directed synthesis of specific prostaglandins in uterus. *Proc Natl Acad Sci U S A.* 1975;72(4):1420–1424. doi:10.1073/pnas.72.4.1420

269 Kim SC, Lee JE, Kang SS, Yang HS, Kim SS, An BS. The regulation of oxytocin and oxytocin receptor in human placenta according to gestational age. *J Mol Endocrinol.* 2017;59(3):235–243. doi:10.1530/JME-16-0223

270 Rucker D, Dhamoon AS. Physiology, Thromboxane A2. [Updated 2020 Sep 13]. In: StatPearls [Internet]. Treasure Island (FL): StatPearls Publishing; 2021 Jan-. Available from: https://www.ncbi.nlm.nih.gov/books/NBK539817/

271 Howarth SR, Vallance P, Wilson CA. Role of thromboxane A2 in the vasoconstrictor response to endothelin-1, angiotensin II and 5-hydroxytryptamine in human placental vessels. *Placenta.* 1995;16(8):679–689. doi:10.1016/0143-4004(95)90012-8

272 Walsh SW. Prostaglandins in Pregnancy. *Glob. libr. women's med., (ISSN: 1756-2228)* 2011; DOI 10.3843/GLOWM.10315

273 Wada M, DeLong CJ, Hong YH, et al. Enzymes and receptors of prostaglandin pathways with arachidonic acid-derived versus eicosapentaenoic acid-derived substrates and products. *J Biol Chem.* 2007;282(31):22254–22266. doi:10.1074/jbc.M703169200

274 Greenberg JA, Bell SJ, Ausdal WV. Omega-3 Fatty Acid supplementation during pregnancy. *Rev Obstet Gynecol.* 2008;1(4):162–169. PMID: 19173020

275 Jacobson JL, Jacobson SW, Muckle G, Kaplan-Estrin M, Ayotte P, Dewailly E. Beneficial effects of a polyunsaturated fatty acid on infant development: evidence from the inuit of arctic Quebec. *J Pediatr.* 2008;152(3):356–364. doi:10.1016/j.jpeds.2007.07.008

276 Swann PG, Venton DL, Le Breton GC. Eicosapentaenoic acid and docosahexaenoic acid are antagonists at the thromboxane A2/prostaglandin H2 receptor in human platelets. *FEBS Lett.* 1989;243(2):244–246. doi:10.1016/0014-5793(89)80137-1

277 Kavanagh J, Kelly AJ, Thomas J. Hyaluronidase for cervical ripening and induction of labour. *Cochrane Database Syst Rev.* 2006;(2):CD003097. Published 2006 Apr 19. doi:10.1002/14651858.CD003097.pub2

278 Kobayashi H, Sun GW, Tanaka Y, Kondo T, Terao T. Serum hyaluronic acid levels during pregnancy and labor. *Obstet Gynecol.* 1999;93(4):480–484. doi:10.1016/s0029-7844(98)00526-2

279 Siiskonen H, Oikari S, Pasonen-Seppänen S, Rilla K. Hyaluronan synthase 1: a mysterious enzyme with unexpected functions. *Front Immunol.* 2015;6:43. Published 2015 Feb 5. doi:10.3389/fimmu.2015.00043

280 Jaya P. Kurup PA. Effect of magnesium deficiency on the metabolism of glycosamino-glycans in rats. *J. Biosci.* 1986;10:487–493 (1986). doi:10.1007/BF02900510

281 Kim SC, Lee JE, Kang SS, Yang HS, Kim SS, An BS. The regulation of oxytocin and oxytocin receptor in human placenta according to gestational age. *J Mol Endocrinol.* 2017;59(3):235–243. doi:10.1530/JME-16-0223

282 Sakai A, Makino T, Kato Y, et al. A uterine muscle contractile substance obtained from a human placental cDNA library. *Gynecol Endocrinol.* 1993;7(2):77–82. doi:10.3109/09513599309152484

283 Kim S, Campbell J, Yoo W, Taylor JA, Sandler DP. Systemic Levels of Estrogens and PGE2 Synthesis in Relation to Postmenopausal Breast Cancer Risk. *Cancer Epidemiol Biomarkers Prev.* 2017;26(3):383–388. doi:10.1158/1055-9965.EPI-16-0556

284 Wilson T, Liggins GC, Whittaker DJ. Oxytocin stimulates the release of arachidonic acid and prostaglandin F2 alpha from human decidual cells. *Prostaglandins.* 1988;35(5):771–780. doi:10.1016/0090-6980(88)90149-9

285 Snegovskikh V, Park JS, Norwitz ER. Endocrinology of Parturition. *Endocrinol Metab Clin N Am.* 2006;35:173–191. doi: 10.1016/j.ecl.2005.09.012.

286 Richard S, Zingg HH. The human oxytocin gene promoter is regulated by estrogens. *J Biol Chem.* 1990;265(11):6098–6103. PMID: 2108152

287 Larcher A, Neculcea J, Chu K, Zingg HH. Effects of retinoic acid and estrogens on oxytocin gene expression in the rat uterus: in vitro and in vivo studies. *Mol Cell Endocrinol.* 1995;114(1–2):69–76. doi:10.1016/0303-7207(95)03643-1

288 Larcher A, Neculcea J, Chu K, Zingg HH. Effects of retinoic acid and estrogens on oxytocin gene expression in the rat uterus: in vitro and in vivo studies. *Mol Cell Endocrinol.* 1995;114(1–2):69–76. doi:10.1016/0303-7207(95)03643-1

289 Cohlan SQ. Excessive intake of vitamin A as a cause of congenital anomalies in the rat. *Science.* 1953;117(3046):535–536. doi:10.1126/science.117.3046.535

290 Lai X, Wu X, Hou N, et al. Vitamin A Deficiency Induces Autistic-Like Behaviors in Rats by Regulating the RARβ-CD38-Oxytocin Axis in the Hypothalamus. *Mol Nutr Food Res.* 2018;62(5):10.1002/mnfr.201700754. doi:10.1002/mnfr.201700754

291 Antoni FA, Chadio SE. Essential role of magnesium in oxytocin-receptor affinity and ligand specificity. *Biochem J.* 1989;257(2):611–614. doi:10.1042/bj2570611

292 Gimpl G, Fahrenholz F. Cholesterol as stabilizer of the oxytocin receptor. *Biochim Biophys Acta.* 2002;1564(2):384–392. doi:10.1016/s0005-2736(02)00475-3

293 Gimpl G, Fahrenholz F. The oxytocin receptor system: structure, function, and regulation. *Physiol Rev.* 2001;81(2):629–683. doi:10.1152/physrev.2001.81.2.629

294 Condon JC, Jeyasuria P, Faust JM, Mendelson CR. Surfactant protein secreted by the maturing mouse fetal lung acts as a hormone that signals the initiation of parturition. *Proc Natl Acad Sci U S A*. 2004;101(14):4978–4983. doi:10.1073/pnas.0401124101

295 King RJ, Ruch J, Gikas EG, Platzker AC, Creasy RK. Appearance of apoproteins of pulmonary surfactant in human amniotic fluid. *J Appl Physiol*. 1975;39(5):735–741. doi:10.1152/jappl.1975.39.5.735

296 Condon JC, Jeyasuria P, Faust JM, Mendelson CR. Surfactant protein secreted by the maturing mouse fetal lung acts as a hormone that signals the initiation of parturition. *Proc Natl Acad Sci U S A*. 2004;101(14):4978–4983. doi:10.1073/pnas.0401124101

297 Mendelson CR, Montalbano AP, Gao L. Fetal-to-maternal signaling in the timing of birth. *J Steroid Biochem Mol Biol*. 2017;170:19–27. doi:10.1016/j.jsbmb.2016.09.006

298 Buckley SJ. Executive Summary of Hormonal Physiology of Childbearing: Evidence and Implications for Women, Babies, and Maternity Care. *J Perinat Educ*. 2015;24(3):145–153. doi:10.1891/1058-1243.24.3.145

299 Doan E, Gibbons K, Tudehope D. The timing of elective caesarean deliveries and early neonatal outcomes in singleton infants born 37–41 weeks' gestation. *Aust N Z J Obstet Gynaecol*. 2014;54(4):340–347. doi:10.1111/ajo.12220

300 Kamath BD, Todd JK, Glazner JE, Lezotte D, Lynch AM. Neonatal outcomes after elective cesarean delivery. *Obstet Gynecol*. 2009;113(6):1231–1238. doi:10.1097/AOG.0b013e3181a66d57

301 Swift-Gallant A, Jordan CL, Breedlove SM. Consequences of cesarean delivery for neural development. *Proc Natl Acad Sci U S A*. 2018;115(46):11664-11666. doi:10.1073/pnas.1816335115

302 Castillo-Ruiz A, Mosley M, Jacobs AJ, Hoffiz YC, Forger NG. Birth delivery mode alters perinatal cell death in the mouse brain. *Proc Natl Acad Sci U S A*. 2018;115(46):11826–11831. doi:10.1073/pnas.1811962115

303 Deoni SC, Adams SH, Li X, et al. Cesarean Delivery Impacts Infant Brain Development. *AJNR Am J Neuroradiol*. 2019;40(1):169–177. doi:10.3174/ajnr.A5887

304 Singh RK, Chang HW, Yan D, et al. Influence of diet on the gut microbiome and implications for human health. *J Transl Med*. 2017;15(1):73. Published 2017 Apr 8. doi:10.1186/s12967-017-1175-y

305 Singh RK, Chang HW, Yan D, et al. Influence of diet on the gut microbiome and implications for human health. *J Transl Med*. 2017;15(1):73. Published 2017 Apr 8. doi:10.1186/s12967-017-1175-y

306 Świątecka D, Narbad A, Ridgway KP, Kostyra H. The study on the impact of glycated pea proteins on human intestinal bacteria [published correction appears in Int J Food Microbiol. 2011 Dec 15;151(3):340. Dominika, Świątecka [corrected to Świątecka, Dominika]; Arjan, Narbad [corrected to Narbad, Arjan]; Karyn, Ridgway P [corrected to Ridgway, Karyn P]; Henryk, Kostyra [corrected to Kostyra, Henryk]]. *Int J Food Microbiol*. 2011;145(1):267–272. doi:10.1016/j.ijfoodmicro.2011.01.002

307 Urwin HJ, Miles EA, Noakes PS, et al. Effect of salmon consumption during pregnancy on maternal and infant faecal microbiota, secretory IgA and calprotectin. *Br J Nutr*. 2014;111(5):773–784. doi:10.1017/S0007114513003097

308 Kim JH, Kwon OJ, Choi NJ, et al. Variations in conjugated linoleic acid (CLA) content of processed cheese by lactation time, feeding regimen, and ripening. *J Agric Food Chem*. 2009;57(8):3235–3239. doi:10.1021/jf803838u

309 Khan S, Waliullah S, Godfrey V, et al. Dietary simple sugars alter microbial ecology in the gut and promote colitis in mice. *Sci Transl Med*. 2020;12(567):eaay6218. doi:10.1126/scitranslmed.aay6218

310 Leeming ER, Johnson AJ, Spector TD, Le Roy CI. Effect of Diet on the Gut Microbiota: Rethinking Intervention Duration. *Nutrients*. 2019;11(12):2862. Published 2019 Nov 22. doi:10.3390/nu11122862

311 Seaward PG, Hannah ME, Myhr TL, et al. International multicenter term PROM study: evaluation of predictors of neonatal infection in infants born to patients with premature rupture of membranes at term. Premature Rupture of the Membranes. *Am J Obstet Gynecol*. 1998;179(3 Pt 1):635–639. doi:10.1016/s0002-9378(98)70056-0

312 Tapiainen T, Koivusaari P, Brinkac L, et al. Impact of intrapartum and postnatal antibiotics on the gut microbiome and emergence of antimicrobial resistance in infants. *Sci Rep*. 2019;9(1):10635. Published 2019 Jul 23. doi:10.1038/s41598-019-46964-5

313 Ohlsson A, Shah VS. Intrapartum antibiotics for known maternal Group B streptococcal colonization. *Cochrane Database Syst Rev*. 2013;(1):CD007467. Published 2013 Jan 31. doi:10.1002/14651858.CD007467.pub3

314 Ursell LK, Metcalf JL, Parfrey LW, Knight R. Defining the human microbiome. *Nutr Rev*. 2012;70 Suppl 1(Suppl 1):S38-S44. doi:10.1111/j.1753-4887.2012.00493.x

315 Lewis FMT, Bernstein KT, Aral SO. Vaginal Microbiome and Its Relationship to Behavior, Sexual Health, and Sexually Transmitted Diseases. *Obstet Gynecol*. 2017;129(4):643–654. doi:10.1097/AOG.0000000000001932

316 Nagpal R, Tsuji H, Takahashi T, et al. Gut dysbiosis following C-section instigates higher colonisation of toxigenic Clostridium perfringens in infants. *Benef Microbes*. 2017;8(3):353–365. doi:10.3920/BM2016.0216

317 Yang NJ, Chiu IM. Bacterial Signaling to the Nervous System through Toxins and Metabolites. *J Mol Biol*. 2017;429(5):587–605. doi:10.1016/j.jmb.2016.12.023

318 Zhang T, Sidorchuk A, Sevilla-Cermeño L, et al. Association of cesarean delivery with Risk of Neurodevelopmental and Psychiatric Disorders in the Offspring: A Systematic Review and Meta-analysis. *JAMA Netw Open*. 2019;2(8):e1910236. Published 2019 Aug 2. doi:10.1001/jamanetworkopen.2019.10236

319 Stokholm J, Thorsen J, Blaser MJ, et al. Delivery mode and gut microbial changes correlate with an increased risk of childhood asthma. *Sci Transl Med*. 2020;12(569):eaax9929. doi:10.1126/scitranslmed.aax9929

320 Smith GCS. Cesarean section and childhood infections: Causality for concern? *PLoS Med*. 2020;17(11):e1003457. Published 2020 Nov 19. doi:10.1371/journal.pmed.1003457

321 Masukume G, McCarthy FP, Russell J, et al. Caesarean section delivery and childhood obesity: evidence from the growing up in New Zealand cohort. *J Epidemiol Community Health*. 2019;73(12):1063–1070. doi:10.1136/jech-2019-212591

322 Chavarro JE, Martín-Calvo N, Yuan C, et al. Association of Birth by Cesarean Delivery with Obesity and Type 2 Diabetes Among Adult Women. *JAMA Netw Open*. 2020;3(4):e202605. Published 2020 Apr 1. doi:10.1001/jamanetworkopen.2020.2605

323 Mola G. Port Moresby General Hospital, Division of Obstetrics and Gynaecology, Annual Report 2016. Port Moresby, Papua New Guinea: Port Moresby General Hospital, National Department of Health. 2017.

324 Guise JM, Denman MA, Emeis C, et al. Vaginal birth after cesarean: new insights on maternal and neonatal outcomes. *Obstet Gynecol*. 2010;115(6):1267–1278. doi:10.1097/AOG.0b013e3181df925f

325 Van Dillen J, Zwart JJ, Schutte J, Bloemenkamp KW, van Roosmalen J. Severe acute maternal morbidity and mode of delivery in the Netherlands. *Acta Obstet Gynecol Scand*. 2010;89(11):1460–1465. doi:10.3109/00016349.2010.519018

326 Aabakke AJ, Krebs L, Ladelund S, Secher NJ. Incidence of incisional hernia after cesarean delivery: a register-based cohort study. *PLoS One*. 2014;9(9):e108829. Published 2014 Sep 30. doi:10.1371/journal.pone.0108829

327 Miseljic N, Ibrahimovic S. Health Implications of Increased Cesarean Section Rates. *Mater Sociomed*. 2020;32(2):123–126. doi:10.5455/msm.2020.32.123–126

328 Diamond J. Bringing Up Children. In: *The World Until Yesterday*. Penguin Group. 2012

329 Institute of Medicine (US) Panel on Dietary Antioxidants and Related Compounds. *Dietary Reference Intakes for Vitamin C, Vitamin E, Selenium, and Carotenoids*. Washington (DC): National Academies Press (US); 2000. Food and Nutrition Board, Institute of Medicine-National Academy of Sciences Dietary Reference Intakes: Recommended Intakes for Individuals. Available from: https://www.ncbi.nlm.nih.gov/books/NBK225472/

330 Bastos Maia S, Rolland Souza AS, Costa Caminha MF, et al. Vitamin A and Pregnancy: A Narrative Review. *Nutrients*. 2019;11(3):681. Published 2019 Mar 22. doi:10.3390/nu11030681

331 Radhika MS, Bhaskaram P, Balakrishna N, Ramalakshmi BA, Devi S, Kumar BS. Effects of vitamin A deficiency during pregnancy on maternal and child health. *BJOG*. 2002;109(6):689–693. doi:10.1111/j.1471-0528.2002.01010.x

332 Bastos Maia S, Rolland Souza AS, Costa Caminha MF, et al. Vitamin A and Pregnancy: A Narrative Review. *Nutrients*. 2019;11(3):681. Published 2019 Mar 22. doi:10.3390/nu11030681

333 Scholl TO, Chen X, Stein P. Maternal vitamin D status and delivery by cesarean. *Nutrients*. 2012;4(4):319–330. doi:10.3390/nu4040319

334 Mulligan ML, Felton SK, Riek AE, Bernal-Mizrachi C. Implications of vitamin D deficiency in pregnancy and lactation. *Am J Obstet Gynecol*. 2010;202(5):429.e1-429.e4299. doi:10.1016/j.ajog.2009.09.002

335 Hollis BW, Wagner CL. New insights into the vitamin D requirements during pregnancy. *Bone Res*. 2017;5:17030. Published 2017 Aug 29. doi:10.1038/boneres.2017.30

336 Julien WE, Conrad HR, Jones JE, Moxon AL. Selenium and vitamin E and incidence of retained placenta in parturient dairy cows. *J Dairy Sci*. 1976;59(11):1954–1959. doi:10.3168/jds.S0022-0302(76)84467-0

337 Rumbold A, Ota E, Hori H, Miyazaki C, Crowther CA. Vitamin E supplementation in pregnancy. *Cochrane Database Syst Rev*. 2015;(9):CD004069. Published 2015 Sep 7. doi:10.1002/14651858.CD004069.pub3

338 Maldonado M, Alhousseini A, Awadalla M, et al. Intrahepatic Cholestasis of Pregnancy Leading to Severe Vitamin K Deficiency and Coagulopathy. *Case Rep Obstet Gynecol*. 2017;2017:5646247. doi:10.1155/2017/5646247

339 Institute of Medicine (US) Panel on Micronutrients. *Dietary Reference Intakes for Vitamin A, Vitamin K, Arsenic, Boron, Chromium, Copper, Iodine, Iron, Manganese, Molybdenum, Nickel, Silicon, Vanadium, and Zinc.* Washington (DC): National Academies Press (US); 2001. 5, Vitamin K. Available from: https://www.ncbi.nlm.nih.gov/books/NBK222299/

340 Gernand AD. The upper level: examining the risk of excess micronutrient intake in pregnancy from antenatal supplements. *Ann N Y Acad Sci.* 2019;1444(1):22–34. doi:10.1111/nyas.14103

341 Hisano M, Suzuki R, Sago H, Murashima A, Yamaguchi K. Vitamin B6 deficiency and anemia in pregnancy. *Eur J Clin Nutr.* 2010;64(2):221–223. doi:10.1038/ejcn.2009.125

342 Hemminger A, Wills BK. Vitamin B6 toxicity. [Updated 2020 Nov 4]. In: StatPearls [Internet]. Treasure Island (FL): StatPearls Publishing; 2021 April 19. Available from: https://www.ncbi.nlm.nih.gov/books/NBK554500/

343 Zempleni J, Mock DM. Marginal biotin deficiency is teratogenic. *Proc Soc Exp Biol Med.* 2000;223(1):14–21. doi:10.1046/j.1525-1373.2000.22303.x

344 Mock DM, Quirk JG, Mock NI. Marginal biotin deficiency during normal pregnancy. *Am J Clin Nutr.* 2002;75(2):295–299. doi:10.1093/ajcn/75.2.295

345 Kummer S, Hermsen D, Distelmaier F. Biotin Treatment Mimicking Graves' Disease. *N Engl J Med.* 2016;375(7):704–706. doi:10.1056/NEJMc1602096

346 Wald NJ, Morris JK, Blakemore C. Public health failure in the prevention of neural tube defects: time to abandon the tolerable upper intake level of folate. *Public Health Rev.* 2018;39:2. Published 2018 Jan 31. doi:10.1186/s40985-018-0079-6

347 Bailey RL, Pac SG, Fulgoni VL 3rd, Reidy KC, Catalano PM. Estimation of Total Usual Dietary Intakes of Pregnant Women in the United States. JAMA Netw Open. 2019;2(6):e195967. Published 2019 Jun 5. doi:10.1001/jamanetworkopen.2019.5967

348 Peng Y, Hu J, Li Y, et al. Exposure to chromium during pregnancy and longitudinally assessed fetal growth: Findings from a prospective cohort. *Environ Int.* 2018;121(Pt 1):375–382. doi:10.1016/j.envint.2018.09.003

349 Kaplan JH, Lutsenko S. Copper transport in mammalian cells: special care for a metal with special needs. *J Biol Chem.* 2009;284(38):25461-25465. doi:10.1074/jbc.R109.031286

350 Overcash RT, Marc-Aurele KL, Hull AD, Ramos GA. Maternal Iodine Exposure: A Case of Fetal Goiter and Neonatal Hearing Loss. *Pediatrics.* 2016;137(4):e20153722. doi:10.1542/peds.2015-3722

351 Correia-Branco A, Rincon MP, Pereira LM, Wallingford MC. Inorganic Phosphate in the Pathogenesis of Pregnancy-Related Complications. *Int J Mol Sci.* 2020;21(15):5283. Published 2020 Jul 25. doi:10.3390/ijms21155283

352 Xu X, Li X, Sun H, et al. Murine placental-fetal phosphate dyshomeostasis caused by an xpr1 deficiency accelerates placental calcification and restricts fetal growth in late gestation. *J Bone Miner Res.* 2020;34(1):116–129. doi:10.1002/bjmr.3866.

353 Wolak T, Sergienko R, Wiznitzer A, Ben Shlush L, Paran E, Sheiner E. Low potassium level during the first half of pregnancy is associated with lower risk for the development of gestational diabetes mellitus and severe pre-eclampsia. *J Matern Fetal Neonatal Med.* 2010;23(9):994–998. doi:10.3109/14767050903544736

354 Wood RJ. Manganese and birth outcome. *Nutr Rev.* 2009;67(7):416–420. doi:10.1111/j.1753-4887.2009.00214.x

355 Vollet K, Haynes EN, Dietrich KN. Manganese Exposure and Cognition Across the Lifespan: Contemporary Review and Argument for Biphasic Dose-Response Health Effects. *Curr Environ Health Rep.* 2016;3(4):392–404. doi:10.1007/s40572-016-0108-x

356 Julien WE, Conrad HR, Jones JE, Moxon AL. Selenium and vitamin E and incidence of retained placenta in parturient dairy cows. *J Dairy Sci.* 1976;59(11):1954–1959. doi:10.3168/jds.S0022-0302(76)84467-0

357 Institute of Medicine (US) Committee on Nutritional Status During Pregnancy and Lactation. *Nutrition During Pregnancy: Part I Weight Gain: Part II Nutrient Supplements.* Washington (DC): National Academies Press (US); 1990. 15, Trace Elements. Available from: https://www.ncbi.nlm.nih.gov/books/NBK235243/

358 Mao C, Liu R, Bo L, et al. High-salt diets during pregnancy affected fetal and offspring renal renin-angiotensin system. *J Endocrinol.* 2013;218(1):61–73. Published 2013 Jun 1. doi:10.1530/JOE-13-0139

359 Razavi AS, Chasen ST, Gyawali R, Kalish RB. Hyponatremia associated with preeclampsia. *J Perinat Med.* 2017;45(4):467–470. doi:10.1515/jpm-2016-0062

360 King JC. Determinants of maternal zinc status during pregnancy. *Am J Clin Nutr.* 2000;71(5 Suppl):1334S–1343S. doi:10.1093/ajcn/71.5.1334s

361 Fosmire GJ. Zinc toxicity. *Am J Clin Nutr.* 1990;51(2):225–227. doi:10.1093/ajcn/51.2.225

Index

1α,25 dihydroxycholecalciferol (calcitriol), conversion, 105
1-α-hydroxylase, expression, 143
2-series prostaglandins
  balance, 225
  forms, 222
3-beta-hydroxysteroid dehydrogenase (3β-HSD) enzyme
  absence, 106, 112
  changes, detection (absence), 105
  function, 100
  importance, 103
  location, 102
3-series prostaglandins, production, 225
5,10 methylenetetrahydrofolate, transformation, 56
5-deoxyadenosylcobalamin, usage, 168
5-methylenetetrahydrofolate (5-MTHF)
  folate methylation, 61
  transformation, 56
11β-hydroxylase, 97
11β-monooxygenase, 97
17,20-desmolase, 97
17,20 lyase, 97
17-beta-hydroxysteroid dehydrogenase (17β-HSD)
  absence, 112
  DHEA-S conversion, 101
17-OH pregnenolone
  CYP17A1, impact, 101
  synthesis, 100
17-OH progesterone
  CYP17A1, impact, 101
  production, 120
  synthesis, 100
  transfer, 110
17α-hydroxylase, 97
17α-monooxygenase, 97
18-hydroxylase, 97
18-monooxygenase, 97
20,22-desmolase, 97
20,22 lyase, 97
21-hydroxylase, 97
21-monooxygenase, 97
21α-hydroxylase, 97
21β-hydroxylase, 97
25(OH)D. *See* Serum 25-hydroxycalciferol
677CT MTHFR mutation, 63

A

A1298C MTHFR SNP, genetic problems, 56
Abraham, Guy E., 130
Acetylation, 64, 288
  increase, 160
Acetylcholine, discovery, 179
Acetyl coenzyme A (acetyl-CoA), 160
  Krebs cycle entry, 77
  presence, 65
  pyruvate breakdown, 77
Acetyl-coenzyme A, formation, 76
Acetyl group, removal, 65
Acetyl-L-carnitine, requirement, 86
Actin (contracting protein), 90
Active labor, catecholamine surge, 242
Acupuncture, 26–27
Adenosine triphosphate (ATP)
  energy, 76
  methionine, binding, 58
Adenosylhomocysteinase, SAH conversion, 59
Adenosylhomocysteine (AdoHcy) (SAH), presence, 59
Adenylation, 64
Adequate Intake (AI), 260

values, choline, 62
Adipose tissue, building, 85
Adrenal glands, 96, 100
  ACTH, impact, 148
  DHEA-S production, 115
  fetal adrenal glands
    cortisol production, 117
    DHEA-S secretion/supply, 101, 110, 112
  hormone production, 82
  maternal adrenal glands, DHEA-S secretion/supply, 112
  steroidogenesis, occurrence, 96
  vitamin D metabolites, formation, 98
Adrenal hormone synthesis, 100–103
Adrenocorticotropic hormone (ACTH)
  fetal pituitary production, 113
  regulation role, 100
  release/production, 117, 148
  sensitivity, increase, 80
  stimulation role, 100, 112
  upregulation, 118
Adrenodoxin, impact, 96
Adrenodoxin reductase, impact, 96
Adulthood
  insulin resistance, 54
  metabolic syndrome, 54
Advanced maternal age (AMA)
  pregnancies, 89
Afternoon fatigue, 152
Agitation, 190
A-ha moments, 24–25
Albumin
  proteins, transport role, 126
  transport protein, 92
  zinc deficiency, impact, 92
Aldosterone, 97
  adrenal precursor, impact, 110
  production, CYP11B1 regulation, 100
  regulation role, 161
  synthesis, 100
Aldosterone synthase, 97
Alistipes levels, increase, 245

Alkaline phosphatase
  formation, zinc (importance), 174
  increase, 175
Allergies
  food allergy testing, 33
  impact, 257
  risk, birth method (connection), 250
Alpha-carotene, 232
Alpha cells, impact, 142
Alpha-linoleic acid (ALA), 224, 226
  acid conversion, 224
Alpha-tocopherol, 102
Aluminum, impact, 79
Alzheimer's disease, oxidative stress (link), 82
American diet, 81, 109
  change, 19
  dysbiosis, relationship, 246
American nutrition, functional nutrition (contrast), 34–36
Amino acid
  anabolism usage, 93
  arginine, breakdown, 203
  base, sugar (binding), 58
  combination, 229
  complexes, 90
  complex protein breakdown, 71
  conditional amino acids, 90–91
  enzyme base, 90
  essential amino acids, 91, 182, 185, 229
  glycine, 160
  L-arginine, 112
  nitrogen
    methyl group, addition, 59
    removal, 91–92
  nonstorage/recycling/breakdown, 92
  nucleotide component, 58
  selenocysteine, 90
  serine, carbon transfer, 56
  synthesis, 91
  tryptophan, 182
  tyrosine, 185

binding, 122
Amniotic cells, CRH expression, 117
Amniotic environment, prostaglandin synthesis (increase), 222–223
Amniotic fluid
  addition/composition, 197
  infection, 248
  surfactants, detection, 238
Amniotic sac, SP-A travel, 238
Anabolic changes, 75
Anabolic metabolism, 93, 288
Anabolic phase (lipid breakdown phase), 85, 93
Anabolic processes, PIGF stimulation, 67
Anabolic states, creation, 93
Anabolism, 92–93
Androgen
  cortex production, 100
  DHEA-S, 115–116
  testosterone, 114–115
Androgen, cortex production, 100
Anemia, 157, 192
  apoptosis, increase (impact), 160
  biomarker, ferritin level assessment, 164
  borderline anemia, presence, 19
  case study, 173–175
  causes, 158–159
  correction, testosterone (impact), 163–164
  functional anemia, 165
  gestational anemia, 158, 169–170
  hypertension, relationship, 196–197
  improvement, 169
  iron-deficiency anemia, 174
  iron deficiency, contrast, 166–170
  malnutrition anemia, 196
  pernicious anemia, 167
  predictor, folate deficiency (impact), 167
  presence, 157, 196
  presentations, 167
  prevention, 172

problems, 197
reasons, 166–167
risk, increase, 158
symptoms, 200
systemic causes, 169
vegan diet, relationship, 158, 170–172
vitamin D status, correlation, 169
zinc-deficiency anemia, 167, 174
Antibiotics, usage, 247–249
Antibodies
  antithyroglobulin antibodies, involvement, 133
  autoimmune antibodies, NIS destruction (association), 133
  protein requirement, 90
  thyroid antibodies, 132–134
  thyroid peroxidase (TPO) antibodies, diagnosis, 122
Antiemetic effects
  P5P blood values increase, association, 150
  vitamin B6, relationship, 149
Antigens
  antigen-presenting cells, vitamin D receptor expression, 133
  processing/presenting, 133
  proteins, thyroid proteins (distinguishing), 132
Anti-inflammatory fatty acids, usage, 222
Antinutrients
  impact, absence, 162
Antinutrients, decrease, 36
Antioxidants, 96
  capacity (vitamin E), 102
  carotenoids, presence, 98, 232
  cell protection, 96
  cellular antioxidant (CoQ10), role, 207
  coenzyme Q10 (fat-soluble oxidant), impact, 88, 89
  demand, increase, 120
  dietary/innate antioxidants, increase (requirement), 205

endogenous antioxidants,
  formation, 81
enzymes, production (decrease), 80
functions (vitamin A), 169
glutathione/methionine, body
  usage, 59
impact, 79, 207, 220
low levels, nutritional problems, 81
nitric oxide function, 203
nutrients, deficiency, 205
presence, 195
ratio, imbalance, 80–81
reactive oxygen species, balance, 204
requirement, 124, 188
selenium role, 128
SOD, manganese cofactor, 205
usage, 222
Antithyroglobulin antibodies,
  involvement, 133
Anxiety, 177, 179
  DHEA, connection, 191
  DHEA-S serum decrease,
    relationship, 115
  maternal depression, relationship, 181
  oxidative stress, link, 82
  physical manifestation, 149, 190
  pregnancy assessment, 191–192
  prenatal depression, connection, 178
  presence (pregnancy/postpartum), 188
  stress manifestation, 149
  symptoms, nutrition (role), 186
Apoptosis, 165
  increase, impact, 160
Appetite
  development, 152
  increase, 66, 93
  problems, 157, 177
Arachidonic acid (AA)
  formation, 225
  prostaglandin derivation, 224
Arginine (conditional amino acid)
  breakdown, 203
  estrogen, interaction, 112

L-arginine, NO synthesis, 112
Aromatase, 97
  activity, vitamin D alteration, 105
  CYP19A1-aromatase enzyme, placenta
    usage, 112
  expression, stimulation, 223
Asthma
  presence, 33
  risk, birth method (connection), 250
Atherosclerosis, oxidative stress (link), 81
Attention deficit disorder
  oxidative stress, link, 82
  risk, Cesarean delivery (impact), 249
Attention deficit hyperactivity disorder
  (ADHD), 179
Autism
  oxidative stress, link, 82
  risk, Cesarean delivery (impact), 249
  risk (increase), folic acid
    supplementation (association), 63
  unmetabolized folic acid,
    relationship, 63
Autoimmune antibodies, NIS
  destruction (association), 133
Autoimmune disease, oxidative stress
  (link), 82
Autoimmune hypothyroidism, 132
Autoimmune paleo diet, 36
Autoimmune thyroid disease, pregnancy
  complication risk (association), 134
Autoimmune thyroiditis (trigger),
  supplemental iodine intake (impact),
  129–130
Autonomic nervous system (ANS),
  178–179
Aztec tribes, legumes (soaking), 72

B
Babies
  adrenal glands (DHEA-S
    production), 115
  alertness/wakeness, increase, 242
  brain, scheduled birth (impact),
    242–243

cesarean-delivered babies, health
    risks, 250
chemical changes, 215f
childbirth preparation, 237–238
    insulin resistance, 55
    pituitary (trigger), estrogen elevation
        (connection), 113
    preconception nutrition, 53
Bacterial dysbiosis (H. Pylori), 146–149
Bacterial infections, 80
    H. Pylori, 147
    impact, 250
Bacteroides levels, increase, 245
Barker, David, 53
Barker's Hypothesis, 54
Beef liver, consumption
    (advantages), 233
Beta-adrenergic (β-adrenergic) receptors,
    increase, 122
Beta-carotene
    birth defects, link (absence), 236
    cell protection, 96
    consumption, 236
    deficiency, impact, 98
    vitamin A form, 232
Beta cells, impact, 142–143
Beta-cryptoxanthin, 232
Betaine
    consumption, 59–60
    sensitivity, increase, 63–64
    trimethylglycine (TMG), 59
Betaine-homocysteine methyltransferase
    (BHMT), homocysteine
    breakdown, 59
Beta-tocopherol, 102
Bicarbonate, 198
Bifidobacterium
    bacteria species, CLA production, 246
    levels, increase, 245
Bile reabsorption, 86
Bilophila levels, increase, 245
Biochemical constitution, 187
Birth

method
    importance, 241
    microbiome, relationship, 249–250
    order, importance, 69
    scheduled birth, impact, 242–243
Birth control, use
    comparison, 144
    nausea, predisposition, 155
Birth defects
    beta-carotene, link (absence), 236
    fear, 233
Bisphenol A (BPA), impact, 59
Blanching, usage, 165
Blood pressure
    elevation, 18
    oxidative stress, link, 81
    improvement, 20
    increase, 17–18, 195–196
    low level, 155
    maintenance, cortisol (impact), 118
    reduction, 198
    regulation, plasma increase
        (impact), 161
    studies, focus, 198
    systolic blood pressure, increase, 206
Blood sugar levels
    increase, 119
    regulation, 152
Body
    fat, gain, 85
    function, nutrient deficiency
        (impact), 45
Body mass index (BMI),
    measurement, 144
Bone malformation, signs, 42
Borderline anemia, presence, 19
Brain
    function, alteration, 181
    oxidative stress sensitivity, 82
Breads, origin, 73
Breathing patterns, changes, 190
Brody, Jane E., 234
Bromine, usage/intake, 131

Brownstein, David, 130
Business of Being Born, The, 217
B vitamins
  consumption, 55
  requirement, 86
  water solubility, 77

C

C677T MTHFR SNP
  genetic problems, 56
  preeclampsia development risk, increase (association), 202
Calcitriol blood concentrations, 106–107
Calcium, 198
  bone entry, 42
  histone modification dependence, 65
  hypocalcemia, 221
  supplementation, 201
  vitamin D, uncoupling, 107
Calf cramps, potassium deficiency, 199
Carbohydrates, 83–84
  breakdown, 76, 83
  complex carbohydrates, 83–84
  digestion, 246
  focus, 34
  simple carbohydrates, 83–84
Carbon dioxide, Krebs cycle byproduct, 79
Carbon monoxide, endothelial production (increase), 112
Cardiovascular disease
  high fats/sugars, link, 46
  oxidative stress, impact, 79
Carotenoids, presence, 98
Catabolic metabolism, 93
Catabolic phase (lipid breakdown phase), 85, 93
Catabolic states, creation, 93
Catabolism, 92–932
Catalase, cell protection, 96
Catecholamines
  oxytocin, balance, 242
  production/secretion, 101–102
  increase, 189
  stability, 190
  surge, 241–243
Cells
  protection, antioxidants (impact), 96
  receptors
    function, 236–237
    protein requirement, 90
Cellular antioxidant (CoQ10), role, 207
Cellular death, pause, 243
Cellular metabolism, 75–76
  proteins, usage, 91–92
Cellular respiration, 76
Central nervous system (CNS), 178
  precursor, 63
Certified nurse-midwives (CNMs), assistance, 122
Cervical remodeling, 230f
  nutritional deficiencies, impact, 220–221
  phases, 219
  premature cervical remodeling, risk (increase), 220
  preterm cervical remodeling risk, correlations, 220
Cervical ripening, 219t
  hyaluronic acid, impact, 227–229
  induction, 216
  prostaglandins, impact, 222–223
  stimulation, estrogen (impact), 214
Cervix, 216–218
  collagen remodeling, 218
  components, 217
  dilation, 219t
  repair, 219t
  softening, 219t
Cesarean delivery
  babies, health risks, 250
  decision, 242–243
  risks, 250–251
Childbirth
  complications, oxidative stress (link), 82

Index

functional childbirth, 211
maternal physiological changes, 241
preparation, 237–238
progression, 216
transitional time, 31
Childhood chronic diseases, increase, 41
Childhood obesity rates (increase), school lunches (relationship), 41
Children, glucose metabolism (changes), 54
Chloride, 198
Chlorine, usage/intake, 131
Cholecalciferol (Vitamin D3), synthesis, 105
Cholestasis, CoQ10 (link), 90
Cholesterol
  functional range, 181
  importance, 86–88
  levels, impact, 88
  requirement, 236–237
  serum cholesterol values, increase, 87–88
  synthesis, 86–87
  transfer, 96–97
  types, 87
Choline
  adequate intake (AI) values, 62
  consumption, 55
  cycles, 57
  dietary consumption, 56
  dietary reference, 275
  forms, 62
Chromatin, breakdown, 159–160
Chromium, dietary reference, 276
Chronic disease, increase, 46
Chronic fatigue, oxidative stress (link), 82
Chronic hypertension, 194
  preeclampsia, superimposition, 194
Chronic stress, impact, 148
Citric acid cycle, 76
Clinical nutrition curriculum, offering, 16

Clostridium levels, increase, 245
Cobalamins, 168
Cobalt, requirement, 58
Coenzyme Q10 (CoQ10), 88–90, 207–208
  characteristics, 89
  deficiency, 205
  histone modification dependence, 65
  presence (decline), aging (connection), 208
  serum levels, increase, 88
Collaboration, importance, 17–20
Collagen
  degrading/remodeling, zinc (impact), 220–221
  fibers, softening, 220
  remodeling, 218–220, 219t
  Type III collagen fibers (degrading), protease enzymes (impact), 219–220
  types, 217–218
Collagenase (stimulation), hyaluronic acid (impact), 228
Complete blood count (CBC), 18–19, 158, 173
Complex carbohydrates, 83–84
Comprehensive metabolic panel (CMP)
  retest, 20
  usage, 19, 174
Conditional amino acids, 90–91
Conjugated linoleic acids (CLAs), consumption/production, 246
Constipation, presence, 152
Contractions
  mildness (false labor), 213
  MLCK prevention, 109
  oxytocin, impact, 214, 216
Copper
  dietary reference, 277
  levels, elevation, 49
  zinc, balance, 167
Cord blood, DHA (presence), 225
Corpus luteum
  carotenoids, presence, 98

estradiol, production, 111
progesterone production, 108
Cortex, corticosteroid/androgen production, 100
Corticosteroids, cortex production, 100
Corticotropin-releasing hormone (CRH) (hypothalamic hormone)
production
increase, 110, 213
initiation, 231
release/secretion, 148, 214
upregulation, 118
Cortisol, 117–119
adrenal precursor, impact, 110
deficiency, 186
elevation, oxidative stress (impact), 82
formation, ACTH stimulation, 112
functions, 118
increase, 188, 241
levels
balance, 101
increase, effects, 182
maternal cortisol, transfer, 112
negative effects, DHEA balancing function, 116
production, 119
regeneration, 188
regulation, magnesium (impact), 118
role, 117, 218
uterine/fetal cortisol, impact, 109
Coupling, 124
COVID-19 shutdowns, 21
Cultural cuisine/food, assessment, 37–38
Cultures, bridging, 29
CYP11A1 (side chain cleavage) enzyme, 97, 105
inactivation, beta-carotene deficiency (impact), 98
MK-4, correlation, 104
CYP11B1, 97, 105
ACTH/potassium regulation, 100
CYP11B2, 97, 105
CYP17A1, 97, 100–101, 105, 112

CYP19A1, 97
CYP19A1-aromatase enzyme, placenta usage, 112
CYP21A2, 97, 105
Cysteine (conditional amino acid), 91
Cytochrome P450 (CYP) enzyme
list, 97
oxidative stress damage, 96
system, 96
Cytokines
levels, increase (effects), 182
serum levels, DHEA (inverse relationship), 116

D

Dairy, complexity, 245–246
Decarboxylation, 77
Deficiency
insufficiency, contrast, 42–43
value, increase, 43
Dehydration
electrolyte balance, relationship, 197–200
occurrence, 198
Dehydroepiandrosterone (DHEA), 96
antidepressant effects, 115
anxiety, connection, 191
conversion, 105
cytokines (serum levels), inverse relationship, 116
production, 87, 101
substrate, 106
supplementation, 191
Dehydroepiandrosterone sulfate (DHEA-S) (androgen), 115–116
levels, increase, 115
production, 101
Deiodinase enzymes (selenium-containing enzymes), 126
Deiodinase, placenta production, 145
Deiodinase, zinc (catalyst role), 151
Delta-tocopherol, 102
Dementia, oxidative stress (link), 82
Deoxyribonucleic acid (DNA)

expression, 64
methylation, 55–60, 63, 66, 202
nucleotide combinations, 58
sequencing/patterning, 53
strands
  creation, 59
  stabilization, 64, 65
transcription, 159
Deoxyribonucleic acid (DNA) methyltransferase (DNMT), stimulation, 59
Depression, 177, 179
  persistence, 189
  pregnancy assessment, 191–192
  presentations, subtypes, 187
  sign, inflammation (relationship), 188–189
  symptoms
    myelin integrity, impact, 181
    nutrition, role, 186
Diet
  assessment, 195
  attention, 36
  impact, 194–196
  importance, 19
  keto diet, popularity, 86
  Mediterranean Diet, 45
  moderation, importance, 45
  mother/father diet, importance, 68–69
  preconception diet, 163
  quality, absence (impact), 81
  western diet, problems, 47
Dietary antioxidants, increase (requirement), 205
Dietary culture, respect, 36–38
Dietary esters, conversion, 232
Dietary fats, impact, 224–227
Dietary folate, absorption percentage, 61
Dietary Guidelines for Americans (CDC), 40–41
Dietary habits (establishment), education system (impact), 40
Dietary intakes
  analysis, 43
  percentage, comparisons, 44
Dietary liver, retinol source, 235
Dietary Reference Intakes (DRI), 260
Dietary vitamin A, birth defects link (absence), 236
Diiodotyrosine (DIT), formation, 124
Dilation and curettage (D&C), 173
Dilation responses, reduction, 202
Dimethyltryptamine (DMT), formation, 182
Disease
  cardiovascular disease, high fats/sugars (link), 46
  nutrition, relationship, 45–47
DNA methyltransferase (DNMT)
  function inhibition, BPA (impact), 59
  stimulation, cortisol (impact), 59
Docosahexaenoic acid (DHA), 224–227
  decrease, impact, 203
  isolated DHA supplementation, 225, 227
Dopamine, regeneration, 188
Doula, presence, 20
Dysbiosis (creation), American diet (impact), 246

E

Eclampsia, 194
Edema. *See* Pitting edema
Education system, meals (availability), 41–42
Eicosapentaenoic acid (EPA), 224–226
Elastin fibers, 217
Electrolytes
  balance, dehydration (relationship), 197–200
  minerals, presence, 197
  ratios, imbalances, 198
  requirement, 114
  types, 198
Embryo viability, decrease, 56
Endocytosis, 124
Endogenous antioxidants, formation, 81

Endogenous stress, 147–148
Endothelial derived hyperpolarizing factor (EDHR), endothelial production (increase), 112
Endothelial dysfunction, 47
Enteric nervous system (ENS), 178
Environmental halogens, thyroid hormones (relationship), 131–132
Environmental toxins, impact, 80–81
Enzymes, changes, 93
Epigenetics, 54, 55, 201–202
  changes, continuation, 68
  stress, impact, 68
Epinephrine, production/secretion, 101–102, 186
Epithelial cells, thyroid hormone production role, 125
Ergocalciferol (Vitamin D2), synthesis, 105
Erythroblasts, 159–160
Erythrocytes (red blood cells), formation, 159–160
Erythroferrone, iron regulation role, 162
Erythropoiesis, 159–160
Erythropoietin, iron regulation role, 162
Essential amino acids, 91, 182, 185, 229
Essential tremors, oxidative stress (link), 82
Estetrol (E4), 110
  production, 111
Estradiol (E2), 110
  blocking, impact, 113
  corpus luteum production, 111
Estriol (E3), 110
  hormone/blood transfer, 111
Estrogen, 96, 110–114
  arginine, interaction, 112
  elevations, baby pituitary (connection), 113
  estrogen-associated chemical changes, 112
  fetal estrogen, ovarian follicular maturity role, 113
  levels, increase, 114, 213
  nausea, association, 144
  production, 87, 106
    increase, 126
  progesterone, balance, 114
  regulation role, 161
  types, 110
Estrogen receptors (ERα/ERβ), binding, 111
Estrogen synthase, 97
Estrone (E1), 110
  production, 111
Exocytosis, 123
Exogenous stress, 147–148
Extracellular matrix (ECM), 217

F

Failed inductions, 229
Fallon, Sally, 13
False labor, 213
Familial dysfunction, pattern, 69
Fast signaling, 82
Fat
  dietary fats, impact, 224–227
  evidence, insufficiency, 46
  protection, 88–90
Father, diet (importance), 68–69
Fatigue, 173, 177, 189
Fat-soluble choline, 62
Fatty acids, balance, 225
Fear, feelings, 190, 192
Ferritin
  adequacy, 163
  assessment, 164
  serum ferritin values, increase, 165
  test, 173–174
Fetal adrenal glands
  cortisol production, 117
  DHEA-S secretion/supply, 101, 110, 112
Fetal brain
  development, DHA studies, 227
  glucose supply, maintenance, 242
Fetal cortisol, impact, 109

Fetal estrogen, ovarian follicular maturity role, 113
Fetal genetics (change), overnutrition/undernutrition (impact), 54
Fetal health, 173
Fetal heart, glucose supply (maintenance), 242
Fetal hormones, dependencies, 106
Fetal insulin resistance, increase, 66
Fetal lung maturation (stimulation), cortisol (impact), 237
Fetal maturation, cortisol levels (balance), 101
Fetal programming, 53–55
　epigenetic process, impact, 55
Fetus
　3β-HSD, absence, 106
　17-OH progesterone, transfer, 110
　placenta, hormone production relationship, 116f
Fight-or-flight response, 101–102, 179, 186, 189, 190
Flavin adenine dinucleotide (FAD) adrenodoxin reductase, usage, 96
Flavoenzymes, 77
Fluoride, toxicity/presence, 132
Folate
　conversion, 58
　cycles, 57f
　deficiency, 167
　　neural tube defects, association, 63
　dietary consumption, 56
　dietary folate, absorption percentage, 61
　food-sourced folate, protein binding, 60
　methylation, impact, 56
　natural folate, functionality, 61
　requirements, increase, 167
Folic acid
　presence, 60
　saturation, 61
　supplementation, autism risk (increase), 63
　synthetic folic acid, impact, 61
　synthetic reduction, 61
　usage, 19
Food allergy testing, 33
Food customs, 36–37
Food Politics (Nestle), 35
Food-sourced folate, protein binding, 60
Forbes, Scott, 146
Fructose, 83
Fruit, consumption, 43
Functional anemia, 165
Functional childbirth, 211
Functional Fertility (Thompson), 60
Functional medicine
　certification, importance, 47
　defining, 31–32
　specialization, 48

G

Galactose, 83
Gamma-tocopherol, 102
Gap junctions, 114
Gastritis, 148, 149
Gastroestophageal reflux disease (GERD), 146
Gene expressions, regulation, 55
Genetic methylation, 57f
Genetic mutations
　expression (inhibition), methyl groups (impact), 55
　impact, 81
Genetic nutrition, 71–72
Genetic programming (epigenetics), 54, 55
Genetic variants, 56
Geriatric pregnancies, 89
Gestational anemia, 158, 169–170
Gestational diabetes, 119
　CoQ10, link, 90
　oxidative stress, link, 82
Gestational disease, placental dysfunction (connection), 66

Gestational hypertension, 193, 194
  complication, HELLP (Impact), 169–170
  development, western diet (impact), 47
  increase, 207
  patterns, 199
  risk, 195
Gestational transient thyrotoxicosis (GTT), impact, 145–146
Ginger usage, peppermint usage (contrast), 153–155
Globulins, 90
Glomerular endothelial swelling, increase, 202–203
Glucagon, function, 142
Glucocorticoid production, increase, 222–223
Gluconeogenesis, triggering, 119
Glucose, 83
  metabolism, changes, 54, 84–85
  supply, maintenance, 242
  thiamine, requirement, 142
  transport/breakdown, 76–77
Glutamate residues, 61
Glutamine (conditional amino acid), 91
Glutathione (antioxidant), body usage, 59
Glutathione peroxidase parallel steroidogenesis, cell protection, 96
Glycine (conditional amino acid), 160
Glycogenolysis, signal, 118–119
Glycoprotein, secretion, 168
Grains, consumption, 72
Gray matter, 180
Group B Strep (GBS), 247–249
  decrease, antibiotics (usage), 248
  lung infection, 33
Growth differentiation factor 15 (GDF-15), importance, 152
Gut
  bacteria, cobalt conversion, 168
  bacteria/yeast, presence, 245
  motility, problems, 152
  pain, 190
Gut microbiome
  change, 247
  impact, 32
  vaginal microbiome, mimicry, 249

H

Hair loss symptoms, zinc (impact), 127
Halogens, exposure, 146
Hashimoto's thyroiditis, 122, 132
Hashimoto's Thyroiditis (Wentz), 133
Headaches, presence, 118
Healthy fats, consumption, 44
Heartburn, 139
Heme iron, antinutrients effect (absence), 162
Heme transport proteins, presence, 164
Hemocytoblast (stem cell), 159
Hemoglobin, 90
  cutoff (homebirth midwife level), 157
  formation, 160
  levels, 174–175
  making, process, 160
  NO, binding, 204
Hemolysis Elevated Liver enzymes Low Platelets (HELLP) syndrome, 169–170, 193, 196
Hepcidin
  decrease, testosterone (impact), 163–164
  estrogen regulation role, 163
  iron regulation role, 162–163
  production (increase), inflammatory cytokines (impact), 165
High blood pressure, oxidative stress (link), 82
High density lipoprotein (HDL), 87
Histidine (essential amino acid), 91
Histone acetylation, 77
  increase, malnutrition (impact), 65–66
Histone acetyltransferases (HATs), impact, 65
Histone deacetylases (HDACs), acetyl group removal, 65

Histone modification, 55, 64–66
  nutrients, impact, 65
Homebirth midwives
  assistance, 12
  hemoglobin cutoff, 157
Homocysteine, 58
  breakdown, BHMT requirement, 59
Hormonal factors, 143–146
Hormones, 95
  changes, 188
  production, oxidative stress
    (impact), 82
  synthesis, 106
Hospitalization rates (increase), viral/
  bacterial infections (impact), 250
H. Pylori (bacterial infection), 146–149
  stress, impact, 148
  ulcer formation, relationship, 147
Human chorionic gonadotropin
  (hCG), 143
  impact, 109
  levels, elevation, 135
  secretion, 120, 143–144, 148
Hyaluronic acid (HA)
  synthesis, estrogen/PGF2α
    (importance), 228
Hyaluronic acid (HA), impact, 227–229
Hydrochloric acid (HCl), 131, 168
Hydroxysteroid dehydrogenases
  (HSDs), 96
Hyperemesis gravidarum (HG)
  development, 140
  experience, 142
  genetic cases, 153
  GTT, impact, 145–146
Hypertension
  anemia, relationship, 196–197
  categories, 194
  causes, 195
  diet, impact, 194–196
  oxidative stress, 203–207
  risk (increase), placental morphology
    (association), 67

treatability, 193
Hypocalcemia, 221
Hypoglycemia, tendency, 152
Hypothalamic-pituitary-adrenal (HPA)
  axis (modulation), magnesium
    (impact), 118
Hypothyroidism
  cause, 133
  development, risk, 132
Hypoxia
  elevated markers, 196
  problems, 197

I
Immature red blood cells
  (reticulocytes), 160
Immune inflammatory responses,
  increase, 204
Immune responses
  increase/avoidance, 33
  suppression, 148–149
Imposter syndrome, 21–22
Indoleamine 2,3 dioxygenase (IDO),
  production (increase), 182
Induction
  failed inductions, 229
  failure, 17
  Pitocin, usage, 217
Infections, 188, 189, 193, 214, 244
  risk, 248
Infertility, explanation (absence), 173
Inflammation, 158, 202
  iron deficiency, relationship, 164–165
  phytochemicals/antioxidants,
    protective effect, 207
  sign, depression (relationship),
    188–189
Inflammatory activity, 47
Inflammatory cytokines, impact, 165
Inflammatory protein, impact, 152
Innate antioxidants, increase
  (requirement), 205
Inorganic selenium, 128
Insomnia, 117–118, 177

Institute for Functional Medicine
(IFM), 17
Insufficiency
  deficiency, contrast, 42–43
  value, increase, 43
Insulin
  dysregulation issues, 141–142
  production, increase, 84–85, 141
  receptors, lactogen (binding), 85
Insulin-like growth factor binding protein 7 (IGFBP7)
  importance, 152
  insulin resistance/metabolic syndrome risk increase, association, 152
Insulin resistance, 119, 142
  adulthood, 54
  IGFBP7, association, 153
  oxidative stress, impact, 82
Intracellular moisture, addition, 228
Intrauterine growth restriction (IUGR), oxidative stress (impact), 79
In vitro fertilization (IVF), 56
Iodination, 124
Iodine
  amount, debate, 127–131
  deficiency, 122, 128
  dietary reference, 278
  iodine-induced autoimmune thyroid disease, risk (increase), 130
  thyroid hormone, importance, 146
  toxicity, 129
Iodine: Why You Need It, Why Can't Live Without It (Brownstein), 130
Iron
  absorption
    decrease/increase, 163
    hepcidin, impact, 163
  accumulation, 160
  characteristics/forms, 162
  dietary reference, 279
  iron-deficiency anemia, 174
  level, 174
  metabolism, shift, 161–164, 175
  regulation, hormones (impact), 162
  supplementation, 164
  increase, 169, 172
  values, adequacy, 163
Iron deficiency
  anemia, contrast, 166–170
  inflammation, relationship, 164–165
  NHANES report, 158
Islets of Langerhans, 142
Isoleucine (essential amino acid), 91

J
Junk food, impact, 81

K
Keto diet, popularity, 86
Ketogenesis, 85–86
  maternal ketogenesis, impact, 86
Ketones, transfer (risk), 86
Kidneys, protein (leakage), 202–203
Krebs cycle, 76–79, 88, 160
  disruption, aluminum (impact), 79
  intermediate chemicals, usage, 92
  nutrient cofactors, display, 78f
Kynurenine
  picolinic acid conversion, 183
Kynurenine pathway
  activation, increase, 183
  tryptophan degradation, 182

L
Labor
  antibiotics, usage, 247–249
  false labor, 213
  Group B strep (GBS), usage, 247–249
  onset, 215f
  oxytocin physiology, 231
  physiology, 213–216
  premature labor, 214
  preparation, 238
  progression, problems, 228–229
  stress, 241–242
Lactobacillus levels, increase, 245
Lactogen

Index

placenta production, 85–86
Lactogen, insulin receptors (binding), 85
L-arginine (amino acid), NO synthesis, 112
LDL, conversion, 113
Legumes, consumption, 72
Leucine (essential amino acid), 91
Linoleic acid (LA)
  conjugated linoleic acids (CLAs), consumption/production, 246
  consumption, 224
Lipid breakdown, metabolic phases, 85
Lipid compounds, production/balance, 223
Lipid metabolism, 85–86
Lipid oxidation inhibition, 204
Lipid peroxidation reactions, 203
Lipoprotein lipase (LPL)
  decrease, 86
  increase, 85
Liver
  consumption, debate/reduction, 233–234
  dietary liver, retinol source, 235
  enlargement, non-alcoholic fatty liver disease (association), 63
Long-chain polyunsaturated omega-3 fatty acids, types, 224
Low density lipoprotein (LDL), 87
  availability, placenta regulation, 113
  cholesterol (availability), pregnenolone production (relationship), 98
  increase, stimulation, 120
Lungs, inflammation (decrease), 33–34
Luteal phase, progesterone (presence), 27
Luteinizing hormone (LH), increase, 108
Lymphocyte proliferation, action (suppression), 109
Lysine (essential amino acid), 91

M
Macronutrients, ratio, 246
Macrophage production (increase), SP-A (impact), 238
Magnesium, 198
  assistance, 68, 203
  deficiency, 118, 199–200
  demand, increase, 113–114, 199
  dietary reference, 282
  histone modification dependence, 65
  nausea, association, 151–152
  requirement, 58, 183, 236–237
Magnesium deficiency, 19
  CRH/ACTH upregulation, association, 118
Malnutrition
  impact, 65–66
  maternal malnutrition, 220
Malnutrition anemia, 196
Manganese
  deficiency, 206
  dietary reference, 283
  SOD, 2096
Manganese, deficiency, 205
Markle, Meghan, 177
Maternal adrenal glands, DHEA-S secretion/supply, 112
Maternal cascades, 237
Maternal cortisol, transfer, 112
Maternal death rate (US), 14
Maternal depression, anxiety (relationship), 181
Maternal gestational diabetes, impact, 54–55
Maternal heritage, importance, 28–29
Maternal hormones, dependencies, 106
Maternal ketogenesis, impact, 86
Maternal malnutrition, 220
Maternal nutritional intake, impact, 55
Maternal outcomes (improvement), iron supplementation (impact), 172
Maternal physiological changes, 199
Maternal stress responses, continuation, 68
Maternal vascular changes, 202–203

Maternity
  care, specialization (advantage), 49
  complications, racial groups (correlation), 47
  healthcare, medicalization, 9
Maternity functional medicine, importance, 31, 71–72, 239
Matrix metalloproteinases (MMPs), 202
Mean corpuscular hemoglobin concentration (MCHC), stability, 161
Mean corpuscular volume (MCV)
  increase, 157–158
  stability, 161
Mediterranean Diet, 45
Melatonin, formation, 182
Menaquinone (vitamin K2), 103
Menses, loss, 163
Messenger RNA (mRNA), translation, 90
Metabolic changes, 75
Metabolic dysfunction, 66
Metabolic imbalances, 188
Metabolic panel. *See* Comprehensive metabolic panel
Metabolic programming, changes, 54
Metabolic regulation, 92–93
Metabolic syndrome
  adulthood, 54
  risk (increase), IGFBP7 (association), 153
Metalloproteinase enzymes
  actions, upregulation, 221
  zinc component, 220–221
Methionine (antioxidant)
  body usage, 59
  creation process, 58
  cycle, entry, 57
  essential amino acid, 91
Methionine sulfate, 58
Methylate, 61
Methylation
  importance, 64, 160
  meaning, 55

Methylcobalamin, usage, 19, 168
Methylenetetrahydrofolate reductase (MTHFR)
  enzyme role, 55
  impact, 56
  mutation, 63, 91
Methylfolate, function, 58
Methyl groups, impact, 55
Microbial fermentation, 244
Microbiome, 243–245
  birth method, relationship, 249–250
  gut microbiome
    change, 247
    impact, 32
  mother, diet (relationship), 245–247
Midwives, 28
  interaction, 24–25
  presence, 20
Migraines, oxidative stress (link), 81
Miscarriage
  estrogen blocking, impact, 113
  oxidative stress, impact, 79
  recurrence, 56, 173
  thyroid antibodies, association, 134
Mitochondria, 207–208
  DNA, presence, 76
  function, abnormality, 208
  oxidative stress, impact, 82
  weakness, increase, 80
MK-4/MK-7, 104
Molybdenum, dietary reference, 284
Monoiodotyrosine (MIT), formation, 124
Monooxygenase reactions, 96
Morning sickness, 139–140, 149, 158, 175
Mother
  cesarean delivery, risks, 251
  chemical changes, 215f
  diet
    importance, 68–69
    microbiome health, relationship, 245–247

malnourishment, 54
preconception nutrition, 53
Motherhood, journey, 15
Motility changes, 190
Myelin
  composition, 181
  importance, 180
Myocin light chain kinase (MLCK) system, contraction prevention, 109
Myosin (contracting protein), 90

N

National Health and Nutrition Examination Survey (NHANES), 43
  dietary failure, 41
  iron deficiency report, 158
National School Lunch Act (1947), 40
Natural folate, functionality, 61
Nature, knowledge, 35
Nausea, 139, 190
  decrease, P5P (impact), 149
  elevation, progesterone (link), 144
  estrogen, association, 144
  genetics, 152–153
  ginger usage, peppermint usage (contrast), 153–155
  hyperthyroid function, connection, 146
  increase, magnesium (association), 151–152
  induction, absence, 146
  metabolic factors, 141–143
  nutritional factors, 149–152
  pathogenesis, 140
  predisposition, 155
  presentation, 141
Neonatal intensive care unit (NICU), lung infection, 247–248
Neonatal units, admission (risk), 243
Nervous system, 178–180
Nestle, Marion, 35
Neural tube defects (NTDs), folate deficiency (association), 63
Neurons, glucose usage, 82
Neurotransmitters
  function, alteration, 181
  increase, 190, 241
  life cycle, 180
  receptors, cholesterol (impact), 181
  release/regulation, 179
Nickel SOD, 205
Nicotinamide adenine dinucleotide (NAD)
  cofactor role, 183
  formation, 182
  function, 103
  metabolic pathway, disruption, 151
  production, 182
Nicotinamide adenine dinucleotide phosphate hydrogen (NADPH), electron transfer, 96
Nicotinamide adenine dinucleotide plus hydrogen (NADH), synthesis, 77
NIS. *See* Sodium-iodine symporter
Nitric oxide (NO)
  hemoglobin, binding, 204
  production, increase, 112, 203
  release, 200
Nitric oxide system (NOS), 179
Nitrogen base, methyl group deposit, 58f
Non-alcoholic fatty liver disease, liver enlargement (association), 63
Nonheme, presence, 162
Norepinephrine, production/secretion, 102, 186
Nourishing Traditions (Fallon), 13
Nucleotide structure, 58f
Nutrient density
  absence, 38
  increase, 36
Nutrient Power (Walsh), 187
Nutrients
  cofactors, impact, 96
  power, 186–188
  RDA level, irrelevance, 187
Nutrition

American nutrition, functional
  nutrition (contrast), 34–36
assessment, inclusion, 16
biochemical role, 47
changes, 48
clinical nutrition curriculum,
  offering, 16
confusion, 11
connection, 43–45
disease, relationship, 45–47
knowledge, attainment, 40
medical school coursework,
  inadequacy, 15–16
moderation, importance, 46
physical degeneration,
  relationship, 69–72
preconception nutrition, 53
prenatal nutrition, research, 25
science, history, 45–46
Nutritional cofactors, requirement, 99f
Nutritional deficiencies, 42, 81, 83,
  167, 192
  cervix remodeling, relationship,
    220–221
  premature labor cause, 214
Nutritional insufficiencies, 81
Nutrition and Physical Degeneration
  (Price), 13
*Nutrition Education in U.S. Medical
  Schools* (National Academy of Science-
  National Research Council), 15

O

OB/GYNs, assistance, 12
Omega-3 fatty acid
  consumption, 224
  supplementation, 225
Omega-6 fatty acid, consumption, 224
Organic selenium, 128
Organ meat, dietary intake
  (vilification), 233
Organ systems, oxidative stress
  (impact), 81–82
Ornithine (conditional amino acid), 91

Ovaries
  aromatase activity, alteration, 105
  hormone production, 82
Overnutrition
  fetal insulin resistance, increase
    (association), 66
  impact, 54
Ovulation (cause), LH (impact), 108
Oxalates (oxalic acid), cultural approach,
  165–166
Oxidative compounds, ratio
  (imbalance), 80–81
Oxidative particles, antioxidant
  neutralization, 79
Oxidative stress, 47, 79–82, 158, 192
  attention deficit disorder, link, 82
  autism, link, 82
  cause, 200
  elevated markers, 196
  hypertension, association, 203–207
  increase, 207
  long-term oxidative stress, impact, 81
  phytochemicals/antioxidants,
    protective effect, 207
  preeclampsia, association, 203–207
  problems, 82
  reduction, 232
    antioxidants, impact, 79
    CoQ10, usage, 88–90
    vitamin E supplementation,
      impact, 205
  signs, 202
Oxygen supplementation/resuscitation
  rates, increase, 243
Oxytocin
  catecholamines, balance, 242
  cell receptors, magnesium/cholesterol
    (requirement), 236–237
  physiology (labor), 231
  prolactin/relaxin, comparison, 229
  protein, relationship, 229, 231
  receptors, expression (increase), 114
  usage, debate, 233–236

P

P5P. *See* Pyridoxal-5-phosphate
Paleo diet, 36
Palpitations, 190
Parasympathetic nervous system, 179, 188
Parasympathetic state, dysfunction, 189
Parkinson's disease, oxidative stress (link), 82
Pathogenic invasion, impact, 244
Patient-physician collaboration, importance, 17–20
Peppermint usage, ginger usage (contrast), 153–155
Peripheral nervous system (PNS), 178
Pernicious anemia, 167
Phenylalanine (essential amino acid), 91
Phosphate, 198
Phosphatidylcholine, 62
Phosphatidylserine (PS), 101
Phosphorus
  dietary reference, 280
  presence, 64
  storage form, 72
Phosphorylation, 64
Phylloquinone (vitamin K1), 103
Physical damage, reversal, 33–34
Physical degeneration, nutrition (relationship), 69–72
Physician
  burnout, The Physicians Foundation survey, 17
  physician-patient burnout, importance, 17–20
Phytates
  cultural approach, 72–73
  impact, 71
Phytonutrients, presence, 195, 246–247
Picolinic acid, production, 182, 183
Pineal gland, melatonin production, 182
Pitocin, usage, 217, 227
Pitting edema
  improvement, 19
  presence, 18
Placenta
  17β-HSD, absence, 112
  blood flow, decrease, 67
  chemical changes, 215f
  development, 66–67, 152, 201–202
  gene alterations, 202
  dysfunction, 207–208
  gestational disease, connection, 66
  signal, 203
  fetus, hormone production relationship, 116f
  function, vitamins/minerals (impact), 68
  health
    importance, 67–68
    magnesium, impact, 112
  hormones, dependencies, 106
  ketones, transfer (risk), 86
  morphology, associations, 67
  oxidation, signs (problems), 82
  oxygenation, 196
  trophoblast cell, function (inability), 67
  type III deiodinase production, 135
Placental cells
  aromatase activity, alteration, 105
  CRH expression, 117
Placental insulin growth factor (PIGF), impact, 67
Plasma, increase, 161, 197
Platelet aggregation, blocking, 226
Plato, 45
Polycystic ovary syndrome (PCOS), 115, 142
Polyphenols, presence, 246–247
Polyunsaturated fats, addition, 34
Postpartum, anxiety (presence), 188
Postpartum depression, oxidative stress (link), 82
Post-traumatic stress disorder (PTSD), impact, 68
Potassium, 198

deficiency, 19
dietary reference, 281
pregnancy RDA, 198–199
regulation role, 100
Pottenger, Francis, 15
Practitioners, answers (search), 11–12
Preconception diet, 163
Preconception nutrition, 53
Predisposed maternal factors, 47
Preeclampsia, 18, 193
  CoQ10, link, 90, 207–208
  maternal vascular changes, 202–203
  mitochondria, relationship, 207–208
  multi-system disease, 200
  nutritional associations, 200–201
  nutritional/chemical prerequisites, 19
  occurrence, 115, 208
  oxidative stress, impact/link, 79, 82, 203–207
  pathogenesis, 47
  placental morphology, association, 67
  risk, 201–202
    increase, C677T MTHFR SNP (association), 202
    increase, vitamin B2 (association), 200
  SOD, connection, 206
  superimposition, 194
  symptoms, 208–209
Preformed vitamin A retinoids, types, 232
Pregnancy
  anemia, 157
  anxiety
    assessment, 191–192
    presence, 188
  autoimmune disease, 132–134
  chronic disease, increase, 46
  complications
    increase, 134
    Vitamin D deficiency, connection, 106
  copper levels, elevation, 49
  cortisol, role, 117
  depression, assessment, 191–192
  metabolic changes, 75, 119
  phases, 93
  nausea, 139
  nutritional habits, impact, 53–54
  oxidative stress, impact, 79, 82
  progesterone production, placenta control, 108
  thyroid hormones, presence/impact, 134–135
  transitional time, 31
  vitamin D
    daily intake recommendation, 43
    metabolism, 106–108
Pregnancy, sustaining (hormonal interactions), 119–120
Pregnancy-Unique Quantification of Emesis (PUQE), vitamin B6 usage assessment, 150
Pregnant women, questions, 11
  answers, 12–14
Pregnenolone
  cholesterol conversion, 97
  conversion, 100
  LDL conversion, 113
  production, LDL cholesterol dependence, 98
  role, 98
Preimplantation embryos, generation, 56
Pre-labor contractions, oxytocin (impact), 214
Premature cervical remodeling, risk (increase), 220
Premature cervical softening/ripening, risk (increase), 220
Premature labor, 214
Prenatal care, focus, 14
Prenatal depression, anxiety (connection), 178
Prenatal dietary reference intakes, 260
Prenatal nutrition, research, 25

Prenatal vitamin A, consumption (Debate), 233–236
Prescription prenatal, usage, 19
Preterm labor, oxidative stress (impact), 79
Price, Weston A., 13–15, 24–25, 29, 35
　family/birth order examination, 69
　nutrition, importance, 212
　nutrition study, 46
　Vaughan, connection, 38
Processed sugars, impact, 81
Progesterone, 108–110
　corpus luteum production, 108
　decrease, 214
　estrogen, balance, 114
　increase, 110, 151–152, 218–219
　luteal phase hormone (yang hormone), 27
　nausea, link, 144
　pregnenolone conversion, 100
　production
　　3β-HSD, importance, 103
　　increase, 108–109
Prolactin, oxytocin (comparison), 229
Proline (conditional amino acid), 91
Prostacyclin (PGI2), 222, 223
　endothelial production, increase, 112
　levels, change, 203
Prostaglandin 2α (PGF2α), 228
Prostaglandin D2 (PGD2), 222
Prostaglandin E2 (PGE2), 222, 223
Prostaglandin F2α (PGF2α), 222, 223
Prostaglandin H2 (PGH2), 222–223
Prostaglandins
　2-series prostaglandins, forms, 222
　derivation, 224
　expression, increase, 114
　formation/function, dietary fats (impact), 224–227
　impact, 222–223
　production increase, estrogen signal, 222

receptor expression (increase), progesterone (impact), 222
　synthesis, increase, 222–223
Protease enzymes, impact, 219–220
Protein
　breakdown/denaturing, 91
　intake, monitoring, 92
　leakage, 202–203
　metabolism, 90–92
　　blood values, monitoring, 92
　oxytocin, relationship, 229, 231
　protein-based transport molecules, cortisol binding, 119
　transport protein, function, 90
　upregulation, EPA (usage), 225
Protein, consumption, 44
Provitamin A carotenoids, types, 232
Pyridoxal-5-phosphate (P5P)
　blood values increase, antiemetic effects (association), 150
　impact, 149
Pyridoxine hydrochloride (pyridoxine HCl), usage, 19, 150
Pyrrole rings, formation, 160
Pyruvate, creation/breakdown, 76–77

Q
Questions/answers, passion, 23–24
Quinolinic acid, production, 182, 183

R
Racial groups, maternity complications (correlation), 47
Rancid fats, impact, 88
Reactive oxygen species (ROS), 79
　neutralization, vitamin E ability, 221
　production, 204
Recommended Daily Allowance (RDA), 260
Recurrent preeclampsia risk (reduction), vitamin D supplementation (impact), 200
Red blood cells (erythrocytes)
　formation (erythropoiesis), 159–160

increase, 161
maturation, 160
reticulocytes (immature red blood cells), 160
Red blood count (RBC), analysis, 173–174
Red-lining, 37
Red meat, avoidance, 34
Refined grains, reduction, 19
Refined/processed trans-fats, impact, 81
Refined sugars, impact, 81, 84
Relaxin
 oxytocin, comparison, 229
 production, 214
Reproductive function, nutrition adequacy, 45
Reproductive organs, 96
Reticulocytes (immature red blood cells), 160
Retinal, 232
Retinoic acid, 232
Retinol, 232
 source, 235
Retinyl esters, 232
Reverse-transcription-polymerase chain reaction (RT-PCR) analysis, 207
Riboflavin, usage, 19

S
S-adenosylmethionine (SAMe) (AdoMet), 182
 conversion, 60
 creation, 55–56, 57f
 impact, 58
 methylation, occurrence, 64
 methyl group deposit/donation, 58f, 186
Safe Childbirth (Vaughan), 38, 69–72
Salt, limitation, 34
Saturated fats, consumption, 44
Schizophrenia, 179
School lunches
 childhood obesity rates, increase (relationship), 41

problems, 39
Science, reliance, 35–36
Seafood, consumption, 47
Selective serotonin reuptake inhibitor (SSRI) medication, 191
Selenate, 128
Selenite, 128
Selenium
 antioxidant role, 128
 characteristics/types, 128
 deficiency, 126
 dietary reference, 285
Selenocysteine (amino acid), 90, 128
Selenomethionine, 128
Serine (conditional amino acid), 91
 carbon transfer, 56
Serine hydroxymethyltransferase (SMT), impact, 56
Serotonin (5-HT)
 formation, 182
 regeneration, 188
Serum 25-hydroxycalciferol [25(OH)D] (25-OH vitamin D)
 cholesterol, conversion, 105
 evaluator role, 106
 maintenance, 107
Serum cholesterol values, increase, 87–88
Serum ferritin values, increase, 165
Serum iron (test), 173
Serum lipid values, increase, 86
Side chain cleavage enzymes, 97
Simple carbohydrates, 83–84
Simple sugars, 83
Single-nucleotide polymorphism (CNP), impact, 56
Six Nation Reservation
 Price visit, 212
 Vaughan visit, 70
Small intestine bacterial overgrowth (SIBO), 154
Sodium, 198
 consumption, 44

dietary reference, 286
Sodium-iodine symporter (NIS)
  destruction, autoimmune antibodies (association), 133
  iodine transport control, 123
Somatic nervous system (SNS), 178
Specialization, importance, 47–49
Stem cell (hemocytoblast), 159
Steroid hormones, impact, 92–93, 222
Steroidogenesis, 96–98
  complexity, 102
  process, enzyme requirements, 99f
Steroidogenic acute regulatory (StAR) protein, requirement, 96–97
Steroid synthesis regulation
  Vitamin D, relationship, 104–105
  Vitamin K, relationship, 104
Stress, 147, 189
  anxiety, physical manifestation, 149, 190
  chronic stress, impact, 148
  endogenous stress, 147
  exogenous stress, 147–148
  hormones, impact, 148
  impact, 68, 244
  maternal stress responses, continuation, 68
Stroke, oxidative stress (link), 81
Stromal extracellular matrix (stromal ECM), 217
Study Links Excess Vitamin A to Birth Defects (Brody), 234
Substrates, appetite (increase), 93
Succinyl coenzyme (succinyl-CoA), 160
Sudden infant death syndrome, 118
Sugar
  amino acid base, binding, 58
  blood sugar levels, 119, 152
  consumption, 44
  processed/refined sugars, impact, 81
  refined sugar, 81, 84
  simple sugars, 83
Superoxide dismutase (SOD)

antioxidants, production, 207
  cell protection, 96
  families, 205
  preeclampsia, connection, 206
Surfactant protein A (SP-A), impact, 238
Surfactants, 237–238
  detection, 238
Sympathetic nervous system, 179, 186
Sympathetic state, dysfunction, 189
Synapse (neuron gap), 179
Synthetic folic acid, impact, 61
Systolic blood pressure, increase, 206

T

T-cell activation, 133
Testes
  aromatase activity, alteration, 105
  hormone production, 82
Testosterone (androgen), 96, 114–115
  maternal blood levels, increase, 115
Tetrahydrofolate (THF), dietary folate conversion, 56
Thiamine. *See* Vitamin B1
Threonine (essential amino acid), 91
Thromboxane, 223
Thromboxane A2 (TXA2), 223
  DHA, binding, 226
  requirement, 203
Thyroglobulin, 123
  iodination, increase, 130
  protein base, 133
Thyroid antibodies, 132–134
  increase, vitamin D levels (correlation), 133–134
  miscarriage, association, 134
Thyroid-binding globulin (TBG), transport role, 126
Thyroid glands
  function, 122–125
  hormone release, 122
  stimulation, 145
Thyroid hormones, 93
  activation, 126–127

environmental halogens, relationship, 131–132
iodine, importance, 146
presence/impact, 134–135
production, 123–126
epithelial cell role, 125
stimulation role, 100
Thyroid peroxidase (TPO)
antibodies, diagnosis, 122
importance, 133
selenium, importance, 128
Thyroid physiology, 121
Thyroid proteins, antigen proteins (distinguishing), 132
Thyroid receptors, types, 127
Thyroid-releasing hormone (TRH), 125
Thyroid-stimulating hormone (TSH)
production, 147
secretion, 125
values, 121
Thyroxine (T4), 123–126
Tolerable Upper Intake Limit (UL), 260
TPRM6 magnesium channels, regulation, 113–114
Traditional Chinese medicine (TCM), 186–187
approach, 10
training, 26–28
Traditional cultures, acknowledgment, 37
Transport proteins, function, 90
Trauma, 192, 214
Trauma survivors, genetic stress (connection), 68
Traumatic birth, 14–15
Tricarboxylic cycle, 76
Triggers, identification, 33
Triglycerides
caloric storage, 87
values, increase, 87–88
Triiodothyronine (T3), 123–126
zinc, requirement, 127
Trimethylglycine (TMG), 59

Trophoblast cells, 66–67
function, inability, 67
hCG secretion role, 143
mitochondrial function, abnormality, 207
Tryptophan (essential amino acid), 91, 182
pathway, 184f
nutrition, impact, 185–186
serotonin synthesis, 182
Tryptophan dioxygenase (TDO)
demand, increase, 150
production, increase, 182
Type 1 diabetes, 141
Type 2 diabetes, 142
oxidative stress, impact, 82
Type I collagen, 217t
Type II collagen, 217t
Type III collagen, 217t
fibers (degrading), protease enzymes (impact), 219–220
Type III deiodinase, placenta production, 135
Type IV collagen, 217t
Tyrosine (conditional amino acid), 91, 185
binding, 122

U

Ubiquinol, 89
Ubiquinone, 89
Ubiquitination, 64
Ulcers, 146
formation, H. Pylori (impact), 147
Ultrasounds, usage, 173
Undernutrition, impact, 54
Unmetabolized folic acid, 60–63
autism, relationship, 63
Uterine cortisol, impact, 109

V

Vaginal birth after cesarean (VBAC) deliveries, 18, 20
Valine (essential amino acid), 91

Index

Vascular function (changes), placental morphology (association), 67
Vasoconstriction, increase, 200
Vasoconstrictors, impact, 223
Vaughan, Kathleen, 38–39, 69–70
　Six Nation Reservation visit, 70
Vegan diet
　anemia, relationship, 158, 170–172
　usefulness, 195
Vegetables, consumption, 36, 43, 45, 47
Vegetarian diet, usefulness, 195
Viral infections, impact, 250
Vitamin A
　antioxidant functions, 169
　characteristics/forms, 232
　consumption, debate, 233–236
　dietary forms, 232
　dietary reference, 262
　solubility, 235
Vitamin B1 (thiamine)
　dietary reference, 266
　insufficiency, 142
　requirement, 77
Vitamin B2 (riboflavin)
　dietary reference, 267
　preeclampsia risk (increase), association, 200
　presence, 77
Vitamin B3
　dietary reference, 268
　histone modification dependence, 65
　requirement, 65
Vitamin B5 (pantothenic acid)
　characteristics, 80
　dietary reference, 269
　histone modification dependence, 65
　presence, 65
　requirement, 77
Vitamin B6 (pyridoxine)
　antiemetic effects, 149
　cofactor role, 150–151
　deficiency, 151
　dietary reference, 270
　histone modification dependence, 65
　SHMT, impact, 56
Vitamin B7 (biotin)
　dietary reference, 271
　enzyme cofactor, 77
Vitamin B9, dietary reference, 272
Vitamin B9, histone modification dependence, 65
Vitamin B12 (cobalamin)
　breakdown/absorption, 244
　characteristics/groups, 168
　dietary reference, 273
　histone modification dependence, 65
　requirement, 58
　increase, 167
Vitamin C
　assistance, 68
　deficiency, 35
　dietary reference, 274
Vitamin D (calciferol), 96
　anemia, correlation, 169
　calcium, uncoupling, 107
　characteristics, 105
　daily intake recommendation, 43
　deficiency, 19, 109, 200
　　pregnancy complications, connection, 106
　dietary reference, 263
　forms, 105
　increase, 66–67
　insufficiency, 42
　metabolites, formation, 98
　receptors, expression, 133
　steroid synthesis regulation, relationship, 104–105
　supplementation, impact, 200
　test usage, 19
　usage, 19
Vitamin D2 (ergocalciferol), 105
Vitamin D3 (cholecalciferol), 105
Vitamin E (tocopherol)
　antioxidant capacity, 102
　assistance, 68

cell protection, 96
characteristics, 102
deficiency, 109
dietary reference, 264
lipid oxidation inhibition, 204
ROS neutralization role, 221
Vitamin K, 89
characteristics, 103
dietary reference, 265
forms, 103
steroid synthesis regulation, relationship, 104
Vitamin K1 (phylloquinone), 103
Vitamin K2 (menaquinone), 103
Vomiting
decrease, P5P (impact), 149
induction, absence, 146

W

Walsh, William, 187
Water-soluble choline, 62
Wentz, Izabella, 133
Western diet
characterization, 195
problems, 47
Western medicine, clinical nutrition (combination), 32
Western nutrition, biases, 34–35
White matter, 180
Whole food ingredients, consumption, 36
Whole grains, consumption, 43
Whole wheat flour, zinc absorption, 73
Winfrey, Oprah, 177

Y

Yang hormone (progesterone), 27

Z

Zinc
absorption, 71, 73
assistance, 68
catalyst role, 151
characteristics, 71

collagen remodeling, relationship, 220–221
copper, balance, 167
deficiency, 92, 126, 151, 205
dietary reference, 287
histone modification dependence, 65
importance, 174
requirement, 57, 65, 91, 127
supplementation, evidence, 221
zinc-deficiency anemia, 167, 174
Zona fasciculata, 100
Zona glomerulosa, 100
Zona reticularis, 100

Resources for Continuing Your Journey

From here, your journey continues. From here, you have many different roads you can take. If the road you choose takes you down a path of continued education and advancement, then it is not the wrong path, no matter which way it takes you. One of the greatest things my father ever told me was, "Keep learning."

Functional Maternity Website

Through my website (*www.functionalmaternity.com*), I offer several options for practitioners and patients alike to continue seeking out more knowledge. The courses, e-books, and opportunities I offer here are designed for people interested in learning more about functional medicine in maternity care or who are looking for resources to help them through their pregnancy journey. There are both free and paid courses and e-books available.

Downloads and e-books

Excited to continue learning about functional medicine and maternity care? Check out the many free e-book downloads and resources I have on my website.

Mentorship

There are few functional medicine practitioners out there who specialize in maternity and pregnancy, and I want those who are treating pregnant mothers to be able to do so with confidence. For years, I've offered mentorship programs for practitioners who would like more one-on-one coaching in their education journey. This program is designed to help practitioners through case studies and individualized question and answer sessions.

Live webinars

Occasionally, I offer live webinars on specific and focused topics related to maternity medicine. During these webinars, participants are able to ask questions and receive handouts and other tools to create an interactive experience. These advanced courses will cover topics not addressed in this book.

Maternity functional medicine training program

I am excited to be offering this new program in the upcoming future. This program will be designed to provide practitioners with the advanced knowledge they need to begin treating maternity patients successfully. The program will be divided into modules that encompass much of what I've discussed in this book but at an even deeper level. These modules will provide the practitioners with case studies, unique conditions, and unique presentations in a program designed to mimic the clinical setting. The program will be a study at your own pace with testing and certification of completion at the end. Many of the modules will be available with continuing education credit from a variety of medical organizations.

Non-medical practitioner continuing education

As a doula myself, I know that doulas are in a fantastic position to provide dietary and lifestyle advice when properly trained. My doula-specific, CEU-approved courses are designed to give doulas usable tools in guiding their clients nutritionally through pregnancy and postpartum. They will be exposed to research-based protocols and trained to support women nutritionally through pregnancy. They will receive the tools needed to guide these women through coaching. Eventually, I would like to have this be a certification program that doulas can use in their practices.

Other training opportunities

There are many other functional medicine programs out there. For many of my courses, having a certification in functional medicine is a must. These programs offer comprehensive functional medicine programs with certifications that are well recognized.

Institute for Functional Medicine (IFM) - IFM is one of the oldest programs for functional medicine in the country. It is considered the most comprehensive program for functional medicine. Many of the educators are world-renowned practitioners. Learn more at ifm.org.

Functional Medicine University (FMU) - FMU is a 100 percent online functional medicine certification program that is done in modules that you can accomplish at your own pace. Webinars and courses are taught by some of the biggest names in functional medicine. Learn more at functionalmedicineuniversity.com.

Future books

No, this is not the last you'll see of me. I have two other books in the works. Stay up-to-date on what is new by subscribing to my email list.

Practitioners

There are so many amazing functional medicine and healthcare practitioners out there with a wealth of knowledge. Many of them have amazing, information-packed websites, programs, courses, and more that cover topics related to functional medicine, women's health, and pregnancy.

Dr. Ben Lynch

Dr. Ben Lynch is the foremost authority on methylation and epigenetic changes and their effects in pregnancy. He's the author of the book *Dirty Genes* and the founder of the Seeking Health Supplement company, which focuses on functional supplement products with a unique pregnancy line.

Dr. Kalea Wattles

Dr. Wattles is a naturopathic physician who specializes in functional medicine fertility. She is a clinical staff member at the Institute for Functional Medicine and helped design their advanced training in male and female fertility support.

Dr. Aviva Romm

Dr. Romm is the face of functional medicine in women's health. A midwife, physician, and herbalist, she has written several books on different aspects of women's health. Her website provides resources for both patients and practitioners looking to increase their knowledge.

Kresser Institute

Chris Kresser is a pioneer in functional medicine and also a fellow acupuncturist. His websites and blogs are a wealth of information. The kresserinstitute.com website is geared toward practitioners and contains advanced articles and research. His chriskresser.com website is geared toward anyone seeking health and wellness information.

Obstetrical Acupuncture Association

The OBAA is an organization of obstetrically trained acupuncturists. The organization is committed to providing up-to-date research, resources, trainings, and mentorship for acupuncturists looking to advance their training in obstetrical acupuncture.

Reading List

Nutrition and Physical Degeneration

This book is a must for anyone in the health and wellness world, or anyone for that matter. Dr. Weston A. Price's book from the 1930s set in motion much of what science is now discovering. His work helped identify missing nutrients in the modern diet and helped shape the understanding that nutrition and deficiency directly affected disease.

Nourishing Traditions (Series)

Sally Fallon has taken the discoveries Dr. Weston A. Price made in the 1930s and has applied it to the modern diet. This series of books gives the reader a general view of traditional foods, recipes, and research to get them started with incorporating Dr. Price's nutritional principles.

Real Food for Gestational Diabetes & Real Food for Pregnancy

Lily Nichols, RDN is one of the best-known prenatal nutritionists in the world. She has written two best-selling books, *Real Food for Gestational Diabetes* and *Real Food for Pregnancy*. Her website is a great spot to pick up her books, schedule a speaking engagement, or download one of her amazing e-books: www.lilynicholsrdn.com.

Nutrient Power: Heal Your Biochemistry and Heal Your Brain

Dr. William Walsh not only wrote this ground-breaking book on nutrient therapy for mental health, but he is also the founder of the Walsh Research Institute, a nonprofit institute dedicated to researching nutrient therapy and functional medicine approaches to mental health conditions.

Food Politics: How the Food Industry Influences Nutrition and Health

Marion Nestle's tell-all book gives a glimpse into the politics behind the nutritional guidelines and why it is so hard to change them even if the research shows they are wrong. She's written many other books, but this one is a must. Also check out her other books, *Unsavory Truth: How Food Companies Skew the Science of What We Eat*, and for all you animal lovers, *Pet Food Politics*.

Iodine: Why You Need It, Why You Can't Live Without It

Dr. David Brownstein, MD, is a family physician and one of the foremost holistic physicians and authors. His book highlights the misconceptions about iodine in the diet and in supplementation. He addresses the connection between inadequate iodine intake with common medical conditions.

Hashimoto's Thyroiditis: Lifestyle Interventions for Finding and Treating the Root Cause

Dr. Isabella Wentz, the thyroid pharmacist, is well-known for her many books related to thyroid disease. This book is a great guide to helping patients identify triggers of autoimmune thyroid disease.

Acknowledgments

The process of writing this book was like the gestation and birth of a child. Like pregnancy and birth, I couldn't do it alone, and creating my ideal "birth" team was crucial. I needed this amazing group of people to coach, encourage, and remind me of the amazing end result I was aiming for. To my husband, Ryan, who encouraged me to take the risk, I couldn't have done it without you. Thank you. You have been my rock and my best friend for the past 20 years. I can do anything in life with you by my side. To my daughters, Mina and Maggie, thank you for being my little cheerleaders and putting up with my intent and sometimes obsessive focus that pulled me away from our normal routines. To Catherine and Nathan, guiding me on this journey, working as my doulas to keep me focused on the end goal, thank you.

Lastly, I would like to acknowledge and thank my patients. I have a saying that when you work with women through this journey of pregnancy, they become family. My little clinic family is amazing. I love and appreciate you all. I am honored that I've been able to walk this path with you, many of you through multiple pregnancies and many of you through the struggle of conception to the beautiful birth of your child. It is a blessing to have fallen into a personal journey that has led me to be a part of so many lives. I wouldn't be me without you.

About the Author
Sarah Thompson

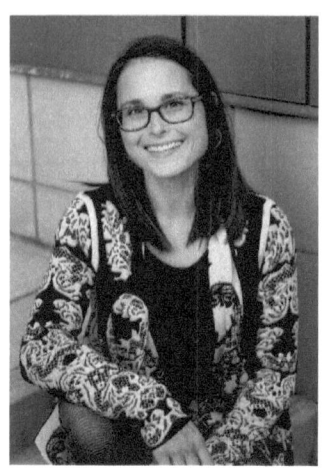

Sarah Thompson, L.Ac., CFMP, Doula, is the founder of Sacred Vessel Acupuncture & Functional Medicine and the creator of www.functionalmaternity.com. She is a certified functional medicine practitioner, licensed acupuncturist, board-certified herbalist, birth doula, and educator with a passion for pregnancy care. She is also known as a leader in the practice and education of maternity functional medicine. Sarah brings together evidence-based research in prenatal and maternity nutrition with the ideas of functional medicine and traditional Chinese medicine. Sarah's clinical experience spans nearly 20 years. When she isn't writing, lecturing, mentoring, or seeing patients in her private practice, she can be found on her small Colorado farm with her husband, two daughters, chickens, miniature cows, dogs, cats, and gardens.

www.ingramcontent.com/pod-product-compliance
Lightning Source LLC
Chambersburg PA
CBHW030115240426
43673CB00029B/484/J